Medical Dosage Calculations FOR DUMMIES®

by Dr. Richard W. Snyder, DO, and
Barry Schoenborn

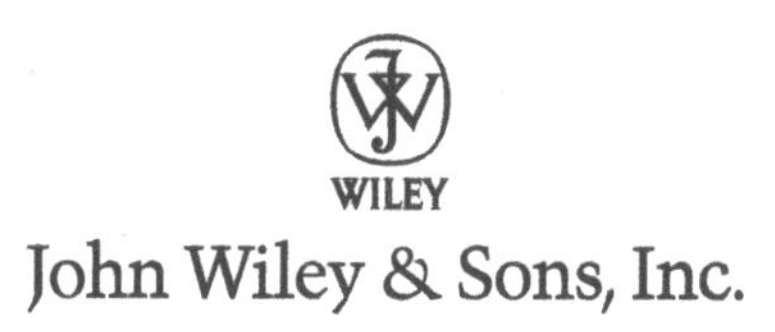

John Wiley & Sons, Inc.

Medical Dosage Calculations For Dummies®

Published by
John Wiley & Sons, Inc.
111 River St.
Hoboken, NJ 07030-5774
www.wiley.com

Library of Congress Control Number: 2011924132

ISBN: 978-0-470-93064-9 (pbk); ISBN 978-1-118-05586-1 (ebk); ISBN 978-1-118-05587-8 (ebk); ISBN 978-1-118-05588-5 (ebk)

Manufactured in the United States of America

SKY10095143_010525

About the Authors

Dr. Rich Snyder, DO, is an osteopathic physician who resides in Easton, Pennsylvania. He's a kidney specialist, board certified in both internal medicine and nephrology. He did his Internal Medicine Residency at Abington Memorial Hospital and completed both clinical and research fellowships in nephrology at the Hospital of the University of Pennsylvania. He also has experience in graduate medical education. As a former associate program director and osteopathic program director at Easton Hospital, he was responsible for both the administration and education of medical residents and medical students.

In addition to maintaining a full time clinical practice at Lehigh Valley Nephrology Associates, he has authored and coauthored several articles in peer-reviewed journals, including the *American Journal of Kidney Disease* and *Kidney International*. He has also presented at national meetings, including the National Kidney Foundation's Annual Meeting. In addition to being a coauthor of *Medical Dosage Calculations For Dummies*, he has written the book *What You Must Know About Kidney Disease: A Practical Guide to Conventional and Complementary Treatments.* He's also been interviewed regionally and nationally on both radio and television about integrative medicine and kidney disease. Beginning in January 2011, he can be heard weekly on his show, *Improve Your Kidney Health,* on VoiceAmerica Radio Health and Wellness Channel.

Barry Schoenborn lives in Nevada City, California. He's a longtime technical writer, with over 30 years' experience. He's written hundreds of user manuals, and (in the early days) worked dozens of part-time jobs that required practical and scientific math. Mathematics and engineering were among his college majors until he abandoned them to earn a degree in Liberal Arts.

He isn't a doctor and tries to avoid being hospitalized. However, he's spent many hours undergoing dental procedures, which sparked an ongoing interest in dentistry and medicine. He's the author of the short stories, "Doc Jones, Frontier Dentist," "Doc Jones, Combat Dentist," and "Murder, She Flossed."

In the past, Barry's technical writing company worked with the State of California agency CalRecycle to teach scientists and administrators how to write clearly. Barry's the coauthor of *Technical Math For Dummies* and *Storage Area Networks: Designing and Implementing a Mass Storage System.*

He was a movie reviewer for the *Los Angeles Herald-Dispatch* newspaper and wrote a monthly political newspaper column for *The Union* newspaper of Grass Valley, California, for seven years. Barry's publishing company, Willow Valley Press, published *Dandelion Through the Crack*, which won the William Saroyan International Prize for Writing.

Dedications

Rich Snyder

This book I dedicate to my mother, Nancy Snyder, herself a registered nurse and constant source of inspiration and encouragement.

I also dedicate this book to every nurse, every healthcare provider, and every caregiver out there. You are the unsung heroes and the ones that inspire hope and healing.

I finally dedicate this book to Dr. Hatem Amer, MD, a kidney specialist and best friend who is himself a rarity: His empathy and compassion is as vast as his brilliance. I consider myself lucky to call him a friend.

Barry Schoenborn

I'd like to dedicate this book to James H. Jones, DDS, my periodontist. Jim recently retired and has been an inspiration for more than 20 years. During that time, I underwent numerous periodontal procedures, fighting the ravages of oral pathogens. I learned a lot of Latin from Jim, and he always explained to me what he was doing and why. He also inspired me to write "dental humor," a funny genre that nobody except a dentist would want to read.

Authors' Acknowledgments

Rich Snyder

I would not have been able to write this book without the heroic efforts of Barry Schoenborn. He is a gifted and talented writer, and I have learned much from him in a short amount of time. I want to thank Erin Calligan Mooney for the opportunity to coauthor this book. I also wish to thank Chrissy Guthrie and Amanda Langferman for their help and support. I also want to thank Matt Wagner for his help and continued support.

Finally, I would like to thank everyone at Lehigh Valley Nephrology Associates for being the great people they are to work with. Many happy years to come!

Barry Schoenborn

This book wouldn't have been possible without the tremendous effort of coauthor Rich Snyder. It's amazing how much he knows! We were supported by a great team at Wiley Publishing (Chrissy Guthrie, Erin Calligan Mooney, and Amanda Langferman), who worked hard to make this book a reality. They're very talented and also happen to be the nicest people you'll ever meet! A big thanks, too, to Matt Wagner of Fresh Books Literary Agency, who presented us to Wiley.

Many thanks to my two favorite family practice physicians. Dr. Sara J. Richey seems to know everything, always listens, and believes in "treating the whole patient." Dr. Jon R. Pritchett also seems to know everything, has an excellent approach to doctoring, and has shared an experience or two from his days as an emergency room doctor.

And, finally, my sincere thanks and apologies to the respiration therapist, nurses, medical assistants, and front office staffs whom I flooded with questions.

Rich and Barry

We would like to acknowledge and thank the following for their help and assistance: Christopher Vancheri and Roche Pharmaceuticals; Marcia Diljak and Eisai Pharmaceuticals; Ron Granish and X-Gen Pharmaceuticals; and Doretta Gray, Cindy Rockoff, et al from Novo Nordisk Pharmaceuticals.

Publisher's Acknowledgments

We're proud of this book; please send us your comments at `http://dummies.custhelp.com`. For other comments, please contact our Customer Care Department within the U.S. at 877-762-2974, outside the U.S. at 317-572-3993, or fax 317-572-4002.

Some of the people who helped bring this book to market include the following:

Acquisitions, Editorial, and Media Development

Senior Project Editor: Christina Guthrie

Acquisitions Editor: Erin Calligan Mooney

Copy Editor: Amanda Langferman

Assistant Editor: David Lutton

Technical Editors: Kathryn E. Humphrey, MSN, RN, and Patricia Roark, RN, BSN

Editorial Manager: Christine Meloy Beck

Editorial Assistant: Rachelle Amick

Art Coordinator: Alicia B. South

Cover Photos: © iStockphoto.com/pixhook

Cartoons: Rich Tennant (`www.the5thwave.com`)

Composition Services

Project Coordinator: Sheree Montgomery

Layout and Graphics: Timothy Detrick, Andrea Hornberger, Lavonne Roberts, Corrie Socolovitch, Christin Swinford

Proofreaders: Sossity R. Smith

Indexer: Ty Koontz

Publishing and Editorial for Consumer Dummies

Kathleen Nebenhaus, Vice President and Executive Publisher

David Palmer, Associate Publisher

Kristin Ferguson-Wagstaffe, Product Development Director

Publishing for Technology Dummies

Andy Cummings, Vice President and Publisher

Composition Services

Debbie Stailey, Director of Composition Services

Contents at a Glance

Contents at a Glance

Table of Contents

Introduction

Whether you're currently working in a healthcare profession or studying in school, you've probably discovered that most healthcare jobs require some math — which is likely why you picked up this book.

Don't panic if you're intimidated by the mere mention of *math.* Most dosing math calculations are simple. At first glance, some dosing problems may seem pretty hard, but look closer. After you read them a few times, you'll see that most seemingly complex problems are really just a combination of simple calculations. After you read through the basics we cover in this book, you'll hit your forehead with the heel of your palm whenever you come up against a challenging-on-the-surface problem and say, "Yes! Of course! I sorta knew that all along, but now I really get it!"

About This Book

This book puts a lot of medical dosing math into just a few chapters and in a very compact form. It's different from other medical dosage math books in four main ways.

- **It's all about dosing in the context of real medical conditions.** Our focus is giving you the right math for real-life situations, not just presenting math problems. We bring up dosing scenarios you just might deal with every day in a medical-surgical unit or in a rehab or homecare setting.
- **It's comprehensive.** It covers *all* the major areas in which you need to do dosing calculations. Other math books often don't give you the broad coverage you need.
- **It offers a great review of math basics and then explains the three main dosing calculation methods.** We begin by looking briefly at numbers, arithmetic, fractions, units, and conversions and then delve deeper into the more dosing-specific math you need to know to be a successful healthcare professional. We also offer many examples of solving dosing problems so you get plenty of practice.
- **It isn't dull (we hope!), as other math books tend to be.** Because it's a *For Dummies* book, you can be sure it's easy to read and includes just enough humor to keep you entertained.

As you start reading, remember: This book is a reference. You can start anywhere you like and jump around as your interest and needs change. But it's also a repair manual; it can help fill voids in your math background.

Some of the chapters are based on an aspect of medicine with particular dosing requirements (for example, pregnancy, insulin, and critical care), while others are based on particular methods of medication administration (for example, oral, injection, and intravenous). Some chapters also cover useful techniques, such as mixing insulin, splitting tablets, and managing an IV line. Regardless of the chapter's particular focus, though, you get plenty of practical, real-life examples to help you hone your dosage calculation skills.

Note: Unlike many *For Dummies* books, this one doesn't have a lot of light, humorous moments because so much in medical dosage calculations is critical. When patients' lives are on the line, we're certainly not going to make any jokes about the topics at hand.

Conventions Used in This Book

We designed this book to be user-friendly, maybe even user-affectionate. The trouble is, we can't come to your school, hospital, or home and do the math for you. If we could, we'd drive right over and bring coffee and donuts!

To make things as user-friendly as possible, we've used the following conventions throughout the book:

- We *italicize* new terms in each chapter; these terms include technical names, slang names, and abbreviations. We follow each one with a short, plain English definition, and we sometimes give you pronunciation cues and word origins when helpful.
- Variables appear as *italics* in formulas (for example, $3a + 4b = 10$).
- Drug names appear with their generic names first, followed by their commercial brand names (where they apply) in parentheses. For example, we say "hydrocodone (Vicodin)" to show you both the generic name and the brand name. In some cases, we use only the generic name. On subsequent references in a given example or section of text, we use only the generic name.
- We abbreviate units of measurement, just as you'll see them every day in your career. For example, we say *g,* not *gram,* and *mL,* not *milliliter,* wherever possible. (See Chapter 4 for more on units of measurement and Chapter 5 for more on appropriate abbreviations.)
- Web addresses appear in `monofont` to help them stand out. They're usually very short and shouldn't break across two lines of text. But if

they do, know that we haven't added any extra characters to indicate the break. Just type what you see into your Web browser.

- We usually begin the first few calculation examples in each chapter with the basic structure of the calculation. That way, you review the basic structure throughout the book and not just in Chapter 4 where we introduce the different methods.
- We usually show the results of a math example to several decimal places. However, we then round the results up or down, using the standard math convention "5 up/4 down." We do this so the dose you give is consistent with the accuracy of the device you use to give it.

What You're Not to Read

We'd love for you to read all the words in this book in the order they appear, but life is short. You don't have to read chapters that don't interest you. This is a reference book, and we've designed it so that you can read only the parts you need. If you get stuck in a chapter, you can go back to a chapter you skipped to get some help.

As you read, rest easy that you can skip the following text without losing anything crucial to the dosage-calculations discussion:

- **Text marked with a Technical Stuff icon:** We've included this text to give you a little history, the origin of a principle, or maybe a formal definition, but this text doesn't provide vital dosage-related info.
- **Text marked with a Did You Know? icon:** This text offers up a little pop culture, a bizarre fact, or maybe some humor, but it's not critical to your understanding of dosage calculations.
- **Text set up in a sidebar:** *Sidebars* are blocks of text that have a gray background. They're interesting (we think), but they aren't critical to your understanding of the main text.

Foolish Assumptions

As we wrote this book, we made the following assumptions about you:

- We assume that you're in a two-year or four-year nursing program. But we also like the idea that you may be a working nurse or a concerned parent or caregiver.
- We assume (or should we say, "hope"?) you learned some basic math in middle and/or high school.

But even if you missed some math concepts in school, you can find the ones you need for medical dosing in the review section of this book (Chapters 1 through 4). It's amazing how little you need to review (multiplying fractions and conversion math) to be caught up on the math you need to do dosing calculations.

- We assume that you'll skip concepts you're already comfortable with. That's perfectly okay because this is a reference book, not a novel.
- We assume that you have access to a computer and the Internet. It's not essential, but it's very handy. Use a good search engine to find out more about any topic in this book — in the worlds of pharmacology, mathematics, and nursing practice.

How This Book Is Organized

This book has five main sections, called *parts,* with about the same number of chapters in the first four sections.

Part I: Getting Up to Speed: Reviewing Math Basics

Part I starts with the math basics that make calculating dosages possible. Go to these chapters if you need to catch up on some math you missed in the past. Chapter 1 gives you the basic concepts covered in this book and describes the need for medical dosage calculations. Chapter 2 is a review of numbers and fundamental arithmetic.

When you get to Chapters 3 and 4, the medical dosing fun begins. Chapter 3 covers the basics of fraction math, which is a core part of the calculations you do in all the other chapters. Chapter 4 reviews the major systems of measurement and shows you how to convert units.

Part II: Minding Your Meds: Administration and Calculation Methods

When you get past Part I (either because you read it or because you already know basic math), you enter Part II, the world of dosage administration and calculation methods. Chapter 5 reviews the basic elements of a prescription, while Chapter 6 focuses on drug labels and patient safety. Chapter 7 deals with the MAR (the very important Medication Administration Record) and explains what you need to know about proper medical documentation. Finally, Chapter 8 walks you through the three classic calculation methods for working up correct dosages. Even if you skip the rest of this part, it's a good idea to review Chapter 8 before moving on to Part III.

Part III: Calculations for Different Routes of Administration

Part III contains "serious math" for dosing calculations. Sounds complicated, but the examples aren't hard to work through. We cover simple oral dosing calculations in Chapter 9 and calculations related to parenteral medication administration (injections, in other words) in Chapter 10. Then we show you how to calculate intravenous dosing in Chapter 11 and reconstitution in Chapter 12. Don't start panicking just yet! The math is simple after you practice it.

Part IV: Dosing in Special Situations

The field of medicine is full of special situations, which is what Part IV is all about. Chapter 13 gives you a rundown on insulin. Chapter 14 is all about administering drugs during pregnancy (the patient's, not yours), and Chapter 15 takes a look at dosing for children. Chapter 16 deals with making dosing changes for patients with different medical conditions (like high or low blood pressure) and shows you how to do multiple calculations for real-life dosage problems. Chapter 17 offers dosing considerations you need to take when dealing with critical care patients, and Chapter 18 covers dosing for enteral and parenteral nutrition.

Part V: The Part of Tens

Part V is the world-famous Part of Tens that appears in all *For Dummies* books. The chapters in this part are very compact and contain handy information. Chapter 19 summarizes the ten most common dosage calculations you're likely to do. Chapter 20 describes ten dosing mistakes and shows you how to avoid them.

Icons Used in This Book

We use several icons in this book to call out special kinds of information.

This icon represents information you definitely don't want to skip over. It'll come in handy as you do the medical dosage calculations throughout this book and in your career as a healthcare professional.

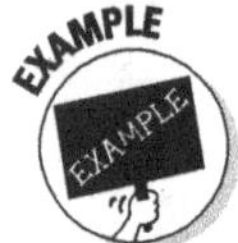

This icon highlights medical dosing problems that appear throughout each chapter. Each example describes a particular situation, asks one or two dosing questions, and then shows you the steps you need to take to get the answers.

This icon points out suggestions or recommendations. Don't skip over the text marked with this icon if you want to know the quick and easy way to get things done.

A warning icon describes a situation where you should exercise care and seek additional advice or instruction. Some dosage situations can be critical to the well-being of the patient, and you need to be aware of them.

The paragraphs next to this icon contain information that's interesting and useful but not vital to your understanding of the topic at hand. This info may include a brief history of a principle, the earliest practitioners, or the origin of a word. This icon also showcases technical points. You can read the text marked with this icon or skip over it. Either is fine.

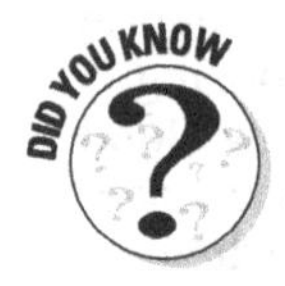

This is our "interesting trivia" icon. The text here usually contains odd facts, pieces of pop culture, bits of history, bizarre terms, or strange findings. You can read the info marked with this icon or skip over it.

Where to Go from Here

You can go to any chapter from here. The book isn't linear, so you can start anywhere.

First, check the table of contents, where you find the names of the parts and the chapters. Then pick any chapter you're interested in.

- If you can't make a choice, begin with Chapter 1. It highlights the broad concepts covered in the book.
- If you have a particular dosing problem you want to work on, find a chapter in the table of contents that deals with it, and go straight to it. You can always check out the index at the back of the book, too.

If, at any time, you get stuck on a concept, look for a cross-reference that tells you which chapter covers that particular topic. Then stop what you're reading, and go visit that chapter.

Part I

Getting Up to Speed: Reviewing Math Basics

The 5th Wave
By Rich Tennant
©RICHTENNANT
EINSTEIN CALCULATES HIS MEDICAL DOSAGE

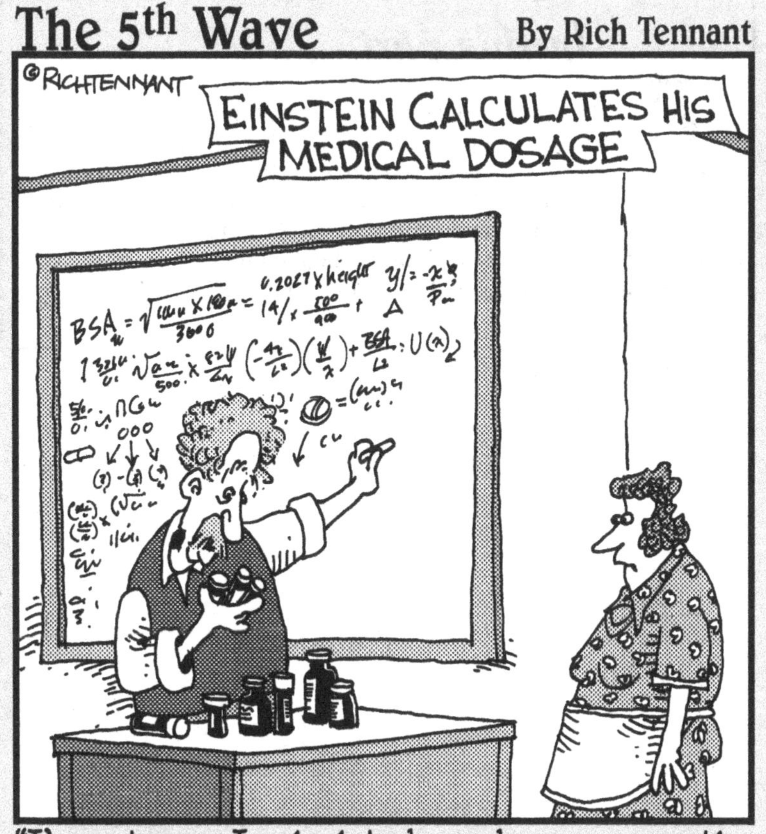

"I'm not sure I calculated my dosage correctly, but I think I'm close to making a breakthrough in time travel."

In this part . . .

Part I is a review of math basics, just in case you missed a concept or two during your education. Chapter 1 stresses the importance of dosage calculations in all healthcare professions. Chapter 2 is a fun and simple review of numbers and arithmetic. In Chapters 3 and 4, you get important basics for medical math — fractions, systems of measurement, and unit conversions.

Chapter 1

Brushing Up on Your Math Skills and Entering the Healthcare Field

In This Chapter

- Looking at the basics of medical math and dosage calculations
- Taking a look at healthcare careers and the need for math
- Remembering the importance of compassion, empathy, and other important skills

If you're a healthcare professional (or planning to be one), you're in one of the most important careers around today. In essence, you help healthy people stay healthy, you help sick people get well, and you help people with critical health conditions live.

Of course, nursing and all health professions involve more than just calculating and administering medications. They're vocations for comforting the sick and injured — clearly they involve much more than just "pushing meds."

However, being a successful healthcare provider means being an able mathematician. After all, the field of medicine relies extensively on administering medications, and you must be able to calculate meds correctly before you dispense them.

In any healthcare education program, medical dosage calculations come up in practically every course (or they should). In addition, most schools of nursing have one course devoted entirely to medical dosage calculations.

In this chapter, we introduce you to the math you need to know to perform basic and complex medical dosage calculations. We also provide an overview of the different careers available in the healthcare field (and show you how they all utilize medical math). Finally, we go beyond math and focus on the other essential components of being a good healthcare provider.

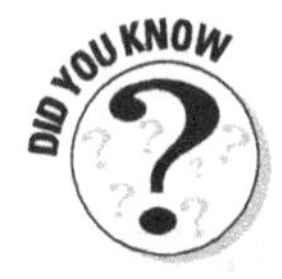

Florence Nightingale had a great gift for mathematics. She was a pioneer in presenting information visually — especially health statistics. She has been recognized for developing a form of the pie chart now known as the polar area diagram.

Knowing What Math You Need to Know in Healthcare

In healthcare, you need to know the following three kinds of dosing math:

- **School math:** The math you learn in order to pass tests while getting an education
- **NCLEX (National Council Licensure Examination) math:** The math you learn to get your license
- **Real-world math:** The math you use to handle your job

It's true; you'll sometimes find questions on tests in school or in practicing for the NCLEX that may never come up in real life, but you still need to be prepared for those questions. Similarly, real life will surely present you with math problems that you never practiced in school. In this section, we cover the math concepts and calculation methods you need to know to be prepared for just about any scenario in healthcare.

Never despair about medical dosage calculations. Each principle in this book is easy if you look at it the right way. Medical dosing math isn't harder than you think; it's actually easier!

Nailing down basic arithmetic

Nursing and related professions require basic math skills, but don't worry if math hasn't always been your favorite subject in school. The best part about medical math is that it's easy to identify just how much math you need to know.

Basic math is essentially just arithmetic — addition, subtraction, multiplication, and division. And you mostly use multiplication and division in your dosage calculations. But don't forget that counting is math, too. For example, when you count out 4 tablets, you're doing addition ($1 + 1 + 1 + 1 = 4$).

In case you missed some of what you need to know math-wise in school, we cover the most important principles in Chapters 2 through 4.

Fiddling with fractions in four forms

Medical dosage calculations use fractions 90 percent of the time (or $\frac{9}{10}$ of the time or in a 9:1 ratio). In case you're wondering, all those phrases mean the same thing.

The four forms a fraction can take are

- **Common fraction (also called a *vulgar* fraction):**

  $$\frac{100 \text{ units}}{50 \text{ mL}}$$

- **Decimal fraction:** 0.56 mL
- **Percent fraction:** 0.9% normal saline (NS)
- **Ratio:** 1:9

Of these four types, you use only two (common fractions and decimal fractions) to do most of the work in your dosage calculations.

Conquering the calculation methods

A word to the wise about the complex math used in this book: There isn't any. All the math used in medical dosage calculations is very simple. For example, one of the most common calculations you see in dosing problems is unit conversion. To convert units, you just have to know how to use some simple formulas, called *conversion factors,* like 1 kg (kilogram) = 2.2 lb (pounds). You use conversion factors mostly to convert mass (weight) and liquid volumes. Chapter 4 explains everything you need to know about units and conversion.

As far as figuring out drug dosage and administration, you use the following three basic calculation methods: the formula method, the ratio-proportion method, and the dimensional analysis method. Chapter 8 walks you through each method and shows you when and how to use it.

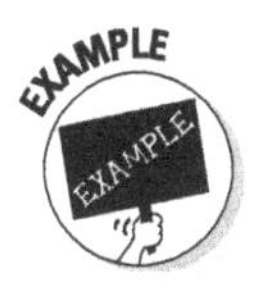

The following problem is an example of some of the math you have to do when calculating medical dosages. It uses the ratio-proportion method (see Chapter 8 for more details).

If 250 mg are in 5 mL and you need to give 333 mg, what's the dose in mL?

To find out, follow these steps:

1. **Set up the following proportion:**

$$\frac{\text{known equivalent}}{\text{known equivalent}} = \frac{\text{known equivalent}}{\text{desired equivalent}}$$

$$\frac{250 \text{ mg}}{5 \text{ mL}} = \frac{333 \text{ mg}}{x \text{ mL}}$$

2. **Cross-multiply and solve.**

   $250x = 5 \times 333$

   $250x = 1{,}665$

   $x = 6.66$

   The answer is 6.66 mL. You'd give 6.7 mL to provide the needed 333 mg.

Calculations with multiple steps may look complex, but they aren't because the math involved in each step is fairly simple. For example, when you calculate a weight-dependent dosage that you must administer intravenously, your calculations typically follow this pattern:

- Convert the patient's weight from lb (pounds) to kg (kilograms).
- Determine the number of mg (milligrams) of the med to give for that body weight.
- Because the med is in a liquid suspension, calculate the mL that contain the number of mg you need to give.
- Because IV meds are often ordered to be dosed per min (minute) but are infused in mL/hr (milliliters per hour), calculate the flow rate by converting from mL/min (milliliters per minute) to mL/hr so you can program an electronic infusion pump.

Living in a metric world

Dosing medications — whether you're working in a hospital, clinic, rehab center, or home setting — is built on the metric system. Don't start panicking, yet. Because the metric system is based on a system of tens, it's easy to learn and to use.

For a long time, medicine used an older system (once called the *English system*) with units like lb (pounds) and fl oz (fluid ounces). Medicine also used the *apothecaries' system* with units such as the grain, dram, and scruple. The United States still commonly uses its household system, which includes units like fl oz (fluid ounces) and Tbsp (tablespoons), but it does so mostly in the kitchen, not the hospital.

Measuring precisely is half the battle

After you calculate a dose accurately, you must dispense it accurately. Sometimes accurate dispensing is as simple as counting out the right number of tablets. However, many doctor's orders call for administering liquid volumes via injections and intravenous (IV) infusions. When administering liquid volumes, accurate dispensing means measuring exactly the amount of the med you need and drawing it up into the syringe.

When you give a med intravenously, you usually dispense it over time. For IV administration, you must calculate accurate IV flow rates and/or drip rates and then set them accurately (see Chapter 11 for details).

Because the older systems haven't disappeared completely, be aware that you sometimes have to convert units from one system to units of another. (See Chapter 4 for tons more details on units and conversion.)

Tools of the Trade for Dosing Meds

This probably goes without saying, but accurate dosing is vital in the healthcare profession. It's a good thing the math isn't hard, because there's no room for error. After all, medicine relies primarily on medications to get healing done, so errors in dosage calculations can mean critical errors in patient health and safety.

Following are three tools of the trade that help you do medical dosing calculations accurately every time:

- **Undivided attention:** Anyone who works in healthcare knows how busy the day can get. When you're dealing with medications, especially when you're performing medical dosage calculations, your undivided attention is paramount to reducing the chance of any dosing error. Take the time to double-check your calculations. The most important mathematical tool you have is your mind.
- **Calculator:** When you're dealing with decimals, percentages, and complex calculations, you often need more than your fingers and a pen and paper. You need a calculator to do more complex calculations. Portable computer-based calculation programs like MedCalc also work well.
- **Medication reference guides:** It's impossible to keep straight all the medications and dosages out there. So you need to use the many excellent reference guides available in book form, smartphone apps, and on the Internet. Use them to research medication names, dosages, possible drug interactions, and clinical applications of the drugs.

Not missing the good ol' days

In the olden days, when Rich (one of the authors) was in medical school, health professionals often walked around with wads of papers and small medical guides stuffed in their pockets. Lucky for you, with modern technology, using a "portable brain" has never been easier. You can download great drug reference guides and computer programs on a smartphone or other small device that can help you do your dosage calculations with just the push of a few buttons. In fact, they're far more efficient than wads of paper and pocket guides that could fall out anytime.

Many hospitals are fully integrating information technology (IT) and becoming fully computerized. With electronic patient records, computerized drug orders, and computer-based patient charting, you're in the forefront of a new medical technology age. In fact, some hospitals even give out small, handheld computer devices that contain patient information as well as various drug references and calculation programs.

All this new technology certainly beats walking around with wads of crumpled-up paper shoved in the pockets of your white coat!

Surveying Healthcare Careers (They All Use Medical Math!)

In this section, we introduce you to various types of healthcare professions. Each of these professions requires knowledge of medical math in some form or another.

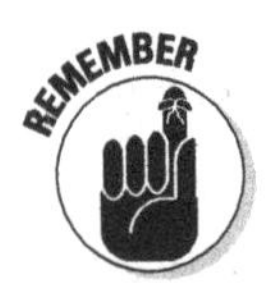

No one is an island. It's important to work as a team. Nurses, doctors, pharmacists, patients, and parents of young patients need to be on the same page. It's not unusual for a nurse or doctor to call a pharmacist for dosing assistance, especially when it comes to giving complicated medications, like those used in chemotherapy. Being on the same page and working as a team are critical to providing both optimal and safe care, with a reduced likelihood of errors.

Looking at the classic nursing careers

A career in nursing takes numerous forms. Some are based on your level of education, while others are based on where you do the work. No matter what initials come after your name, however, you still need to know all about medications and to be able to do dosing calculations.

Each type of nurse needs education, testing, and usually licensing. The basic types are

- **Registered nurse, or RN:** An RN usually has a degree (an AS, ASN, AAS, or AND) or a diploma from a hospital-based school of nursing. But you can also obtain other nursing degrees, including Bachelor of Science in Nursing, Master of Science in Nursing, Doctor of Nursing Science, and Doctor of Nursing Practice. To be an RN, you must pass exams and be licensed. Education and other requirements vary widely, and state law regulates what you can do as an RN. RNs are the largest healthcare occupation in the United States; according to the U.S. Bureau of Labor Statistics, there are about 2.3 million registered nurses.
- **Nurse practitioner, or NP:** If you're an NP, you're an RN with an advanced education. NPs are certified and licensed, but the duties permitted vary according to different states. Often, NPs do many tasks that doctors do (for example, they take histories and manage chronic conditions, such as diabetes). The NP's ability to prescribe drugs varies according to state law. These days, NPs are very common in the offices of family practice physicians. In fact, it's almost essential for the doctors to have one.
- **Public health nurse, or PHN:** Public health nursing is a specialized form of nursing that combines nursing and public health principles. A PHN knows about community health, health maintenance, and disease prevention. Counties and school districts employ one or more PHNs.
- **Licensed practical nurse, or LPN:** An LPN is known as a *licensed vocational nurse* (LVN) in California and Texas. If you're an LPN/LVN, you're well-educated, you've passed exams, and you're licensed. You work under the supervision of an RN. You do many nursing tasks, but you can't do other tasks, depending on what the law and hospital policy allow. The U.S. Bureau of Labor Statistics estimates that about 700,000 persons are employed as LPNs/LVNs.
- **Certified nursing assistant, or CNA:** This certification lets you assist patients with activities of daily living and give care under the supervision of an RN or an LPN/LVN. According to law and hospital policy, this care may include answering patients' call signals, observing patients' conditions, measuring and recording food and liquid intakes and outputs, taking vital signs, and reporting changes to the nursing staff. After the CNA completes a certificate training program (sometimes just one course at a community college), he's required to take a state certification exam.

  In the United States, a certified nursing assistant may be called a *nursing assistant certified* (NAC), *patient care assistant* (PCA), *state tested nurse aid* (STNA), or *nursing assistant-registered* (NA/R).

The Nightingale Pledge

The Nightingale Pledge is the oath nurses take, usually when they graduate from nursing school. The graduating class at Harper Hospital in Detroit, Michigan, was the first to use it in the spring of 1893. Its creator, Lystra Gretter, graduated from nursing school in 1888. Here's what the oath says:

> "I solemnly pledge myself before God and in the presence of this assembly, to pass my life in purity and to practice my profession faithfully. I will abstain from whatever is deleterious and mischievous, and will not take or knowingly administer any harmful drug. I will do all in my power to maintain and elevate the standard of my profession, and will hold in confidence all personal matters committed to my keeping and all family affairs coming to my knowledge in the practice of my calling. With loyalty will I endeavor to aid the physician, in his work, and devote myself to the welfare of those committed to my care."

Similar to the Nightingale Pledge, the Hippocratic Oath that doctors pledge reminds coauthor Rich and his fellow doctors why they become doctors. It's much, much more than just "doing no harm". It means to "benefit the patient" and to "preserve the sanctity of life." The Oath reminds doctors that there's no more rewarding job in the world.

Probing other medical careers

In addition to nursing, several other medical careers, including the following, require an understanding of medical dosage math:

- **Physician assistant, or PA:** Like the NP, a PA is a midlevel practitioner who can work in a physician's office, hospital, or rehabilitation center. PAs are licensed and work under the supervision of a physician. California requires PAs to complete an American Academy of Physician Assistants accredited, formal education program and pass a national exam to get a license. PAs can prescribe medications and other medical treatments. You can bet they need to know their math!
- **Medical assistant:** A medical assistant typically works in a physician's or other health practitioner's office. Medical assistants are tested and certified. You find them in the offices of virtually any specialty, from family practice and internal medicine to *cardiology,* the heart doctor, and *nephrology* (ne-*frall*-a-gee), the kidney doctor. In an office setting, they're often multitasking — recording heights and weights, taking vital signs, recording and trending blood chemistries, and reviewing patient medication dosages and frequency.
- **Pharmacist, or PharmD (Doctor of Pharmacy):** Pharmacists know pharmacology (drugs and drug action) and are also excellent mathematicians. They're responsible for filling prescription orders from doctors

and other healthcare professionals. In the United Kingdom, pharmacists are called *chemists*. In a hospital setting, pharmacists use basic math, different systems of measurement, conversions, and more as they make up many medications.

- **Physician, or MD (Doctor of Medicine) or DO (Doctor of Osteopathic Medicine):** When physicians, also called *doctors,* write prescriptions, they're doing basic math calculations. Some specialties require more math than others. For example, an *oncologist* (ahn-*kall*-a-gist) — a doctor who specializes in cancer — needs to do math calculations when dosing chemotherapy. The calculations are often based on the patient's *body mass index* (or BMI), a vital mathematical calculation based on height and weight. One of the authors, Rich, is an internist and nephrologist. Because nephrology relies a lot on numbers, he's always doing math.

  Doctors come in many varieties. For example, a dentist (DDS) is a Doctor of Dental Surgery. A foot doctor (DPM) is a Doctor of Podiatric Medicine.

- **Home healthcare aide, or HCA:** HCAs, also called *home health aides (HHAs),* are not nurses. They're in a special category. HCAs must complete a certificate training program and pass an examination from the National Association for Home Care. They're usually certified by the state. HCAs usually help in elder care settings and convalescent hospitals. They often assist disabled people in their homes. See the section "Offering help at home" for more details.

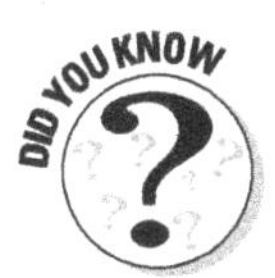

The exciting field of *biomedical engineering* combines engineering math and medical science. This specialty takes concepts studied in engineering and applies them to medicine. Many of the great new inventions in medicine (for example, the artificial heart, artificial hip joints, prostheses, and medical imaging) can be attributed to the wonderful work of biomedical engineers.

Examining emergency medicine

You probably know that a hospital's emergency room (also called the *ER*) has doctors and nurses who specialize in emergency medicine. The ER may also have LPNs/LVNs working in it, depending on state law or hospital policy. But what about those who do emergency medicine outside of the ER?

The emergency medical technician (EMT) takes an examination, is certified and, in some states, is licensed. Television shows have popularized this particular medical position, and sometimes people call EMTs *paramedics*. However, whether that term applies depends on the EMT's level of training. To add to the mix, EMT designations are different in different states, and Canada, the United Kingdom, and Ireland are all different from the United States and from each other.

In the United States, the National Highway Traffic Safety Administration has four levels of EMT, and only one is called a paramedic:

- EMT-B (Basic)
- EMT-I/85 (Intermediate)
- EMT-I/99 (Intermediate)
- EMT-P (Paramedic)

The major difference among EMT levels is the kind of treatment each level can provide. Very broadly, a basic EMT is allowed to assess the patient, control bleeding, monitor the patient, and do cardiopulmonary resuscitation (CPR). At the other end of the spectrum, an advanced paramedic EMT can do intubations, start IVs, and administer a wide range of drugs. The allowed tasks vary according to state law.

Offering help at home

Nurses and other healthcare professionals can and do visit patients at their homes. This aspect of nursing is especially valuable, given the cost of treatment in a hospital and the fact that some hospitals discharge patients quite soon after procedures are done.

The three main types of healthcare professionals (or lay people, in the case of caregivers) who spend a lot of time in the patient's home are

- **Visiting nurse:** This type of nurse is an RN who comes to the patient's home to provide vital nursing assistance. Home care can involve helping with diabetes management, giving injections, and working as part of a team that may include physical therapists or speech therapists.
- **Home health aide, or HHA:** An HHA (also known as a home healthcare aide, or HCA) cares for patients (often elderly, convalescent, or handicapped people) in their homes. The HHA may help the patient bathe, dress, and groom, as well as prepare meals and change the bed linens. She may also administer oral medications under supervision. To work as an HHA in California, you need to earn a certificate issued by the Department of Health Services, which requires that you complete 120 hours of specialized training.
- **Caregiver:** A caregiver is a family member or a friend who helps take care of a patient at home. The caregiver's job includes a lot of daunting and exhausting work, especially when the patient is recovering from a stroke or has a progressive disease, such as multiple sclerosis (MS) or Alzheimer's. Caregivers are better able to do their work when they're familiar with medical dosing and calculations, and they benefit from getting instructions from a nurse.

Beyond the Math: Remembering the Human Side of Healthcare

Nursing is a comprehensive discipline. A successful nurse is

- Well-educated
- Knowledgeable about medications, procedures, and equipment
- Sensitive to reading the state of the patient
- Sensitive to patients, families, and caregivers
- A great time manager
- An able administrator
- Experienced (a quality that comes with time on the job)

In *Notes on Nursing*, Florence Nightingale said, "I use the word nursing for want of a better. It has been limited to signify little more than the administration of medicines and the application of poultices. It ought to signify the proper use of fresh air, light, warmth, cleanliness, quiet, and the proper selection and administration of diet — all at the least expense of vital power to the patient."

Nursing and healthcare careers, in general, can be very demanding. Because you're taking care of the sick and injured, it's more than a job — it's a vocation (from the Latin word *vocáre*, meaning "a calling"). Any healthcare professional will tell you it's a lot of work, too, and (as Rich can attest) it requires a lot of working hours and many sacrifices. But it's rewarding as well. Helping someone heal and being an integral part of the process is one of the most rewarding things anyone can do. Being a nurse or other healthcare professional is essentially the giving of oneself to help another.

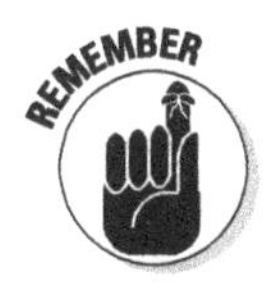

Two major criteria for any healthcare professional are empathy and compassion. If you don't have these qualities, maybe you should rethink a decision to go into nursing or any career that involves patient care. While good organizational and math skills are important, being both empathetic and compassionate is essential.

With the world's population getting older, you'll find yourself taking care of patients with many complex, chronic conditions. Translation: You have to administer more medications, do more medical calculations, and have a lot more empathy and compassion.

When you're sensitive to patients (and their families and caregivers), you're doing your job right. Sensitivity is vital and very much in keeping with the Nightingale Pledge, which states "I endeavor to . . . devote myself to the welfare of those committed to my care." (See the sidebar "The Nightingale Pledge" for more details.)

Great nursing moments in fact and fiction

Nursing has been an essential part of people's lives since before civilization, but the profession wasn't formalized until the 19th century. Here's a rundown of nursing in fact and fiction:

- In prehistory, every band of humans had to take care of the sick and injured among them, which led to the evolution of healers (sometimes called *shamans* or *witch doctors*), who acted as primary care physicians. You can assume that the patient's family handled nursing.
- Over the next several thousand years, you find evidence of doctoring but little or no evidence of nursing. The ancient Egyptians were great doctors, and they knew lots about hygiene and diet, but where were the nurses?
- As long as there have been battles, there have been wounded. You can figure that every army had first responders (EMTs) to collect the wounded, but you can't find much about how the wounded were healed.
- Fast forward to modern times. Florence Nightingale was famous for her nursing during the Crimean War in 1854. Then she opened the first nursing school in London in 1860.
- In 1861, Clara Barton tended to wounded soldiers in the U.S. Civil War and took medical supplies to the front lines. In 1881, she founded the American Red Cross.
- In the 1870s, Linda Richards was the first professionally trained American nurse. Florence Nightingale mentored her, and Richards started the first system of individual medical record keeping.
- Nursing entered the world of fiction in a big way in the 1930s. Helen Dore Boylston was a nurse in World War I and later helped the Red Cross in Europe. She wrote seven books about the fictional Sue Barton between 1936 and 1952. Sue Barton started as a student nurse and went on to work in many settings. At the time, nurses were role models and heroes.
- Nursing in fiction got even bigger in the 1940s. Grosset & Dunlap published 27 books about the fictional Cherry Ames. Cherry started as a student nurse, went to war, and later solved many mysteries while she was on nursing assignments. These books are prized by collectors today.
- In current times, nurses don't get as much exposure. In *Grey's Anatomy,* Season 4, Lauren Stamile plays Rose, a scrub nurse, and that's about it. In nine seasons of *Scrubs,* the only main nurse you see is the head nurse, Carla Espinosa; one episode includes a male nurse, Paul Flowers.
- The TV show *ER* ran for 15 seasons. The only nurse who was a main character was Nurse Carol Hathaway, and she came back from the dead! She "died" from a drug overdose in the pilot but somehow appeared later as a regular. To be fair, over the years, *ER* had its share of nurses in the background.

Chapter 2

Using Numbers and Arithmetic

In This Chapter

- Looking at the different numbers and numeral systems used in healthcare
- Reviewing basic arithmetic — addition, subtraction, multiplication, and division
- Working through some real-world dosing applications of basic math

In medicine, you use math daily. It doesn't matter whether the initials after your name are DO, MD, RN, LVN, PA, or CNA (and that's not the whole list by any means). Every professional in healthcare uses math.

Your ability to do medical math well is essential in a hospital, but it also helps your patients and their caregivers when they're discharged and, of course, the parents of your patients in pediatric cases. All these people rely on your medical dosing instructions.

So you're not exactly great at math? Don't worry! This chapter offers you a quick look at the different number systems you'll see in healthcare and walks you through a quick review of arithmetic — that is, addition, subtraction, multiplication, and division.

If you already have a firm grasp of the arithmetic we cover in this chapter, jump to Chapter 3 for more on fractions or Chapter 4 for more on systems of measurement and conversions. Then turn to Chapter 8 for specifics on the three methods of doing dosage calculations.

If you find that the math in this chapter is incomprehensible, consider getting a good, inexpensive math book, or just spend some time working on math on the Internet. Then come back to this chapter; the extra practice will help you get a better handle on the arithmetic basics that we cover here.

Healthy Numbers: Surveying the Numeral Systems Used in Healthcare

Healthcare professionals encounter two different numeral systems in their day-to-day lives: Arabic and Roman. Arabic numerals are the modern numbers (0–9) you're likely familiar with. Roman numerals, which are more classical and more difficult to work with, make their way into medicine and real life, too. The following sections take a closer look at these two numeral systems and explain where they fit in healthcare.

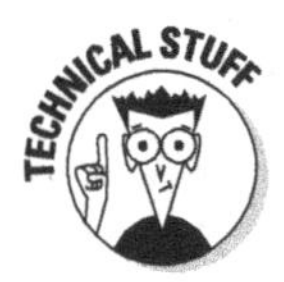

What's the difference between a *number* and a *numeral?* Well, at their simplest, numbers represent a basic quantity of something. Numerals, on the other hand, are the symbols or characters that represent the numbers.

Representing the classics: Roman numerals

Roman numerals are actually letters that represent numbers. The following list shows the common set of Roman numerals and the numbers they represent:

I	1
II	2
III	3
IV	4
V	5
VI	6
VII	7
VIII	8
IX	9
X	10
L	50
C	100
D	500
M	1,000

The Roman numeral system is decimal. It's based on the concept of 10, 100, 1,000, and so on. But it's not positional, meaning there's no zero to serve as a placeholder. (See the section "Zeroing in on Zero: It's really nothing" for details on zero's place in math.)

Although Roman numerals are no fun doing math with, they still have a place in medicine and real life. For instance, you see them on the faces of older clocks, on cornerstones of old buildings, in music chords, and as suffixes to kings' names (for example, Pippin IV) and football games (for example, Super Bowl XLIX). You also hear them in modern numbers and terms. For example, a $100 bill is often called a *C note* (which makes sense because the Roman numeral *C* stands for 100), and the U.S. mile derives its name from the Latin word *mille*, which means 1,000 (and the Roman numeral *M* stands for 1,000).

Modern medicine uses Roman numerals to describe dosages in *grains,* a unit of measurement in the apothecaries' system (see Chapter 4 for more details). Roman numerals also describe coagulation factors in the clotting system. For example, a Factor VIII (eight) deficiency is a primary cause of hemophilia. (In many cases, it's a genetic disorder where the body doesn't make clotting proteins like it's supposed to.)

Making math a lot easier: Arabic numerals

Hindus likely invented Arabic numerals in about 500 CE. By 1000 CE, this new number system had made its way to Europe, and, by the 1200s, mathematicians like Leonardo Fibonacci of Pisa were big fans.

Arabic numerals have several advantages over Roman numerals. First of all, large numbers are much easier to write and calculate with. A single Arabic digit in the correct position can represent a very large number; whereas, you need 15 Roman numerals to represent a relatively small number like 3,888,000. Second, arithmetic is clumsy with classical numerals. In fact, math lore says that if the ancient Greeks had used Arabic numerals, they would have invented calculus centuries before Sir Isaac Newton.

The Arabic numeral system has ten digits: 0, 1, 2, 3, 4, 5, 6, 7, 8, and 9. Like Roman numerals, the Arabic numeral system is decimal, but unlike its classical counterpart, it's also positional. In a *positional system,* you have a ones column, a tens column, a hundreds column, and so on. Zero (0) is a placeholder when no value appears in a column.

You use Arabic numerals for the arithmetic calculations in this chapter and all the dosage calculations throughout the rest of the book. They work very nicely for all number types and all calculations (see the section "Ingesting a Dose of Numbers" for details on the main number types).

Two Hippocrates for the price of one

As you know, Hippocrates of Cos is considered to be the father of modern medicine. After all, he not only founded a medical school but was also responsible for the Hippocratic Oath that physicians today still swear to uphold after graduating from medical school. But he's not the only famous Hippocrates to come out of Greece in the fifth century BCE. Hippocrates of Chios was a mathematician who was and still is famous for his theorems and work in early geometry.

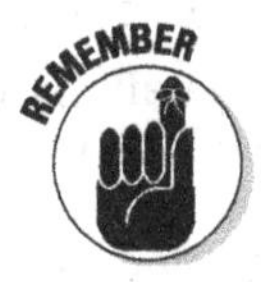

The *metric system* is a special set of Arabic numbers and is a heaven-sent gift to medical dosing calculations. In this system, each unit of weight or volume is a multiple of ten of another unit. Check out Chapter 4 for more on units of measurement and conversion.

Looking at where you see numbers in medicine

Numbers are everywhere in medicine, and, in general, they have the following three functions:

- **Reporting function:** Numbers describe patient basics — height, weight, pulse, and blood pressure. These measurements tell you a lot about the patient's condition, and you make clinical decisions based on them. Numbers also indicate vital signs on a patient's monitor. Knowing the significance of these different reporting numbers is essential in your work.
- **Identification function:** Patient numbers identify patients, and medication numbers identify medications. Identification numbers are vital in dosing meds because you must always give the right medication to the right patient.
- **Calculation function:** Numbers (and this is quite important) explicitly describe the amounts of medications that you administer to patients. Dosing calculations use relatively simple math, while the calculations used in disease research and the development of pharmaceuticals are considerably more complex.

Ingesting a Dose of Numbers

For a system with only ten digits, Arabic numbers sure have a lot of names. In case you don't remember everything you learned during your middle school days, here's a quick look at the main types of numbers you need to know:

- **Natural numbers:** All the positive whole numbers (also called *counting numbers*), beginning at 1 and going on forever
- **Integers:** All the natural numbers, as well as zero and negative numbers
- **Rational numbers:** All the integers, as well as all numbers that can be expressed as a ratio of two numbers, including all common and decimal fractions (see Chapter 3)
- **Irrational numbers:** All the numbers that can't be expressed as ratios, including the square root of 2 ($\sqrt{2}$) and pi (π)
- **Real numbers:** All rational and irrational numbers
- **Imaginary numbers:** A special number type, dealing with the square root of –1 ($\sqrt{-1}$), developed by Gerolamo Cardano and other Italian mathematicians in the 16th century to determine the roots of cubic and quartic polynomials; currently useful in fluid dynamics, quantum mechanics, and relativity

The following sections describe a number line (a way of visualizing numbers) and zero (a fundamental concept in mathematics).

Visualizing numbers on the number line

A *number line* is a graphic representation of the array of real numbers. A number line has 0 in the center, positive numbers at the right of 0, and negative numbers at the left of 0.

The number line in Figure 2-1 shows the full set of integers. (Fractions and irrational numbers fall between the integers on the number line.) It stretches to infinity at both the left and the right. The farther to the right of 0 on the number line you go, the larger the numbers get in value. The farther to the left of 0 you go, the more the numbers decrease in value.

–9 –8 –7 –6 –5 –4 –3 –2 –1 0 1 2 3 4 5 6 7 8 9

Figure 2-1: A number line.

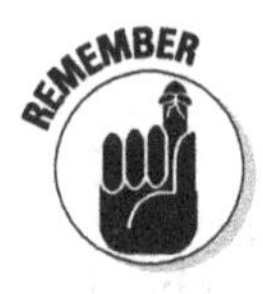

When it comes to numbers, looks can be deceiving. For example, the 9 in *–9* has a larger *magnitude* (the value without the sign, also called *absolute value*) than the 8 in *–8,* but the minus sign (–) tells you that –8 is actually larger than –9. A "larger" negative number has less value than a "smaller" negative number.

Zeroing in on zero: It's really nothing

Zero is an abstract concept. For example, you can't have zero bananas (or any other object). Well, if you have one banana and somebody takes it, you have the concept of zero — even though you no longer have the banana. As the old song goes, "Yes, we have no bananas."

Zero is also a placeholder in positional numeral systems, like the Arabic numeral system (see the earlier section "Making math a lot easier: Arabic numerals" for details). When you see a number with 0 (for example, 103), the 0 represents a column with no number in it. The number 103 has 1 in the hundreds column, 0 in the tens column, and 3 in the ones column.

When you write fractional decimals, be sure to write a zero before the decimal point. It's better notation in medical dosing to describe half a mL as 0.5 mL rather than .5 mL.

In medicine, the term *zero-order kinetics* applies to the rate equation for a chemical reaction; it means that no matter how much of a substance is in your body, your body metabolizes and eliminates it at the same rate. Alcohol (or booze, to use the common term) is a common example of a substance with zero-order kinetics. You can drink a lot, but, for the most part, your body eliminates the alcohol at a constant rate.

Using Addition to Make Everything Add Up

Addition is the process of adding one or more quantities to another quantity. In addition, you can add the terms in any order, thanks to the mathematical property called *commutativity,* which means that changing the order of something does not change the end result. For example:

$$a + b = b + a$$

$$a + b + c + d + e = e + c + b + a + d$$

Take this with a grain of salt

Congestive heart failure (CHF) is one of the most common reasons people are admitted to the hospital. When patients diagnosed with CHF leave, their doctors tell them to watch their sodium intake carefully as part of their daily "homework." So for the CHF patient, adding up salt intake is a regular and constant addition problem.

A patient on a limited sodium diet should take in no more than 2,000 mg of sodium a day. Because NaCl (the chemical formula for salt) is approximately 39 percent sodium by weight, it takes 5.128 g (5,128 mg) of salt to get 2,000 mg of sodium. This equates to approximately 0.85 teaspoon of salt.

The National Institutes of Health suggest that "normal" U.S. citizens consume less than 2.4 g (2,400 mg) of sodium per day. That amounts to 6 g of salt (which contains precisely 2,375 mg of sodium), about a teaspoon. Although a teaspoon may sound small, it's actually a lot of salt.

To do simple addition, first put the numbers in a column. Start by adding the numbers in the first column (the one on the far right). You can add a column of numbers from the top to the bottom or from the bottom to the top. The result is the same.

If the sum of the numbers in one column exceeds ten, you must *carry* the left digit of the two-digit answer to the next column. In other words, write the right digit of the two-digit answer beneath the column you're adding, and write the left digit above the next column to the left like so:

```
 1
428
186
---
??4
```

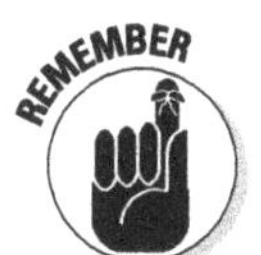

To make addition a little easier, keep in mind the following mathematical facts of life:

- **You can add negative and positive numbers together.** When you see an equation, such as $x = 5 - 4$, you can view it as either subtracting a positive number or adding a negative number. You can also write the equation as $x = 5 + (-4)$.
- **When you add zero to a number, the result is unchanged.** For example, writing $x = 5 + 0$ is the same as writing $x = 5$.
- **When you add two negative numbers together, the result is a larger negative number.** For example, $(-2) + (-8) = (-10)$.

Seeing Subtraction in Action

Subtraction is the process of removing a quantity from a quantity. (The result of a subtraction problem is called the *difference.*)

Unlike addition, subtraction doesn't have the property of commutativity. If you change the order of the terms, you change the result. You can express this concept algebraically as $a - b \neq b - a$, as in the following example:

$$4 - 3 \neq 3 - 4$$

By the way, in case you forgot, the symbol ≠ is the "not equal to" sign.

Do be a borrower and a lender

In Hamlet, Polonius says, "Neither a borrower nor a lender be." Well, in arithmetic, things are different; it's okay to be a borrower and a lender.

In subtraction, the term *borrowing* means converting 1 from the column to the left of the column you're working with and converting it into the units you're working with. As you know, the positions of the numbers are the ones column, the tens column, the hundreds column, and so forth.

To see how borrowing works, consider this subtraction problem:

$$\begin{array}{r} 43 \\ -\ 6 \\ \hline ?? \end{array}$$

Look at the ones column. You can't subtract 6 from 3, so you have to borrow. To do so, look at 43 as a combination of tens and ones:

$$\begin{array}{rr} 40 & 3 \\ & -6 \\ \hline ??? & ??? \end{array}$$

Borrow a 10 from the tens column, and lend it to the ones column. Then subtract:

$$\begin{array}{rr} 30 & 13 \\ & -6 \\ \hline 30 & 7 \end{array}$$

Combine the difference of the tens column (30) with the difference of the ones column (7) to get the answer to the problem — 37.

Working with positive and negative numbers

You can subtract positive numbers from positive numbers, positive numbers from negative numbers, negative numbers from positive numbers, or negative numbers from other negative numbers. To help you keep all these combinations straight, consider the following:

- **When you subtract a positive number from a larger positive number, the result is a positive number.** For example, 5 – 2 = 3.
- **When you subtract a positive number from a smaller positive number, the result is a negative number.** For example, 3 – 4 = –1.
- **When you subtract a positive number from a negative number, the result is a larger negative number.** For example, –7 – 9 = –16.
- **When you subtract a "smaller" negative number from a "larger" negative number, the result is a "less negative" number.** For example, –8 – (–3) = –5.

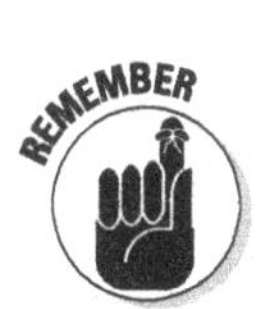

  Subtracting a negative number is like adding a positive number. In algebra, you express such a subtraction as $(-a) - (-b)$ and you can express it better as $(-a) + b$.

- **When you subtract a "larger" negative number from a "smaller" negative number, the result is a positive number.** For example, –3 – (–9) = 6.
- **When you subtract 0 from a positive or a negative number, the result is unchanged.** For example, 9 – 0 = 9.
- **When you subtract a positive number from 0, the result is a negative number.** For example, 0 – 7 = – 7.

In a hospital setting, nurses and doctors pay close attention to a patient's *input* (any fluids the patient is taking in, either intravenously or orally) and *output* (urinary and stool excretion, as well as any output from surgical tubes or drains). Nurses record the total amount of input and the total amount of output for a patient and use subtraction to calculate the difference, which can be either net positive or net negative. They then record the difference in milliliters (mL) in an 8- or 12-hour time period, corresponding to a typical nursing shift. The difference of input and output measurements is important because it alerts the doctors and nurses to changes in the patient's fluid status (that is, too much or too little fluid in the body).

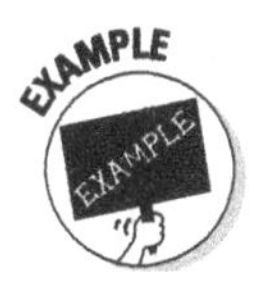

A patient's input is 1,000 mL. Her output is 2,600 mL. What's the net fluid balance for this patient?

To find out, subtract the output from the input, like so:

$$1{,}000 \text{ mL} - 2{,}600 \text{ mL} = -1{,}600 \text{ mL}$$

The patient is net negative 1,600 mL.

For patients with congestive heart failure, doctors in the hospital setting like to keep *I & Os* (the difference of input and output measurements) net negative. They feel positive about the patient being negative. Keeping the patient in a negative fluid balance helps the patient's heart failure get better. When the patient is discharged, she must watch her sodium intake closely. To help her do so, you instruct the patient to dutifully record her body weight at home on a daily basis. If her body weight increases or decreases, the patient may be in positive or negative fluid balance, respectively. The physician closely follows the patient's weight and condition.

Managing Multiplication

Multiplication and division play a much bigger role in medical dosing calculations than do addition and subtraction. In fact, they form the foundation of all your calculations. After all, fractions, decimals, percents, ratios, and proportions, all of which you deal with in dosing calculations, require multiplication and division.

You can describe multiplication as repeated adding. For example, $3 \times 4 = 12$, and you say this equation as "three times four equals 12." But you can also get the answer using repeated addition:

$$3 + 3 + 3 + 3 = 12$$

Multiplication, like addition, is commutative, meaning that the end result doesn't change when you change the order of the terms. For example, $a \times b = b \times a$ and $3 \times 4 = 4 \times 3$.

The commutativity of multiplication is incredibly valuable when you do dosing calculations because it allows you to rearrange terms in an order that makes calculating easier. Rearranging terms is common in elementary algebra.

The basic math isn't hard. Calculators, spreadsheets, smartphones, and the Internet make it easy to multiply big numbers and many numbers in a sequence.

Making multiplication easier with a few shortcuts

To make multiplication a little easier, keep the following shortcuts in mind:

- **When you multiply a number by 0, the result is zero.** For example, 9,567 × 0 = 0.
- **When you multiply a number by 1, the result is that number.** For example, 15.4799 × 1 = 15.4799.
- **When you multiply by 10, 100, or 1,000, to get the answer, simply add 1, 2, or 3 zeroes to the number you're multiplying.** For example, 57 × 100 = 5,700.

  If the number you're multiplying by 10, 100, or 1,000 has a decimal in it, simply move the decimal point to the right based on the number of zeros. For example, 2.33 × 10 = 23.3. (This shortcut also works when you're multiplying by 10,000, 100,000, and so on.)

  When you use a calculator to multiply, check for reasonableness. It's easy to lose track of the decimal point on a small display.

Getting the lowdown on metric units

There's magic in the metric system. The following two "tricks" make dosing calculations in metric units fast and easy:

- **Units are multiples of 10 of other units.** For example, 10 milligrams (mg) equal one centigram (cg), 10 centigrams equal 1 decigram (dg), and 10 decigrams equal 1 gram (g).
- **The units have names (based on Latin) that imply how big or small they are.** For example, *micro, milli,* and *deci* describe increasingly large units, and metric prefixes apply equally to units of liquid volume, weight, and distance.

To go from a larger unit of measurement to a smaller one, multiply. To go from a smaller unit of measurement to a larger one, divide. For example: 1,000 milligrams (mg) equal 1 gram (g). If you have grams and you want to know the equivalent number of milligrams, then multiply by 1,000. If you want to convert milligrams to grams, then divide by 1,000.

For more info on converting units, take a look at Chapter 4.

Doing Division: Divided We Stand

Division is the opposite (or *inverse*) of multiplication. You can describe division as repeated subtraction. For example, $12 \div 3 = 4$, and you say this equation as "twelve divided by three equals four." But you can also get the answer using repeated subtraction:

$$12 - 3 - 3 - 3 - 3 = 0$$

You've subtracted 3 from 12 four times.

Division in medical dosing calculations comes up in each of the traditional methods of dosage calculating: formula method, ratio-proportion method, and dimensional analysis method. See Chapter 8 for all the info about these three methods.

Division for medical dosing calculations generally requires representing terms as fractions to be used in multiplication. It's still division, but you can think of it as "multiplying by the inverse." Find out more about fractions in Chapter 3.

To see what we mean, consider the expression $250 \div 5$, which is better written as

$$\frac{250}{5}$$

You can view this expression not as "250 divided by 5," but as "250 multiplied by $\frac{1}{5}$," like so:

$$\frac{250}{1} \times \frac{1}{5}$$

Calculating division this way is often handy for working with numbers, and it also allows you to cancel out units, thus making dosing math easier. For example, here's a tabs/day calculation using the dimensional analysis calculation method (see Chapter 8 for more details):

$$\text{desired units} = \frac{\text{unit factor}}{\text{unit factor}} \times \frac{\text{unit factor}}{\text{unit factor}}$$

$$x \text{ tabs/day} = \frac{1 \text{ tab}}{250 \cancel{\text{mg}}} \times \frac{750 \cancel{\text{mg}}}{1 \text{ day}}$$

$$x = 3 \text{ tabs/day}$$

From the equation, you see that one tablet contains 250 mg and that you must administer 750 mg per day. Setting up the division problem using the inverse of multiplication causes the milligrams to cancel out, leaving tabs/day.

Two traditional types of division

The two traditional types of division you do by hand are

- **Short division:** This form of hand-calculated division is limited in its capabilities. Nobody uses it anymore because you can do simple division in your head.
- **Long division:** This form of division is the classic method of doing division by hand that you learned in elementary school. Although long division is a useful skill to master, calculators and spreadsheets have largely replaced it.

When you do dosing division, you can round your answer up or down instead of including a chain of decimals. For example, to find the hourly rate for dosing 1 L of a fluid in 3 hours, you divide 1 by 3. The result is 0.333333333 L/hr. To convert to mL/hr, multiply by 1,000. The answer is 333.3333333 mL/hr (see Chapter 4 for more on converting units). You can round that number down to 333 mL/hr.

To make division a little easier, be sure to take advantage of the following shortcuts:

- **Metric units:** With the metric system, the number you divide by is almost always 10, 100, or 1,000. To go from a smaller unit of measurement to a larger one, you simply divide. For example, to convert 3,000 mcg to mg, divide by 1,000 (because 1,000 mcg are in every 1 mg). The answer is 3 mg. (See the earlier section "Getting the lowdown on metric units" and Chapter 4 for more details.)
- **Spreadsheets and calculators:** When you do division calculations in a spreadsheet, you can see the full answer and all the terms used to develop it. Calculators are also handy for division because they are very portable and do a lot of the work for you. Just make sure you don't lose track of the decimal point!

Real-Life Practice: The RN and the Meds

You're a registered nurse (RN) who's providing in-home care for a patient who was recently released from the hospital. The patient had a serious infection and you must help her get a handle on her pills. You look at the discharge medication form and see two meds and the following dosing information:

- Cephalexin (Keflex): 3 pills, 4 times a day, for the next 12 days
- Metronidazole (Flagyl): 2 pills, 3 times a day, for the next 12 days

How many pills of each medication should the patient take each day? What's the total number of pills she has to take over 12 days?

Follow these steps to find out:

1. **Calculate the number of cephalexin tablets she has to take each day.**

   3 pills × 4 times a day = 12 pills each day
2. **Calculate the number of metronidazole tablets she has to take each day.**

   2 pills × 3 times a day = 6 pills each day
3. **Calculate the number of cephalexin tablets she has to take over 12 days.**

   12 × 12 = 144 pills of cephalexin for the 12 days
4. **Calculate the number of metronidazole tablets she has to take over 12 days.**

   6 × 12 =72 pills of metronidazole for the 12 days
5. **Add the two totals to get the total number of pills she has to take over 12 days.**

   72 + 144 = 216 pills total

This example may at first appear trivial, but it's not. It's a common at-home dosing scenario, and the simple math you use to solve it shows the following:

- You can sometimes use very simple arithmetic to answer dosing calculation questions.
- Any dosing problem is easier when you break it into parts.

A handy (and also dandy) way to organize pills at home is to use a *pill organizer* (also known as a *pill box*). A pill organizer is a box for storing daily doses of pills, and it usually has one or more compartments for each day of the week. The box can help the patient take the right number of pills each day, including taking pills at multiple times during the day. Using a pill box can help reduce medication errors, such as missing a dose or doubling a dose. Figure 2-2 shows a pill box.

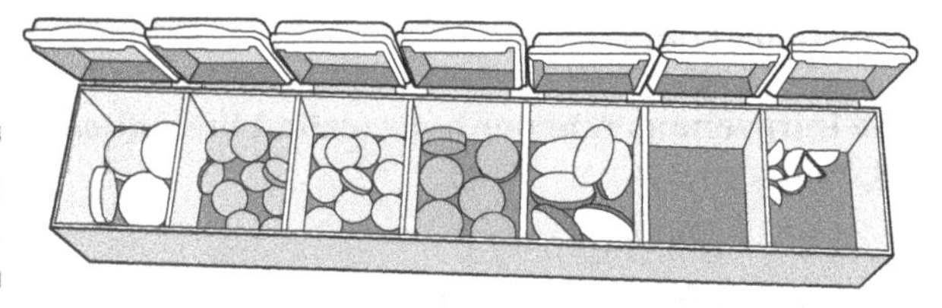

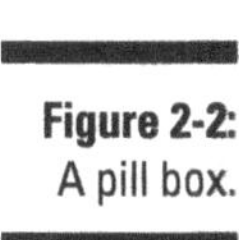

Figure 2-2: A pill box.

Real-Life Practice: A Fluid Approach to Fluids

To help keep a patient from getting dehydrated, you must give him fluids through a type of feeding tube called a PEG tube. You're asked to administer 250 mL every 3 hours. How much will you give him over the course of 24 hours?

To find out, follow these steps:

1. **Divide 24 by 3 to determine how many times you're giving the patient fluid in 24 hours (in other words, how many dosing intervals are in one day).**

   24 hours ÷ 3 hours = 8 dosing intervals

   There are 8 intervals in one day.

2. **Multiply the 8 intervals by 250 mL to determine the total amount of fluid you have to give over 24 hours.**

   250 mL × 8 = 2,000 mL

   You must administer 2,000 mL over the course of 24 hours.

Real-Life Practice: Liquid Assets

You're working in a hospital, and you need to calculate a patient's input of fluids for the day. He's getting 2,000 mL over 24 hours through a PEG feeding tube. You note that he's also getting fluids intravenously at a rate of 50 mL/hr. How much in total fluids is the patient getting in 24 hours?

Follow these steps to find out:

1. **Multiply the intravenous rate per hour (called the *infusion* or *flow rate*) by 24 hours.**

   50 mL/hr × 24 hr = 1,200 mL

   The total from intravenous input is 1,200 mL daily.

2. **Calculate the total input for the patient for the day by adding the volume from both the feeding tube and the intravenous fluids together.**

   2,000 mL (oral) + 1,200 mL (intravenous) = 3,200 mL (total)

   The answer is 3,200 mL daily.

Chapter 3

Getting Familiar with Fractions and Their Fanatic Forms

In This Chapter

- Understanding the different types of fractions
- Converting between fractions, decimals, and percentages
- Calculating percentages
- Putting fractions to work with some simple practice problems

Knowing how to work with common fractions, decimals, percentages, and proportions is crucial when you're dosing medications. But don't panic if you don't remember these names, much less how to use them in math. They're all *fractions* (numbers whose values are between 0 and 1), and they're all easy to work with as long as you know the fundamentals. If you're up to speed on fractions, head on over to another chapter. But if you're looking for a compact review, this is the place for you.

In your work, you may need to calculate a full dose, ¾ (three-fourths) of a dose, or ½ (one-half) of a dose of a medication. In dosing a liquid medication, you may need to give 0.2 mL (two-tenths of a milliliter). Or you may need to give only 25% (twenty-five percent), or ¼ (one-fourth), of a particular medication; that's saying the same thing.

Just as a boxer (or any athlete) needs to know the essentials of speed, coordination, and footwork, you need to know the essentials of fractions. Knowing fractions not only makes you more efficient but also reduces your chances of error and improves patient care. In this chapter, we review the basics of common fractions, decimals, percentages, and proportions and help you do simple (but very important) conversions. After working through this chapter, you're sure to be a fanatic (instead of frenetic) about fractions.

Using Fractions to Probe between Integers

A *fraction* is a number that represents a part of a whole number. A fraction falls between two whole numbers, 0 and 1, on a number line. (To see more about number types and the number line, refer to Chapter 2.)

In the medical field, fractions are considered "good news" numbers because

- All fraction math is pretty easy.
- All forms of fractions are useful in dosing medications.
- You can easily convert fractions from one form to another.

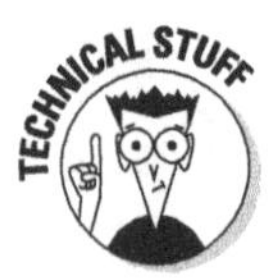

The word *fraction* comes from the Latin verb *frangere,* meaning "to break," which makes sense because a fraction is a small number that has "broken off" from a whole number. The term *fraction* is also related to the word *fracture,* which is a broken bone.

The traditional fraction you probably grew up with in school is called a *common* (or *vulgar*) *fraction* (½ and ¾, for example), but fractions have other forms, as well.

The following numbers are all fractions. They're just written in different ways.

- ⅓
- 0.25
- 50%
- 7:10

The sections that follow take a closer look at these four types of fractions and their roles in medical dosage calculations.

Common fractions

A common fraction has one number (called the *numerator*) written above or to the left of another number (called the *denominator*). The two numbers are separated by a line. For example, in the fraction ⅝, 5 is the numerator and 8 is the denominator:

$$\frac{5\ (\text{numerator})}{8\ (\text{denominator})}$$

You see common fractions like the following examples all the time in real life:

$$\frac{1}{3},\ \frac{1}{4},\ \frac{1}{2},\ \frac{3}{7},\ \frac{4}{5},\ \frac{99}{100}$$

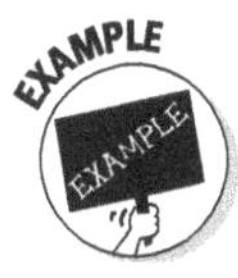

For your personal health and well-being, you have to eat a big slice of apple pie, or about ⅛ of the pie. What do the numbers in ⅛ mean?

- The *8* (the denominator) means that the pie has a total of eight slices.
- The *1* (the numerator) is the portion of the pie you eat. That's one out of eight pieces, or ⅛.

Figure 3-1 shows a pie with eight pieces; ⅛ of the pie is white.

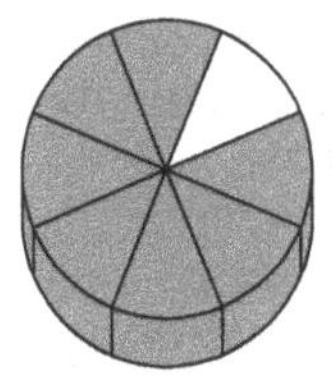

Figure 3-1: A pie with eight pieces.

This example may seem childish, but the $\frac{\text{numerator}}{\text{denominator}}$ definition applies to all fractions. The following sections cover the four types of common fractions.

Mixed fractions

A *mixed fraction* contains both a whole number and a fraction. An example of a mixed fraction is 1½.

Improper fractions

Don't worry; there's nothing immoral about an improper fraction. An *improper fraction* is just a top-heavy fraction, in which the numerator is larger than the denominator. If the fraction were a house, it would collapse. Some examples of improper fractions are

- $\frac{11}{7}$
- $\frac{3}{2}$
- $\frac{160}{4}$

To convert an improper fraction to a mixed number, all you have to do is calculate the whole number component and the remaining fractional component. Here's an example:

$$\frac{11}{7}=\frac{7}{7}+\frac{4}{7}$$

$$\frac{7}{7}=1 \text{ and } \frac{4}{7}=\frac{4}{7}$$

The result is $1\frac{4}{7}$.

When converting an improper fraction to a mixed number, or vice versa, the denominator never changes. Not surprisingly, being a denominator can sometimes be very boring.

Unreduced fractions

Sometimes when you do arithmetic with common fractions, you end up with intermediate results. They're intermediate because you usually have to reduce them to their lowest possible terms before you use them in your dosing calculations. Hence, the term *unreduced fractions.*

Dosage calculations are easier to calculate when you reduce fractions to their simplest forms. Reducing fractions before you do your calculations also cuts down on possible mistakes.

Here are two examples of unreduced fractions:

- $\frac{4}{16}$
- $\frac{120}{6}$

Both are legitimate fractions, but they're far more useful and easier to work with after you reduce them. To do so, simply divide the top and bottom numbers by the largest number that goes into both evenly (also known as the *greatest common factor*). For the first example, divide the top and bottom by 4; for the second example, divide by 6. The reduced results are

- $\frac{1}{4}$
- 20

Fractions in unity

When the numerator and denominator of a common fraction are the same, you have *unity*. That is, any fraction with a numerator that's the same as its denominator equals 1. Here are some examples of fractions with unity:

> ## A little fraction humor . . .
>
> The only reason common fractions are also called *vulgar* fractions is because *vulgar* is the Latin word for "common." They aren't coarse or crude. In fact, they're clean and decent. And the fact that they're some part of a whole number makes them "whole some." (A little fraction humor for you!)

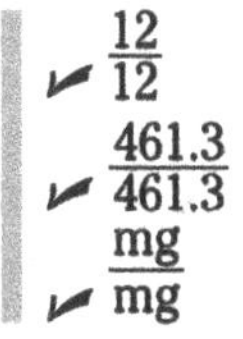

- $\frac{12}{12}$
- $\frac{461.3}{461.3}$
- $\frac{mg}{mg}$

In each case, the identical numerators and denominators cancel each other out. As a result, they're all equal to 1.

Hey! What about that last one, mg/mg? Yes, unity in fractions works for units, too. In fact, it's what drives many dosing calculations. You count on certain units to "fall out" of the calculation because they're equal to 1.

The real value of common fractions is in their structure, which you use in practically all dosage calculations — whether you're applying the formula method, the ratio-proportion method, or the dimensional analysis method. (Find out more about these methods in Chapter 8.)

Decimal fractions

Decimal numbers are all around you, and the decimal system is used worldwide for measurement and calculation. For instance, decimal numbers appear on your grocery receipt, on the instruments on your car's dashboard, on measuring tapes, and in the math you learn in school. Decimal fractions are just a special form of decimal numbers.

A *decimal fraction* has a value of more than 0 but less than 1. The distinguishing marks of a decimal fraction are the decimal point and the decimal places. The following are examples of decimal fractions:

- 0.1
- 0.557
- 0.9999999999999999

A *mixed number*, by the way, is a combination of a whole number and a decimal fraction. Here are some examples of mixed numbers:

- 23.1
- 100.557
- 999,999,999.9999999999999999

Everyone measures and calculates with decimal numbers and decimal fractions. Even American money is expressed in decimal units and fractions, known as dollars and cents. But decimal fractions have enormous advantages in the world of healthcare, too:

- **The *metric system*, which medicine, nursing, and related healthcare professions use almost universally, is a decimal system based on units that are multiples of ten of other units.** Among the fractional units, 10 milligrams (mg) equal 1 centigram (cg), 10 centigrams equal 1 decigram (dg), and 10 decigrams equal 1 gram (g). So 1,000 mg equal 1 gram.
- **In healthcare, the metric units themselves have "implied math," which makes calculating even easier.** *Implied math* simply means that the prefixes for units (for example, *micro-*, *milli-*, *centi-*, and *deci-*) indicate how relatively large or small they are. So when you dose a medication in milligrams (mg), you know 1 mg is 1/1,000 or 0.001 g. Although the math is the same, it's less confusing to dispense a 325 mg aspirin tablet (for example) rather than a 325/1,000 g tablet or a 0.325 g tablet — even though they all mean the same thing.
- **Arithmetic (addition, subtraction, multiplication, and division) is easy to do with metric units.** For doctors and nurses, the metric system is a big improvement over the apothecary units (drams, scruples, grains, and so on; see Chapter 4) used in the early 19th century, which didn't have simple conversion rates. (For example, there are 7,680 minims in a liquid pint, and that's no easy conversion.)

Percentages

A *percentage* is a fraction whose denominator never changes. It's always 100. A number like 33%, for example, refers to 33 parts in 100, or $^{33}/_{100}$, or 0.33. (*Percent* or *per cent* means "per centum," which is from the Latin phrase meaning "by the hundred.") Mathematicians and medical professionals alike use percentages to explain how large or small a quantity is, compared to another quantity.

Percentages compare quantities in the following two ways:

- **By comparing a quantity to the whole:** A normal saline IV solution is 0.9% sodium chloride (NaCl) — 9 grams of sodium chloride dissolved in 1 L (1,000 mL) of water. (For this IV, you have to memorize that *normal* means 0.9%.)
- **By comparing one quantity to another:** A D5NS IV (5% dextrose in normal saline) shows the relative amounts of dextrose and NaCl by its name (5% dextrose in 0.9% sodium chloride). We recommend that you use a drug reference guide or consult a pharmacist if you have any questions concerning the quantity of glucose and other electrolytes in a particular solution.

Impress your friends by telling them that a percentage is a *dimensionless proportionality*. When they say, "Huh?" tell them that a quantity is dimensionless when it doesn't have a physical unit. For example, the comparison of sodium chloride to water in an IV will be the same (say 0.9%) whether the IV comes in a 1 L bag or a 1,000 L tank.

Proportions (and ratios)

A *ratio* is a relationship between two quantities. Ratios are commonplace in everyday life. For example, Greek architecture is said to employ the *golden ratio* — a special relationship of height to width. The format of a motion picture is the *aspect ratio* — again, a special relationship of height to width.

A *proportion* is a relationship between four quantities. You use proportions a lot in doing medical dosage calculations.

Proportions

In a proportion equation, the first quantity (a) divided by the second (b) equals the third (c) divided by the fourth (d).

Proportions take the following form:

$$\frac{a}{b} = \frac{c}{d}$$

When you know three of the quantities, you can solve for the fourth. You simply set up a proportion for the three *known* quantities, or *equivalents* as they're called in medical dosage calculations, and solve for the *desired* quantity, like so:

$$\frac{\text{known equivalent } (a)}{\text{known equivalent } (b)} = \frac{\text{known equivalent } (c)}{\text{desired equivalent } (d)}$$

To solve for the desired equivalent (or d), follow these steps:

1. **Multiply $a \times d$ and $b \times c$ to get a cross-product.**
2. **Divide to solve for x (or d, the desired equivalent).**

Sorry, but it's no more complicated than that! To see how this simple proportion can help you solve medical dosage calculations, consider the following example.

If there are 40 g of magnesium sulfate in a 1,000 mL (1 L) IV, how much solution (in mL) contains 1 g of magnesium sulfate?

To solve this problem, follow these steps:

1. **Set up the following proportion:**

$$\frac{\text{known equivalent } (a)}{\text{known equivalent } (b)} = \frac{\text{known equivalent } (c)}{\text{desired equivalent } (d)}$$

$$\frac{40 \text{ g}}{1{,}000 \text{ mL}} = \frac{1 \text{ g}}{x \text{ mL}}$$

2. **Cross-multiply.**

   That is, multiply $a \times d$ and $b \times c$ to get a cross-product, like so:

   $40x = 1{,}000$

3. **Solve for x.**

   That is, divide 1,000 by 40.

   $x = 25$

   The answer is 25 mL. In other words, 25 mL of solution contain 1 g of magnesium sulfate.

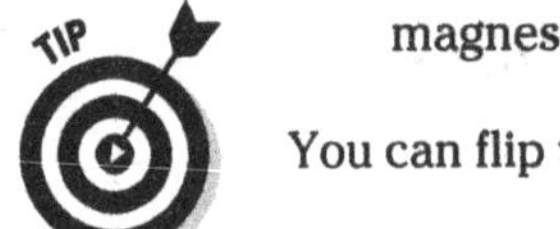

You can flip the right side of the equation upside down, like so, if you prefer:

$$\frac{\text{known equivalent } (a)}{\text{known equivalent } (b)} = \frac{\text{desired equivalent } (c)}{\text{known equivalent } (d)}$$

You still multiply $a \times d$ and $b \times c$ to get a cross-product.

Proportions may just be the handiest tool in the medical dosage calculation handbook! You use proportions as a fast way to calculate weights, volumes, flow rates, and times. It's the Swiss army knife of dosing math. (Check out Chapter 8 for more details on using proportions to calculate dosages.)

Ratios

Ratios are expressions that show the relationship between two quantities. Although they aren't prominent in dosage calculations, ratios are fairly common in healthcare, and they're invaluable for seeing relationships.

A *convenience ratio* looks like a ratio, but it isn't one in the mathematical sense. It's a notational convention that shows a relationship between two quantities.

For example, you typically write a blood pressure measurement as two numbers that look like a ratio, like so:

$$\frac{\text{115 systolic (mmHg)}}{\text{75 diastolic (mmHg)}}$$

You say this ratio as "115 over 75." Although the two numbers are related — since they're both blood pressure measurements — they aren't a real ratio. However, together they tell the healthcare professional a great deal about the patient's condition.

Some meds show two numbers that suggest a ratio but aren't really a ratio. For example, Vicodin may be labeled "5/500," since it contains 5 mg hydrocodone and 500 mg acetaminophen. To avoid confusion, this name should be labeled "5-500."

Humulin 70/30 insulin is a true ratio acting as a convenience ratio. It contains a mixture of 70% intermediate-acting insulin (isophane) and 30% short-acting insulin (regular). However, no calculations are required. When Humulin 70/30 is ordered, the only requirement is to dispense it correctly.

Conquering Fraction-Related Conversions

You can do much more with fractions than simply labeling them according to their forms. Ha! 'Tis nothing! 'Tis but child's play! (We could be doing *Hamlet* here, or perhaps it's Monty Python's *Spamalot*.)

Fractions don't have to stay in any one form. You can convert them, at your will, to other forms. As a medical professional, you need to be flexible enough to convert fractions between common, decimal, percentage, and proportion forms. Lucky for you, the following sections show you how to do just that.

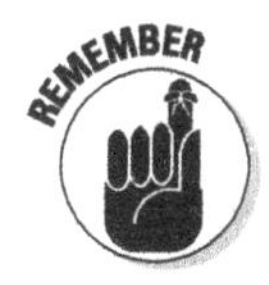

Conquering conversions is paramount to successful medical dosage calculations. As with everything in life, find what manner of calculation works best for you, and then practice it to build confidence. Maintaining the "I can do it" attitude throughout that practice is what keeps you energetic and competent.

Converting fractions into decimals

Turning a fraction into a decimal number is easy. In fact, you probably know some basic conversions, like those that follow, by heart:

- $\frac{1}{4} = 0.25$
- $\frac{1}{2} = 0.5$
- $\frac{3}{4} = 0.75$

The rule for converting fractions to decimals is to simply divide the denominator into the numerator to get the answer. In the first example, divide 1 by 4 to get 0.25. Use a calculator or smartphone, a spreadsheet program, or pencil and paper to practice with the other two examples.

Converting decimals into fractions

Converting a decimal number into a fraction is just as easy as converting a fraction into a decimal (see the preceding section). Maybe easier. The conversion rule is simple: Set the decimal up as a fraction and reduce it to its simplest terms. For example, to convert 0.75 to a fraction, set up the fraction as follows:

$$0.75 = \frac{75}{100}$$

The intermediate answer is $^{75}/_{100}$. To reduce the fraction, divide both the top and bottom numbers by a common factor (see the section "Unreduced fractions" for details). Decimal fractions always have 10, 100, 1,000, 10,000, and so forth as a denominator, so try dividing by factors of 10, such as 5 or 2. If you divide 75 and 100 by 5, you get $^{15}/_{20}$. But wait! That's another intermediate answer. You can do even more division to get to the simplest terms: Divide both terms by 5 again, and you get $^{3}/_{4}$, which is the most reduced answer. (Note that you could've divided 75 and 100 by 25 in the first place to get $^{3}/_{4}$.)

Converting percentages into decimals

The rule for going from percentages to decimals is simple: Divide the percentage by 100. The result is a decimal number because the denominator in a percent is always 100. So, for example, 67% becomes $^{67}/_{100}$, or 0.67.

If you need 20% of a 1 L solution, you need $^{20}/_{100}$, or 0.2 L (also known as 200 mL). You don't even have to plug the numbers into a calculator. To divide by 100, you just move the decimal point two places to the left of its original position. The number 20 really is 20.0. When you move the decimal to the left, the result is 0.200 L, or 0.2 L — the same answer you get with actual division.

Converting decimals into percentages

Converting from a decimal number into a percentage is just the opposite of converting from a percentage into a decimal (see the preceding section). When it comes to decimal conversions, you're faster than any calculator or spreadsheet.

To make this conversion, multiply the decimal by 100 and add a percent sign. The result is a percent. For instance, if you want to make 0.67 a percentage, multiply 0.67 by 100 to get 67 and then slap a percent sign next to it. As a shortcut, you can simply shift the decimal point two places to the right, which is the same as multiplying by 100.

Converting percentages into fractions

Converting percentages into fractions is so fast it'll make your head spin! The rule is to drop the percent sign and put the number over 100 in a fraction. The result is (naturally) a fraction. Then just reduce as necessary (see the section "Unreduced fractions" for details).

For example, to convert 26% to a fraction, follow these steps:

1. **Drop the percent sign and use the numerical portion of the term.**

   26% becomes just 26.

2. **Set the percentage number as a numerator over the denominator 100.**

   $$\frac{26}{100}$$

   The denominator is always 100 for percentages.

3. **Simplify the fraction.**

   $$\frac{26}{100} = \frac{13}{50}$$

   The answer is $\frac{13}{50}$.

Converting fractions into percentages

This conversion is the reverse of the conversion of percentages into fractions (see the preceding section). The rule for converting a fraction to a percentage is to convert the fraction into a decimal and then multiply by 100. The result is a percentage. For example, if you have $\frac{33}{100}$ of something, you divide 33 by 100 to get 0.33 and then multiply by 100 to arrive at 33%.

What if you have $\frac{5}{8}$ of something? What percentage is that? First, divide 5 by 8 to get the decimal 0.625. Then multiply by 100. The result is 62.5%.

Playing the Percentages

Playing the percentages isn't just for gamblers in Las Vegas. A basic math skill is to increase and decrease quantities by percentages, as you see in the following sections.

Calculating percentage increases

To increase a number by a percentage, multiply the original number by the percentage and then add the result to the original number. Consider the following example.

You have a 1 L (1,000 mL) bag of solution. What would the total quantity be if the total volume were increased by 65%?

This example is simple because it starts with a 1,000 mL bag. Just follow these steps:

1. **Multiply the original number (1,000 mL) by 65%.**

   $$1{,}000 \text{ mL} \times 65\% = 1{,}000 \text{ mL} \times \frac{65}{100} = \frac{65{,}000}{100} \text{ mL} = 650 \text{ mL}$$

2. **Add the result to the original number.**

   $$1{,}000 \text{ mL} + 650 \text{ mL} = 1{,}650 \text{ mL}$$

   The answer is 1,650 mL.

Note: The order we use in this example would never be a real doctor's order. It's just an exercise to help you understand percentage increases in a clinical context.

Percentage increases are very useful for expressing changes like percentage weight gain or weight loss, but you should never see a medication order to "increase the dose by 25%" (or any other percent, for that matter). Good orders for IVs, pills, and all other meds should describe exactly what the new higher doses need to be.

Calculating a 100% increase

You know that a percent is a fraction with 100 in the denominator. Well, 100% has 100 in the numerator, too. So 100% looks like this:

$$100\% = \frac{100}{100} = 1$$

The result is the number 1 (or *unity,* as we hot math people sometimes call it; see the section "Fractions in unity" for details). So what do you do when you need to increase a quantity by 100%? You obviously can't multiply it by 1, or you won't get any increase at all. Instead, you have to take the base quantity and add 100% of that quantity to it. Mathematically, a 100% increase in a quantity looks like this, where x is the original quantity:

$$x + \frac{100}{100}x = x + x = 2x$$

To put this equation in shorthand: To calculate a 100% increase in something, simply double the base amount. To calculate a 200% increase in something, simply triple the base amount.

Calculating percentage decreases

Percentage decreases are useful for calculating decreases in patient weight and decreases in patient calorie consumption. But they aren't used in changing the dosages of medications.

For example, the doctor tells you to stop an infusion of 2 mg/hr for one hour and then restart the infusion at 1 mg/hr. Those infusion rates are precise numbers that don't require a dosage calculation to figure out the final rate.

Keep in mind that you do need to recalculate the flow rate, but that's another story. (Turn to Chapter 11 for details on how to do so.)

But if you ever need to calculate a percentage decrease to determine a patient's percentage weight loss, for example, here's what you do: Take the base amount, multiply by the percentage decrease to get the decrease amount, and subtract it from the base amount.

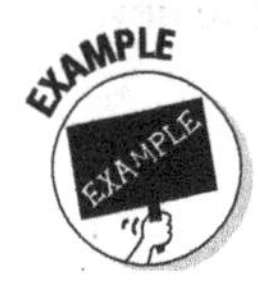

A patient formerly weighed 100 kg (220 lb). Because of a supervised weight loss program, he now weighs 80 kg (176 lb). What's the percentage decrease in weight?

To find out, do the following:

1. **Determine the difference in weight by using subtraction.**

   100 kg – 80 kg = 20 kg

2. **Express the weight loss as a percentage of the original weight, like so:**

   $$x = \frac{20}{100}$$
   $$x = 0.20$$
   $$x = 20\%$$

   The patient has had a 20 percent loss in body weight.

Real-Life Practice: Chow Down to Heal Up

Nutrition is a very important part of healing. It means much more than just putting meat on the bones. In a hospital setting or at home, you may need to closely monitor how much a patient eats. As you do so, you may record (for example) a number like ½, meaning that a patient ate only one-half of a whole patient meal. Sometimes the doc consults a dietitian to closely watch the caloric intake of a particular patient.

You find out that a patient ate only 800 calories in a day when she needed to eat 2,400 calories. What portion of the total amount of needed calories did she consume?

Set this problem up as a simple fraction. Plug in the values and reduce the fraction, like so:

$$x = \frac{\text{calories consumed}}{\text{calories needed}}$$

$$x = \frac{800}{2{,}400}$$

$$x = \frac{1}{3}$$

In terms of calories, the patient ate only ⅓ of what she was supposed to eat. Record the intake, and alert the doctor.

The amounts that patients eat, especially in the hospital, may vary, but you need to try to encourage them to "eat up." Healing can be hard to do without a good meal.

Real-Life Practice: Measuring the Mass

The *body mass index* (or BMI, for short) is a very common calculation that medical professionals use to approximate a patient's total body fat. It's a way to calculate how healthy the patient is, and it appears on many doctors' charts.

The BMI is a fraction: The numerator contains the patient's weight in pounds, and the denominator contains the patient's height in inches. The formula for calculating BMI is as follows (703 is a constant):

$$\text{BMI} = \frac{(\text{mass lbs})}{(\text{height in})^2} \times 703$$

A patient weighs 200 pounds and is 6 feet (72 inches) tall. What's the patient's BMI?

Set up the formula by plugging in the patient's weight and height and then solve for BMI as we do here:

$$\text{BMI} = \frac{200}{72 \times 72} \times 703$$

$$\text{BMI} = \frac{200}{5{,}184} \times 703$$

$$\text{BMI} = 0.03858 \times 703$$

$$\text{BMI} = 27.12$$

The answer is that the patient has a BMI of 27.

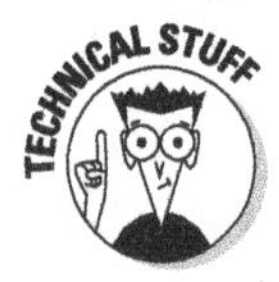

You can use many different equations to calculate the BMI; many involve using special computerized programs like MedCalc. Regardless of which equation you use, though, a BMI of greater than 30 is considered the definition of obesity, which is an epidemic in the United States. So the patient from the preceding example would be classified as *overweight* but not *obese class I.* The doctor would likely tell this patient to eat healthy, watch his caloric intake, and exercise.

Chapter 4

Getting Familiar with Systems of Measurement and Unit Conversions

In This Chapter

- Surveying the measurement systems used in medicine
- Converting from one unit to another in different measurement systems
- Getting some real-world practice with measurements in medical dosing

Measurement has been an essential part of civilization for a very long time. As many math books proclaim, the first farmers and craftspeople used measurement to lay out their fields and establish trade agreements. But did you know that measurement has even older roots in healthcare? Ancient tribal healers had to remember and measure the correct dosages of the correct ingredients to make medical concoctions that would cure their tribe members.

Like ancient healers, today's medical professionals use measurement to help them cure their patients. For instance, they need to know a patient's weight, height, and age to make the right clinical decisions. They also need to know how much of what substance to prescribe.

Although measuring often involves just reading the numbers you see in hospitals and other medical centers — on scales, thermometers, labels, instruments, and so on — it's not always that simple. You also have to count pills, draw up solutions for injections, dilute concentrates, set infusion pumps, and much more, all in specified units of measurement. And to make things even more complicated, you have to do all that using several different measurement systems.

In this chapter, we walk you through these different systems of measurement and help you get familiar with the most common units you'll use in the medical field. We also show you how to convert from one unit to another, whether the units are in the same or different systems. As an added bonus, we include a table at the end of the chapter with a summary of the most useful conversion factors.

By knowing what's what in measurement, you set yourself up for clarity and accuracy in all your medical calculations. (To get some practice with the different dosing calculation methods, turn to Chapter 8.)

Looking at the Main Measurement Systems Used in Medicine

To do medical dosage calculations really well, you need to be familiar with the following four measurement systems:

- **Metric system:** The standard measurement system used throughout the world
- **United States customary system:** A measurement system that's common outside of science and medicine in the United States
- **Household system:** A subset of the United States customary system that's common in kitchens and other areas of home life
- **Apothecaries' system:** An old system whose units still show up in modern life

Review each of these measurement systems carefully. Even though most of what you see in the medical field is metric, the other systems are also important because their units still figure in some medication dosing scenarios.

Metric system

The *metric system* is the most common measurement system used in medicine. Its units are multiples of ten compared to smaller units. When converting from one unit to another, you almost always multiply or divide by 10 or 1,000.

Metric units have Latin prefixes. For example, *kilo* means 1,000, so 1 *kilogram* (kg) equals 1,000 grams (g). Similarly, *milli* means $\frac{1}{1,000}$ (0.001), so a *milliliter* (mL) is $\frac{1}{1,000}$ of a liter (L).

Table 4-1 shows some common metric prefixes and abbreviations used in healthcare. The Prefix column shows the full prefix that comes before the metric base units, such as grams, liters, or meters, to indicate size. The Abbreviation column shows the corresponding abbreviations you apply to the abbreviated base units. (For example, the abbreviation for kilogram combines *k* with the abbreviation *g* to become *kg*.) The Multiply Base Unit by column shows how many base units are in larger or smaller units, and the Exponent column shows the same number in scientific notation.

Table 4-1 Metric Prefixes and Abbreviations

Prefix	*Abbreviation*	*Multiply Base Unit by*	*Exponent*
kilo-	k	1,000	10^3
hecto-	h	100	10^2
deca-	da	10	10^1
base unit (no prefix)		1	
deci-	d	0.1	10^{-1}
centi-	c	0.01	10^{-2}
milli-	m	0.001	10^{-3}
micro-	mc	0.000001	10^{-6}

The following sections take a quick look at the metric units you need to know for weight, volume, length, area, and temperature.

Weight

The following table shows the most important metric units for measuring weight in the medical field.

Unit	*Abbreviation*	*Equivalent*
Microgram	mcg	$\frac{1}{1,000,000}$ g
Milligram	mg	$\frac{1}{1,000}$ g
Gram	g	
Kilogram	kg	1,000 g

Weight is the common term for a mass under the influence of the force of earth's gravity. *Mass* is the scientific term for the weight of an object regardless of the forces acting on it. Because the moon has ⅙ of the earth's gravity, an object with a mass of 6 kg (which weighs 6 kg on earth) weighs only 1 kg on the moon. Unless you have immediate plans to visit the moon, though, you can use *weight* when you're talking about how heavy patients, objects, and substances are.

Fun facts about the metric system

The official name of the metric system is *International System of Units,* or *SI system.* (*SI* stands for système international d'unités.) The metric system is a *decimalized* system, which means each larger unit of length, area, volume, or weight is ten times the size of the previous smaller unit.

Length, area, volume, and weight each have a *base unit,* which is the fundamental unit that other units are related to. Other units are multiples of the base unit. The meter (m) is the base unit of length, but millimeters (mm) and centimeters (cm) are also commonly used. The cubic meter (m^3) is the base unit of volume.

The kilogram (kg) is the base unit of weight, but many meds are dosed in grams (g) and milligrams (mg). An odd fact is that the gram *was* the base unit of weight in the original metric system. The unit was changed, presumably because any variability in the standard kilogram (called the International Prototype Kilogram, or IPK) is less significant than variability in the much smaller standard gram. The IPK is made of a platinum-iridium alloy and is stored in a vault in Sèvres, France.

Can you believe it? The liter (L) is not an official SI unit of volume! It once was part of the metric system (and was based on the amount of water that weighed one kilogram), but the standard was abandoned, because the density of water changes slightly with temperature and pressure. Even so, using SI prefixes and abbreviations with the liter is a standard convention. You use liters (L) and milliliters (mL) all the time in the hospital and in the laboratory. In countries other than the United States, people also use these measurements in cooking.

Here are some interesting equivalents: 1 L of water weighs about 1 kg, and when you divide both units by 1,000, you see that 1 mL weighs about 1 g.

But wait, there's more! The United States is the only industrialized nation that doesn't use metric for standard activities. It uses metric in medicine, science, industry, and the military but not in common, everyday measurements, like the ones used in cooking and sports. Burma (Myanmar) and Liberia are the only other countries that haven't adopted the SI system.

Liquid volume

The following table shows the most important metric units for measuring liquid volume in the medical field.

Unit	*Abbreviation*	*Equivalent*
Milliliter	mL	$\frac{1}{1,000}$ L
Liter	L	1,000 mL

Figure 4-1 shows a typical use of metric units for volume (mL) on a drug label.

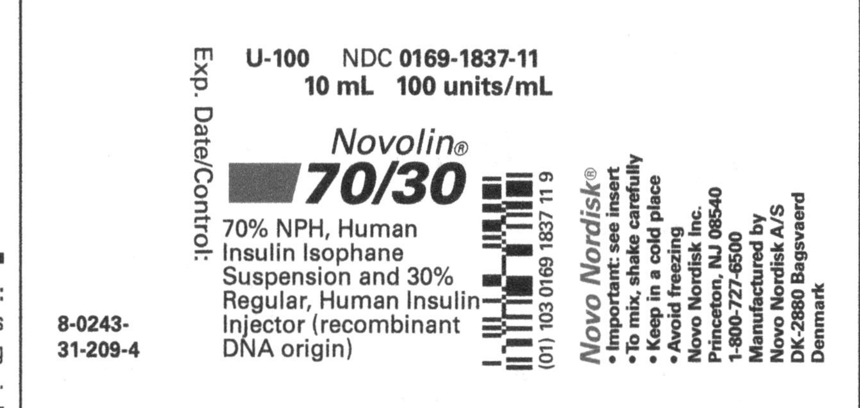

Figure 4-1: Metric units on a drug label.

Reprinted with permission from Novo Nordisk Pharmaceuticals.

Length

The following table shows the most important metric units for measuring length in the medical field.

Unit	*Abbreviation*	*Equivalent*
millimeter	mm	$\frac{1}{1,000}$ m
centimeter	cm	$\frac{1}{100}$ m
meter	m	

Area

The most important metric unit for measuring area in the field of medicine is the square meter (m^2). You use this unit when you're measuring body mass index (BMI) and body surface area (BSA).

Temperature

The most important metric unit for measuring temperature in the field of medicine is degrees Celsius. (But if you want to split hairs, the official metric unit of temperature is called the *kelvin* and is abbreviated *K*.)

The *kelvin* unit of temperature starts at absolute zero. Scientists also use it to measure color temperature and noise in electronic circuits. And 0 kelvin is equal to -273.15 degrees Celsius.

United States customary system

The *United States customary system* is also called the *American system.* Back in the American colonial days, it was called the *English system.* In the United Kingdom, the English system evolved to become the Imperial system. Today's American system is similar, but not identical, to the Imperial system.

You know from everyday life that the American system is traditional and popular in the United States. American units include feet, yards, miles, quarts, and gallons, just to name a few.

Here are the American units (and what they measure) that you may encounter in the field of medicine:

- **Weight:** Pound (lb) and ounce (oz)
- **Liquid volume:** Fluid ounce (fl oz), pint (pt), quart (qt), and gallon (gal)
- **Length:** Inch (in), foot (ft), and yard (yd)
- **Area:** Square inch (in^2) and square foot (ft^2)
- **Temperature:** Degrees Fahrenheit

See the section "Household system" for other American units that are common in the home, especially in the kitchen.

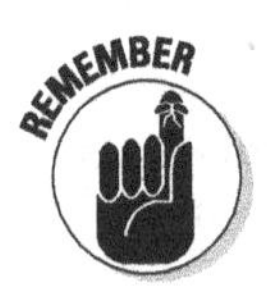

The United States has been slow to go metric. (By the way, the official name for changing to metric is *metrication.*) So even though metric is essential in the lab and in the hospital, your patients won't appreciate some metric measurements. For example, they're not ready to hear their height and weight measurements in meters and kilograms. This is especially true for infants; Mom wants to know how much her baby weighs in pounds and ounces. (Check out the later section "Converting metric to American" for details on how to convert dosages into units your patients will be familiar with.)

Household system

The *household system* is an informal term that describes the set of units that are common in American homes, especially kitchens. Your patients and their families are probably more familiar with this system of measurement than any other, so you need to use it when teaching patients about taking meds.

Here are the household units (and what they measure) that you may encounter in the field of medicine:

- **Weight:** Pound (lb) and ounce (oz)
- **Liquid volume:** Cup (cup), fluid ounce (fl oz), tablespoon (Tbsp), teaspoon (tsp), and drop (gtt)

Teaspoons were once used (and still are) for stirring tea and coffee. A tablespoon is a large serving spoon (or you can think of it as a soup spoon). With everyday teaspoons and tablespoons, volumes vary wildly, but in the kitchen, measuring spoons are precise. In fact, some measuring spoons (and measuring cups, too) have marks for metric equivalents on them.

Figure 4-2 shows a handy volumetric measuring glass that shows tablespoons, teaspoons, and milliliters. It's a home and kitchen variant of a medicine cup, and it's excellent for home dosing of liquids.

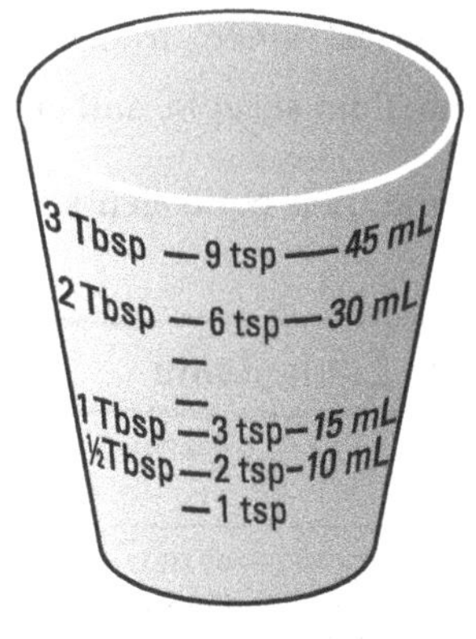

Figure 4-2: A volumetric measuring glass with household and metric units.

The abbreviation *gtt* stands for *guttae*. The term *guttae* is Latin for "drops."

Figure 4-3 shows a typical medicine dropper (officially called a *Pasteur pipette*), which you use to dispense drops. Although gtt is a household unit, some eye droppers have mL marks on them, which allow you to dispense by the mL as well as by the drop.

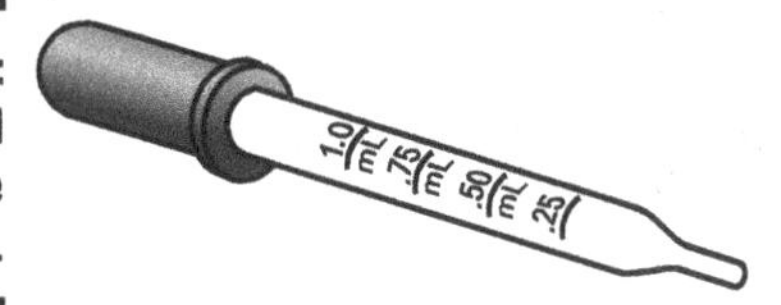

Figure 4-3: Typical medicine dropper.

Apothecaries' system

The *apothecaries' system* of measurements is a very old system that has its roots in Roman times. The system was wildly popular from the start of medieval medicine (about 1,000 CE) and was the standard for dispensing meds through the early 20th century. The United States replaced the apothecaries' system with the metric system in 1971.

The only apothecaries' unit that you may encounter somewhat frequently in the field of medicine is the grain (gr), which measures weight and is the unit on which the whole system is based.

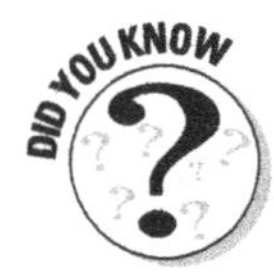

What exactly is a grain? Way back when, traders used wheat or barley grains to define weight. In the 13th century, King Henry III of England declared that an English penny was to be equal to 32 grains of wheat.

Other apothecaries' units that you'll rarely see include the following:

- **Weight:** Apothecaries' pound, apothecaries' ounce, dram, and scruple
- **Liquid volume:** Fluid ounce, fluid dram, fluid scruple, and minim

Table 4-2 shows some apothecaries' units and their equivalents.

Table 4-2 Apothecaries' Unit Equivalents

Apothecaries' Unit	*Apothecaries' Equivalent*	*Metric Equivalent*
1 gr		65 mg (64.8 mg precisely)
0.015432 gr		1 mg
15 gr (15.432 gr precisely)		1 g
5,760 gr	1 lb Troy	
60 gr	1 dram	
8 dram	1 oz	

In medical dosing calculations, you sometimes see doctor's orders in grains because some drugs, including codeine, opium, and phenobarbital, have been in the United States Pharmacopeia (USP) for many decades (and, thus, were once dosed in grains). You usually need to convert gr to mg.

For example, an aspirin tablet may be called a 5 gr (or gr v) tablet. That's the equivalent of 325 mg (because 1 gr = 65 mg and 65 × 5 = 325). So if a doctor writes *ASA gr v,* she's using *ASA* for aspirin, *gr* for grains, and *v* as the Roman numeral for 5.

Be sure to read prescriptions very carefully whenever you're dealing with grains (or any other measurement, for that matter!). After all, it's easy to read prescriptions wrong because sometimes the *gr* looks a lot like a *g*. Worst-case scenario: A patient could receive phenobarbital 0.5 g instead of 0.5 gr (0.03 g) if you read the prescription wrong. Obviously, 0.5 gr is precisely 32.4 mg and 0.5 g is 500 mg. The dose of 500 mg is 15.43 times the prescribed dosage!

Examining the Rules of Conversion

Converting units isn't hard. You just need to know the tricks and basic ground rules and then practice them a bit. The two main rules of converting from one unit to another are

- Know the conversion factor.
- Convert to identical units before doing the remaining math in a problem.

If you do these two things every time you work through a dosing calculation, you'll be well on your way to finding the right answer. The following sections take a closer look at these two rules of conversion.

Knowing the conversion factor

To convert from one unit to another, you need to know the *conversion factor* (or formula) for those two units. For example, *1 kg = 2.2 lb* is the conversion factor for converting from kg to lb, or vice versa. You can look up conversion factors in this chapter, on the Internet, in a smartphone application, or in another book. (Many pocket-sized reference guides contain the main conversion factors you need to know.) But don't forget your very capable brain and memory! Many formulas are so simple that you probably have them memorized already (and if you don't, you soon will!).

To do a conversion, you simply plug the appropriate conversion factor into the following equation:

desired unit = given unit × conversion factor

For example, to convert kg to lb, insert the given unit (for example, 10 kg), multiply by the conversion factor, and solve for the result, like so:

$$x = 10\text{ kg} \times \frac{2.2\text{ lb}}{1\text{ kg}}$$

$$x = 22\text{ lb}$$

The answer is 10 kg = 22 lb.

The longer you work in the field of medicine, the more conversions you'll know by heart. If you're just starting out, don't try to cram too many formulas in your head. For now, focus on the following simple but important conversion factors:

- 1,000 milligrams (mg) = 1 gram (g)
- 1,000 micrograms (mcg) = 1 mg
- 1,000 milliliters (mL) = 1 liter (L)

Other conversions, even those between two different systems, can be almost as simple. For example, 1 tablespoon (Tbsp) in the household system equals 15 mL in the metric system. Going between these two units isn't much harder than multiplying or dividing by 10, as you would do with metric-to-metric conversions. (See the section "Putting It All Together — A Conversion Chart for Healthcare" for other useful conversion factors.)

Converting to identical units

When you do math with different units of length, weight, or liquid volume, you first have to make the units the same.

For example, you can't add mg directly to g. First, you must convert g to mg or mg to g so the units are the same. The same is true with volumes. You can't add 100 mL + 0.5 L because the units aren't the same. You first have to convert the 0.5 L to mL. The preceding section tells you that 1 L equals 1,000 mL, so 0.5 L equals 500 mL (0.5 × 1,000 = 500). After you convert everything to one unit, you can add 500 mL to 100 mL, like so:

500 mL + 100 mL = 600 mL

Sometimes the quantities you get in dosing calculations are accurate but very inconvenient to work with in real life. It's okay to convert these quantities to more manageable units. For example, if you need to dispense 0.375 L of a fluid, it's more convenient to think of it as 375 mL.

Doctors can write orders using different units that mean the same thing. Often the units a doctor uses are based on personal preference. For example, a doctor orders 1 L 0.9% saline IV to be given over four hours. She could also write the order as 1,000 mL 0.9% saline IV over four hours. The doses are identical.

Converting Units in Different Measurement Systems

In healthcare, the most common conversions are metric-to-metric; however, metric-to-American and American-to-metric conversions come up as well — mainly in figuring patient height and weight and sometimes in dealing with temperature. You also see American-to-American conversions when you're dealing with household units.

We cover all these conversions in the following sections. Because you occasionally have to convert from apothecaries' units to metric, we include a section on that as well.

Converting metric to metric

Although the metric system includes many different units and conversion factors, only a few conversions dominate dosing math.

Table 4-3 shows common metric-to-metric weight conversion factors.

Table 4-3 Metric-to-Metric Weight Conversion Factors

Unit	*Equivalent*
1,000 mcg	1 mg
1,000 mg	1 g
1,000 g	1 kg

Table 4-4 shows common metric-to-metric liquid volume conversion factors.

Table 4-4 Metric-to-Metric Liquid Volume Conversion Factors

Unit	*Equivalent*
1,000 mL	1 L
100 mL	1 dL

In case you're curious, deciliters (dL) are used in the lab. For example, the level of cholesterol in a patient's blood is expressed in mg/dL

EXAMPLE

You're asked to give 250 mL of normal saline intravenously. What percentage of 1 L is this?

To solve this problem, use the basic conversion formula and follow these steps:

1. **Use the conversion factor 1 L = 1,000 mL to set up the following equation and solve for *x*:**

   desired unit = given unit × conversion factor

   $$x = 1\text{ L} \times \frac{1{,}000\text{ mL}}{1\text{ L}}$$

   $$x = 1{,}000\text{ mL}$$

2. **Divide 250 mL by 1,000 mL to get a decimal fraction.**

   $$x = \frac{250\text{ mL}}{1{,}000\text{ mL}}$$

   $$x = 0.25$$

3. **Convert the decimal fraction 0.25 to a percent by multiplying by 100 and adding the percent sign.**

   $$x = 0.25 \times 100$$

   $$x = 25\%$$

   The decimal fraction 0.25 is equal to 25%. You must give 25% of 1 L. (See Chapter 3 for details on converting from decimals to percentages.)

Converting metric to American

You can find many metric-to-American and American-to-metric conversion factors out there, but you need to know only a few for most dosing calculations.

Table 4-5 shows common metric-to-American weight conversion factors. You often express a patient's weight to him or her in pounds (lb), not kilograms (kg).

Table 4-5 Metric-to-American Weight Conversion Factors

Metric Unit	*American Equivalent*
454 g	1 lb
0.454 kg	1 lb
1 kg	2.2 lb (2.20462262 lb, precisely)
1 g	0.035 oz (0.0352739619 oz, precisely)

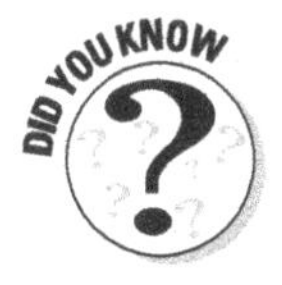

Some hospital beds have a built-in scale, with zeroing, pounds-to-kilograms conversion, total weight retention calculation, and equipment subtraction.

Table 4-6 shows common metric-to-American liquid volume conversion factors. You use American units mostly to instruct patients about how to administer liquids.

Table 4-6 Metric-to-American Liquid Volume Conversion Factors

Metric Unit	*American Equivalent*
1 mL	20 gtt
5 mL	1 tsp
15 mL (14.8 mL precisely)	3 tsp
15 mL	1 Tbsp
30 mL (29.57 mL precisely)	1 fl oz
30 mL	2 Tbsp
237 mL (customary) 240 mL (legal, for nutrition labeling)	8 fl oz
237 mL	1 cup

Table 4-7 shows common metric-to-American height conversion factors. You use American units mainly to let patients know how tall they are and how their waistlines are trending.

Table 4-7 Metric-to-American Length Conversion Factors

Metric Unit	*American Equivalent*
1 m	39.37 in
0.3049 m	1 ft
2.54 cm	1 in

Converting American to American

American unit conversions are common for people who grew up in the United States, but they occur fairly rarely in medical practice. To be fair, in hospital administration, desks are still sized in inches, printer paper is 8.5 in x 11 in, and you may ask a nursing assistant to move a bed a couple of feet (rather than 0.6096 m) closer to a wall. But most dosage calculations deal with metric units.

Even so, you need to be familiar with the common American-to-American conversion factors shown in Table 4-8 because those are the units your patients will likely know. Two of the most common American-to-American conversions are from ounces to pounds and from pounds to ounces.

Table 4-8 American-to-American Conversion Factors

Unit	*Equivalent*
12 in	1 ft
3 ft	1 yd
36 in	1 yd
16 oz	1 lb
3 tsp	1 Tbsp
2 Tbsp	1 fl oz
8 fl oz	1 cup
2 cup	1 pt
2 pt	1 qt

Your patient tells you he drinks four pints a day at home. How many fluid ounces is this?

Follow these steps to find out:

1. **Use the conversion factor 1 pt = 16 fl oz to set up the following equation:**

   $$x = 4 \text{ pt} \times \frac{16 \text{ fl oz}}{1 \text{ pt}}$$

2. **Multiply and solve.**

   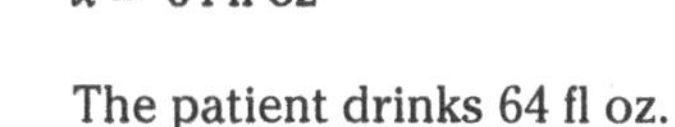

   $$x = 64 \text{ fl oz}$$

   The patient drinks 64 fl oz.

An infant weighs 120 ounces. What's that in pounds and ounces?

To answer this question, follow these steps:

1. **Use the conversion factor 1 lb = 16 oz to set up the following equation:**

   $$x = 120 \text{ oz} \times \frac{1 \text{ lb}}{16 \text{ oz}}$$

2. **Multiply and solve.**

   $$x = \frac{120}{16} \text{ lb}$$

   $$x = 7.5 \text{ lb}$$

   The result is 7.5 lb.

3. **Convert the fractional 0.5 lb back to oz, like so:**

   $$x = 0.5 \text{ lb} \times \frac{16 \text{ oz}}{1 \text{ lb}}$$

   $$x = 8 \text{ oz}$$

   The fractional part of the infant's weight is 8 oz. The final answer is 7 lb 8 oz.

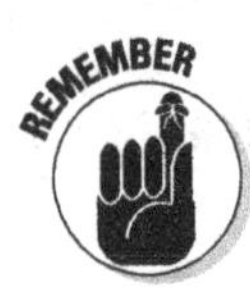

Conversions between mL, tsp, and Tbsp are common. Over time, you'll be able to do them in your head.

Converting American to metric

From time to time, you need to convert from American to metric units. This particular conversion comes up most often in converting weight and height. You use weight and height in body mass index calculations and weight by itself in weight-based dosing of several medications.

Table 4-9 shows the common American-to-metric conversion factors you need to know.

Table 4-9 American-to-Metric Conversion Factors

American Unit	*Metric Equivalent*
1 in	2.54 cm
1 yd	0.9144 m
1 lb	0.454 kg
1 oz	28.35 g
1 tsp	5 mL
1 Tbsp	15 mL
1 fl oz	30 mL
1 cup	237 mL (customary) 240 mL (legal, for nutrition labeling)

Converting apothecaries' units to metric

With the exception of one unit (the grain), the apothecaries' system of weight and liquid measurement is no longer used in medicine. Table 4-10 shows common apothecaries' conversion factors with the grain.

Table 4-10 Apothecaries' Conversion Factors

Apothecaries' Unit	*Metric Equivalent*
15 gr (15.4323584 gr precisely)	1 g
1 gr	0.06479891 g
1 gr	65 mg (64.8 mg precisely)

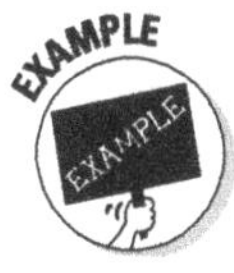

How many mg are in $\frac{1}{6}$ gr?

Follow these steps to find out:

1. **Use the conversion factor 1 gr = 65 mg to set up the following equation:**

$$x = \frac{1}{6}\text{gr} \times \frac{65\text{ mg}}{1\text{ gr}}$$

2. **Multiply and solve.**

$$x = \frac{65}{6}\text{ mg}$$

$$x = 10.83\text{ mg}$$

The answer is 10.83 mg. You can round that up to 11 mg.

Converting temperature

In the nonmetric United States, a patient takes her temperature at home with a thermometer that measures it in degrees Fahrenheit (F), but, at the hospital, docs and nurses measure temperatures in degrees Celsius (C). The expected "normal" core body temperature is 37.0 degrees C or 98.6 degrees F. Actually, an under-the-tongue reading can be a little lower.

To convert degrees F to degrees C, use this formula:

$$C = \frac{5}{9} \times (F - 32)$$

To convert degrees C to degrees F, use this formula:

$$F = \left(\frac{9}{5} \times C\right) + 32$$

Real-Life Practice: Filling Up on Fluids

You document that your patient ate only 50% of his meal and drank only half a cup of fluids. What's the equivalent fluid consumption in tablespoons?

There's no direct correlation between cups and tablespoons, so you have to improvise. Do so by following these steps:

1. **Convert cups to fl oz by using the conversion factor 1 cup = 8 fl oz.**

   $$x = 0.5 \text{ cup} \times \frac{8 \text{ fl oz}}{1 \text{ cup}}$$

2. **Multiply and solve.**

   $$x = 0.5 \times \frac{8}{1} \text{ fl oz}$$

   $$x = 4 \text{ fl oz}$$

   After multiplying, you see that 0.5 cup is 4 fl oz.

3. **Convert fl oz to Tbsp by using the conversion factor 2 Tbsp = 1 fl oz.**

   $$x = 4 \text{ fl oz} \times \frac{2 \text{ Tbsp}}{1 \text{ fl oz}}$$

4. **Multiply and solve.**

   $$x = 4 \times \frac{2}{1} \text{ Tbsp}$$

   $$x = 8 \text{ Tbsp}$$

   The final answer is 8 Tbsp.

Real-Life Practice: Sipping on Syrup

You're administering a med in syrup form at a dose of 600 mg every 12 hours. It comes in a strength of 100 mg/5 mL. What's the equivalent dose in tablespoons?

To solve this problem, you first have to use the ratio-proportion method (which we cover in Chapter 8) to convert the dose from mg to mL. After that, all you have to do is covert mL to Tbsp. Follow these steps:

1. **Plug the numbers you know from the problem into the ratio-proportion equation, like so:**

$$\frac{\text{known equivalent}}{\text{known equivalent}} = \frac{\text{known equivalent}}{\text{desired equivalent}}$$

$$\frac{100 \text{ mg}}{5 \text{ mL}} = \frac{600 \text{ mg}}{x \text{ mL}}$$

2. **Cross-multiply and solve.**

$$100x = 3{,}000$$

$$x = 30 \text{ mL}$$

The answer is 30 mL.

3. **Use the conversion factor 1 Tbsp = 15 mL to convert from mL to Tbsp.**

$$x = 30 \text{ mL} \times \frac{1 \text{ Tbsp}}{15 \text{ mL}}$$

$$x = 30 \times \frac{1}{15} \text{ Tbsp}$$

$$x = 2 \text{ Tbsp}$$

The answer is 2 Tbsp. If, by chance, you needed the answer in teaspoons, all you'd have to do is use the conversion factor 1 Tbsp = 3 tsp. The answer, in teaspoons, is 6.

Part II

Minding Your Meds: Administration and Calculation Methods

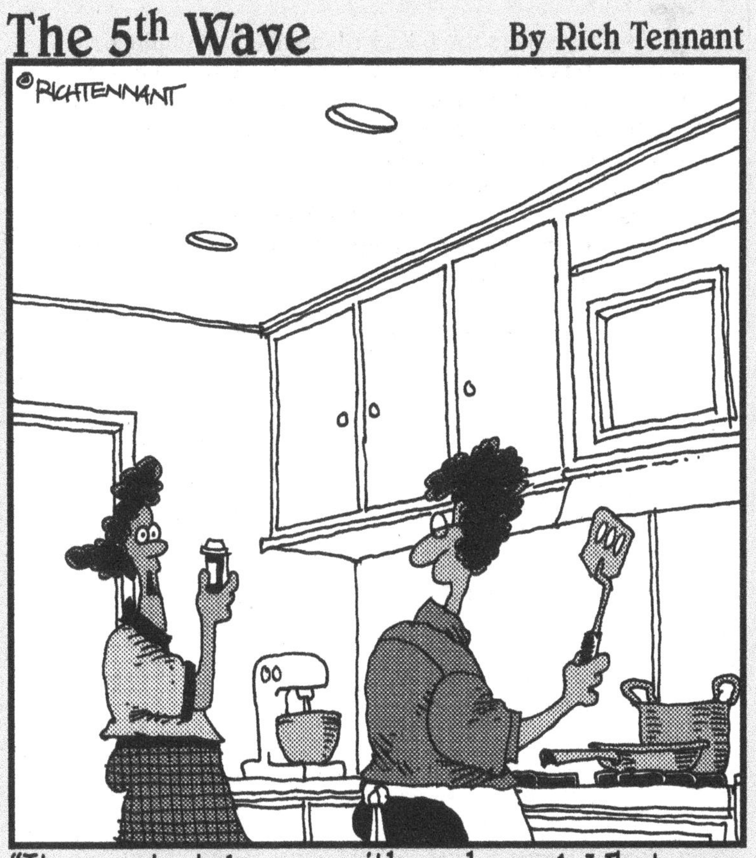

"It says to take one with each meal. What goes well with phenylephrine?"

In this part . . .

This part covers the basics of medication administration and calculations. In Chapter 5, we take a close look at exactly what makes up a prescription. Similarly, Chapter 6 examines the important information you find on every drug label. Chapter 7 deals with the MAR (the Medication Administration Record) and other essential documentation forms you need to be familiar with. The last chapter in this part, Chapter 8, is all about the three classic methods of calculating dosages.

Chapter 5

The Prescription: Just What the Doctor Ordered

In This Chapter

- Looking at the main elements of a good prescription, whether it's written or electronic
- Including the route of administration and time-related details on all prescriptions
- Individualizing prescriptions with patient-specific restrictions
- Dealing with verbal orders and the problems that can accompany them
- Getting some real-life prescription practice with two example problems

The *prescription* (or *doctor's order* as it's sometimes called) is the main way physicians formulate and document their plans to take care of patients. Doctors and other providers who write medication orders — including certified registered nurse practitioners (CRNPs) and physician assistants (PAs) — prescribe many different kinds of medications, but the main components of every prescription are the same.

All prescriptions have to be clear, concise, readable, and easily understood. Although it's the doctor's responsibility to make sure every prescription meets those requirements, you have an obligation to the patient to make sure the doctor's order is right at each step, from the initial writing of the prescription to the medication's administration. Because your number-one commitment is to patient safety and reduction of medical errors, you must always be on the lookout for prescription-related errors. When you find one, you must do everything you can to correct it right away.

If you plan to become a nurse or work in a related field, you will likely be responsible for dispensing medications, so it's vital that you get totally familiar with prescriptions. This chapter is here to help you do just that. It gives you all the tools you need to decipher and administer prescriptions and to deal with errors when they occur. Specifically, it helps you get familiar with the essential components of a truly perfect prescription and the problems with a less-than-perfect prescription.

Comparing Written versus Electronic Prescriptions and Patient Charts

All prescriptions come in one of two basic flavors: written or electronic. The traditional form is written, and the new form is electronic (as in *electronic medical record,* or EMR). Although written prescriptions may be going out of style in some medical settings, both forms serve the same purpose — to display the details of the doctor's order.

In a hospital setting, the patient's information appears either in a written chart in a ringed binder or on a computer (via electronic charting). Hospitals and other medical facilities often keep written patient charts in a designated area, usually at the nurse's station.

In an outpatient clinic, the system may be a little different. The doctor enters the exam room with the patient's chart in hand, or the room has a computer monitor that gives the doctor access to patient history.

Both written and electronic charts usually contain a section labeled *Physician Orders* or *Doctor's Orders,* in which you find all the patient's prescriptions. Written charts have tabs either on the side or at the bottom of the chart to help you find the orders section quickly.

The following sections take a closer look at written and electronic prescriptions so that you're prepared to work with either form.

The ancient and honorable prescription

Although no written records prove when the first prescriptions came about, they have no doubt been around since people began to walk upright. Imagine the ancient Medicine Man or Healer Woman saying, "Well, Og, there's a lot of this going around. Chew on two of these leaves and see me in the morning."

Fast forward to Sumeria in the third millennium BCE. Archeologists have found a clay tablet specifying water, wine, beer, branches, oil, bread, and wool in the pharmacopeia. Now that's prescribing the old-fashioned way!

Fast forward again to the 1500s when Latin was the written language of the doctor. The prescription symbol *Rx* appears in numerous medical documents from that time and is from the Latin verb *recipere,* meaning "to take." The order, or prescription, named the ingredients needed to compound the prescription. The word *prescription* roughly translates into *pre* (meaning "before") and *script* (meaning "writing"), which makes sense since the prescription is what the doctor has to write down before the pharmacist (or, in the old days, the apothecary) can compound the needed medication.

If you're a student, you probably don't know where you'll work when you finish school, but you can learn about the various forms and charting practices that different medical centers use by asking medical professionals about their workplace practices. If you're working right now, you're already familiar with the system your facility uses for doctor's orders.

The traditional written word

The written word of the doctor is still present in abundance at the nurse's station in the hospital, in large collections of manila files in a private practice or clinic, and in the handwritten prescriptions doctors write for patients who want to drop off prescriptions at pharmacies or mail them in to prescription services. But the world of written orders has its drawbacks.

For one, the paper records in the order section of patient charts are usually 8.5-x-11-inch pieces of paper covered with the Egyptian hieroglyphics that make up the doctor's orders. Prescriptions written for a patient can seem to be indecipherable. No wonder famous newspaper columnist Earl Wilson said, "You may not be able to read a doctor's handwriting in a prescription, but you'll notice that his bills are neatly typewritten."

Another problem with handwritten orders and patient charts is that the contents of a manila folder or binder can easily spill. And there's nothing like a spontaneous game of "fifty-two card pickup" when a patient's binder bursts open or his folder spills.

Even more important than issues with readability and organization is the fact that the contents of paper charts don't transmit electronically. The ability to transmit medical information electronically will be essential in the emerging field of telemedicine, and it shows great promise in other areas, including interdepartment hospital communications, remote radiological evaluation, and EMT-to-emergency-room communications. Transmittable medical information may also improve patient safety and lower healthcare costs.

In your profession, you may encounter the semiautomated world for handwritten prescriptions. For example, a dental practice phones in a prescription — often for a pain-management med like hydrocodone 5/500 (Vicodin) — to a local pharmacy while the patient is undergoing an oral surgery. The office follows up with a fax. Of course, the patient could also take the handwritten prescription directly to the pharmacy itself.

But time marches on. With the advent of the electronic medical record, changes are coming to the way doctors and other medical professionals prescribe meds. In the next few years, in both the outpatient and inpatient settings, the EMR and electronic prescribing will likely be mandatory for all healthcare providers, which means prescriptions will be no longer be handwritten.

The electronic medical record

If a hospital uses an electronic medical record (EMR) system, order management should be smooth sailing. The doctor enters the required information directly into a computer (see the section "Identifying the Essential Ingredients of a Good Prescription" for what info needs to be part of every prescription). This information then goes electronically ("down the wire") to the hospital pharmacy, as well as to the unit or floor where the patient is located.

Note: Some patients report that they've received "written" prescriptions, but they are printed by the computer. In the semiautomated world of handwritten documents, expect to see some digitizing. That is, expect to see handwritten medical documents scanned for storage in a computer system. These aren't true digital records, but such scanned documents can be stored, retrieved, and transmitted. One of the authors (Barry) wrote the manuals for such a system for medical documents for the Pelican Bay supermax prison in California.

EMR systems have advantages, but they're not perfect. For example, it's possible to enter an order incorrectly, and sometimes information doesn't get enough scrutiny, because you may think "it's in the computer, so it can't be wrong." Many systems, however, have built-in "safety nets" for prescribing professionals. For example, some systems notify doctors about medication interactions at the time the medication is ordered to allow the doctor to change the medication if she wishes. If the doctor does change the order, she needs to document a reason for doing so. In addition, computer systems are subject to system failures and power outages.

Identifying the Essential Ingredients of a Good Prescription

A good prescription includes everything that the pharmacy needs to know to fill it and everything the medical professional (or patient) needs to know to administer it safely and correctly. The prescription must be accurate, legible, and totally unambiguous. Such a prescription isn't hard to achieve when the doctor takes the time to write the prescription correctly and the support staff takes the time to verify the information.

All prescriptions, whether they're electronic or handwritten, must be accurate and unambiguous, which is where the following sections come in.

Patient identification

Our program of presenting medical information now pauses for patient identification: name, date of birth (DOB), and medical record number. Every prescription must clearly and precisely identify the patient associated with the order by listing the following required patient information:

- **Patient name:** As you probably expect, the patient name includes the first name, last name, and middle initial (if applicable). After all, a hospital or clinic may have two patients with the same name or similar-sounding names, which increases the chances for potentially catastrophic errors. The patient name is a starting point for preventing such errors.
- **Date of birth (DOB):** Date of birth is a big help in ensuring that an order is for the correct patient. Even if a hospital has two John A. Does, the chances that they share the same birth date are pretty slim.
- **Medical record number:** The order must also have a medical record number or patient account number. This number helps prevent mix-ups because every patient has his or her own identification number.

Here's a scenario that reiterates the importance of proper patient identification on med orders: Many written charts include paper order sheets that don't have an imprint of the patient's nameplate (which contains the patient's ID information). If you don't write the patient ID info on the order sheet and if the order sheet is barely hanging onto the ringed binder containing the patient's chart, it can easily fall to the floor. If it does, the nurse or unit secretary has no way of knowing whom the order belongs to! Of course, this isn't a problem if the hospital uses an electronic order-entry system.

Correct spelling

On all prescriptions, the spelling of the medication must be correct. Correct spelling is especially important for meds that have very similar names. If you find that the spelling on a prescription is confusing or just plain unreadable, call the doctor for clarification. Correct spelling may seem obvious, but you'd be surprised how often confusion occurs because of the name of a med.

Will the real medication please step forward?

Every medication has a brand name (also called a *trade name*), a generic name, or both. But to make things more confusing, many medications have more than one brand name. For example, labetalol (luh-*bet*-el-all), a commonly prescribed medication used to treat high blood pressure, has two brand names — Trandate (*tran*-date) and Normodyne (*norm*-a-dine). Some medications have more than two brand names. Can you believe that? How many names does a medication need anyway?

Always pay particular attention to medications with multiple brand names. If you're not familiar with the name of the med on the prescription, don't hesitate to call the doctor.

As a rule, the doctor writes either the brand name of the medication or its generic equivalent on each prescription. Sometimes, to make the prescription as clear as possible, the doctor includes both names. For example, *hydrocodone 5/500 (generic for Vicodin)* expresses the name of the medication completely enough to eliminate any ambiguity.

Beware of meds with confusing similar names

Many medications sound alike or have similar spellings but are completely different. Inserting or deleting just one or two letters in a drug name can literally mean the difference between life and death for your patients. The official name for these similar-sounding names in the field of linguistics is *false friends*.

For example, Celebrex (*cell*-a-brex) is a common anti-inflammatory medication used in the treatment of arthritis. Cerebyx (*sair*-a-bicks), in contrast, is an antiseizure medication. Obviously, these two drugs do very different things, although they sound similar. As you look at prescriptions, remember that clarity is your friend and ambiguity and confusion are the enemies!

Table 5-1 shows a brief list of some similar-sounding pharmaceutical names.

Table 5-1 Meds with Confusing Similar Names

This med	*with this property*	*isn't*	*this med*	*with this property*
Amicar	postoperative bleeding treatment		Omacor	lowers high triglyceride levels
Benadryl	antihistamine		Bentyl	treatment for Irritable Bowel Syndrome (IBS)

This med	*with this property*	*isn't*	*this med*	*with this property*
Cerebyx	epileptic seizure treatment		Celebrex	arthritis, pain, and colon/ rectal polyp treatment
Clonidine	antihypertensive to lower blood pressure		Klonopin	anticonvulsive
Lamictal	epilepsy and bipolar disorder treatment		Lamisil	fungal nail infection treatment
Phenobarbital	anticonvulsive		Pentobarbital	pre-op sedative; seizure treatment
Ritalin	attention-deficit hyperactivity disorder treatment		Ritodrine	used to stop premature labor
Selegiline	early-stage Parkinson's disease and senile dementia treatment		Salagen	glaucoma treatment
Zantac	gastric ulcer, duodenal ulcer, gastroesophageal reflux disease treatment		Zyrtec	antihistamine used to treat hay fever, allergies, and Kimura's disease

Although your math skills are very important in computing medical dosages, they won't matter a bit if the med is wrong. So you absolutely must double-check the spelling of the medications on all the prescriptions you work with to make sure they're correct and that they leave no room for confusion. If you have any question about a medication, call the prescribing physician or pharmacist.

Use the Internet or drug reference guides to clear up any concerns you have about drug names. The following Web sites, printed books, and apps offer plenty of accurate, clear drug information:

- Epocrates free smartphone app (available from the Apple iTunes app store)
- Physicians' Desk Reference (available as a printed book, a pocket guide, or a CD at www.pdr.net)
- RxList (www.rxlist.com)
- Medscape (www.medscape.com)
- Drugs.com (www.drugs.com)

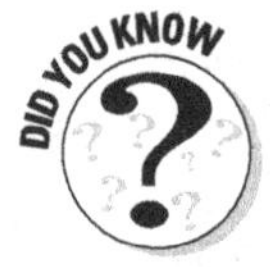

Brand names are essential to modern pharmaceutical firms, but they aren't a recent phenomenon. The "modern" concept of brand-name drugs originated in the 19th century. In 1853, Charles Frederic Gerhardt, a French chemist, prepared acetylsalicylic acid, and, by 1899, the drug company Bayer called this drug *Aspirin.* (Yes, it was a brand name, folks!). By the way, so was *Heroin.* Figure 5-1 shows an early ad for Bayer Aspirin.

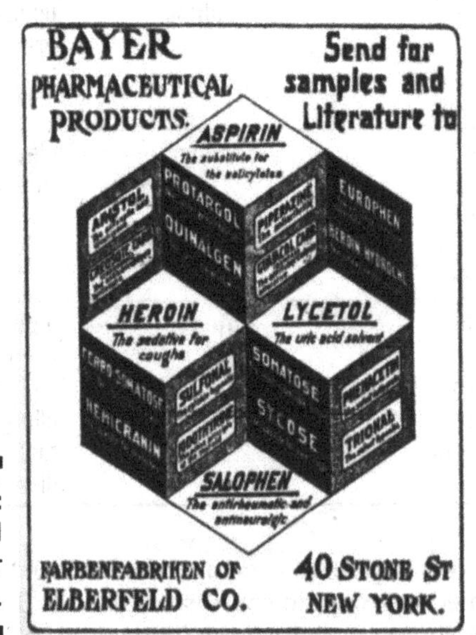

Figure 5-1: Early ad for Bayer Aspirin.

Don't cut a medication short

Sometimes doctors abbreviate drug names on medication orders to speed things up. But doing so only generates confusion and increases room for error. So don't let the doc shortchange a medication.

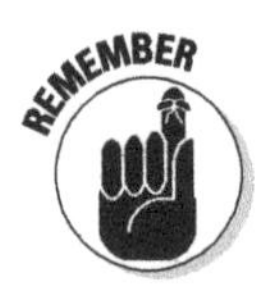

Expect and insist that all medication orders include fully written out, correctly spelled drug names. Doing so won't always make you best friends with the doctor, but it's very good medical practice. For instance, a commonly abbreviated med is magnesium sulfate. The trouble is that the abbreviation $MgSO_4$ (magnesium sulfate) looks a lot like the abbreviation MSO_4 (morphine sulfate). The two are, of course, completely different medications!

Clear, correct dosage

For a prescription to be accurate, the medication name must be correct, but the prescription must also contain very clear dosage instructions that include the right numbers and abbreviations related to units, frequency, and route of administration.

The following sections explain the importance of writing clear numbers and using common, unambiguous abbreviations for dosage instructions on prescriptions. (For more on the route of administration, head over to the section "Location, Location, Location: Knowing the Route of Administration," and for more on frequency and other time-related details, check out the section "Timing Is Everything: Knowing When and How Often to Give a Med.")

Checking numbers for clarity and accuracy

You have to know how much of a prescribed medication to give the patient before you start administering it. Seems intuitive, right? It may seem that way, but sometimes the numbers on a prescription can be downright difficult to decipher. For example:

- The number 3 may resemble a 5 or 8.
- The number 2 may look like a 7.
- Decimal points may be missing or misplaced (which can have dastardly consequences, depending on the medication prescribed).

  To make sure decimal points appear where they're supposed to appear, the prescriber must write (for example) *.4* as *0.4* so it's clear that she intended to use a decimal point.

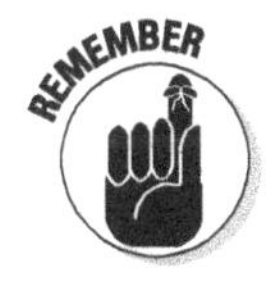

Look at the numbers on the order. Observe the number of mg, mL, or insulin units specified in the order. Observe the numbers indicating frequency of dosing. If the numbers seem ambiguous or inconsistent with drug references, consult the doctor or the pharmacist. If you have an electronic order-entry system, in many cases, the background of the medication is already listed, and all you do is click on a particular dosage or frequency. For example, if you order furosemide (Lasix), your screen will ask you to choose from a variety of dosage options, including 40 mg, 80 mg, and so forth. The doc then needs to choose the frequency (once daily, twice daily, and so forth). The order usually includes a section where the doc can write more restrictions or clarifications, if needed.

The doc or midlevel practitioner places the order unless it's a verbal order, in which case it's taken by a registered nurse (RN). With EMR systems, the doses of many medications are already typed in the program by the time you see them. Sometimes, however, you have to physically type a med's dose; when you do, be sure to double-check the numbers in the dose to make sure they're accurate.

Using acceptable dosage abbreviations

Paradoxically, it's okay to abbreviate certain words and phrases on prescriptions. Some abbreviations, like the ones listed in Table 5-2, are unambiguous and widely accepted in the medical field. Expect to see these abbreviations on the medical orders you work with.

Table 5-2 Common and Accepted Dosage Abbreviations

Abbreviation	Meaning	Abbreviation	Meaning
mg	milligram	SL	sublingual
kg	kilogram	STAT	NOW! This is an emergency!
mcg	microgram	ASAP	as soon as possible
mL	milliliter	subq	subcutaneous
L	liter	BP	blood pressure
mEq	milliequivalents	HR	heart rate
NG	nasogastric tube	RR	respiratory rate
IM	intramuscular	NKDA	no known drug allergies
IV	intravenous	ac	before meals
KVO	keep the vein open	pc	after meals
PO	by mouth	bid	twice a day
NPO	nothing by mouth	tid	three times a day
PR	per rectum	q3h	every 3 hours
PRN	as needed		

Avoiding unacceptable abbreviations

Just as some abbreviations are unambiguous and widely accepted, other abbreviations are not. These unacceptable abbreviations are a shortcut to trouble because they cause ambiguity and confusion (the enemies of patient safety and quality healthcare!). For this reason, you don't want to see them on any medical orders you work with.

The Joint Commission (formerly the Joint Commission on Accreditation of Healthcare Organizations) is an organization designed to improve healthcare quality and patient care. Because the use of abbreviations is so important to both issues, the Joint Commission came up with a list of unacceptable abbreviations. Table 5-3 lists some of these unacceptable abbreviations. (Find the full Joint Commission list at www.jointcommission.org/Do_Not_Use_List_of_Abbreviations/.)

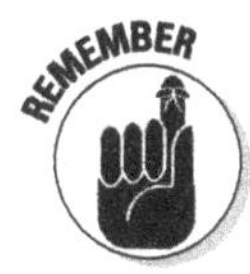

If you see the abbreviations in Table 5-3 in a doctor's order, don't hesitate to question the doctor for clarification.

Table 5-3 Unacceptable Abbreviations

Abbreviation	*Mistaken Meanings*	*Better Choice*
DC or D/C	Does it mean "discontinue" or "discharge"?	Write *discontinue* or *discharge*.
HS	Does it mean "half-strength" or "at bedtime"?	Write *at bedtime* or the designated time.
QD	Does it mean "every day" or "right eye"? *QD* looks like *OD*, which means "right eye." (*OS* means "left eye.")	Write *every day*.
QOD	Does it mean "every other day" or "daily"?	Write *every other day*.
MSO_4 or $MgSO_4$	Does it mean "magnesium sulfate" or "morphine sulfate"?	Write *magnesium sulfate* or *morphine sulfate*.
U or IU	Does it mean "unit" or "zero"?	Write *units*.
IV	Does it mean "intravenous," "international units," or "4"?	*IV* is an acceptable abbreviation for "intravenous," but the doc could write *international units* or *intravenous* to be clearer.
SQ or SC	Does it mean "subcutaneous," or could it be mistaken for "5Q" ("5 every")?	Write *subq, subcut, subcutaneous*, or *5 every*.
TIW	Does it mean "twice a week" or "three times a week" (the real meaning)?	Write *twice a week* or *three times a week*.
cc	Does it mean "cubic centimeter" or "milliliter"?	Write *milliliter* or *mL*.
Ug or µg	Does it mean "microgram" or "Ugh"? Could it be mistaken for *mg*?	Write *microgram* or *mcg*.
OD	Does it mean "once daily" or "right eye"?	Write *once daily* or *right eye*.

Timed and dated legible signature

Every doctor's order on a patient's chart must have a legible signature. In fact, a doctor's order on a patient chart isn't complete until it has a legible signature that's dated and timed. Some written prescription orders are stamped with the date and time; some include written dates and times. Either way, every prescription needs to have a time and date.

If the written signature is illegible, expect a legible printed or stamped version of the doctor's signature to appear below it. Reading prescriptions shouldn't be a game of "Guess which doc wrote this?"

The signature should also include a way to contact the physician or other healthcare provider if you have any questions. It may be a pager number (what doctor doesn't love getting paged?) or a cellphone number. When you have a legible, dated, and time-stamped signature with some contact info, you indeed have a super signature!

Location, Location, Location: Knowing the Route of Administration

The *route of administration* is the path a prescription takes to get into the body. All prescriptions must explicitly state the route of administration for the prescribed med.

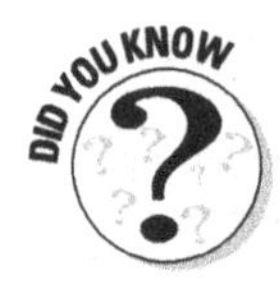

The route of administration doesn't apply only to life-sustaining pharmaceuticals. Murder-mystery fans and toxicologists are quick to say that it also refers to how a poison gets into a victim.

Doctors can prescribe at least 16 different routes of administration. So after you know the medication and the dosage you need to administer, find out how or where to give it. The nine most common routes are

- **Oral:** The patient chews or swallows the medication. Oral administration is the most common way of administering medications. The doctor either writes out the word *orally* or uses the abbreviation *PO,* which means "by mouth." (Check out Chapter 9 for more on oral administration.)
- **Subcutaneous:** Now don't get squeamish. *Subcutaneous* means "under the skin," which is where a syringe enters the picture (as well as the skin). Knowing where (and how) to administer a subcutaneous injection is very important. (Find out more by jumping to Chapter 10.) Doctors write *subq, subcut,* or *subcutaneous* on prescriptions to designate this delivery method.

Doctors often prescribe a subcutaneous administration of heparin to bedridden patients to prevent blood clots from forming.

- **Intradermal:** *Intradermal* means "into the skin," and it's a good method for conducting allergy tests or getting the tuberculosis (TB) inoculation you must have every year when you work in healthcare. Doctors usually write *ID* when they order this form of delivery.
- **Intravenous:** After oral, intravenous is probably the most common route of administration a doctor orders. *Intravenous* means "within the vein," and this administration method sends the med directly into the bloodstream. The doctor usually just writes *IV* on prescriptions that require this delivery method. (See Chapter 11 for more details on IV administration.)

Don't confuse *IV*, meaning intravenous, with the Roman numeral for the number 4. Sounds a little silly, but people have been known to do so.

- **Sublingual:** The patient puts the pill under the tongue, which makes sense since *sub* means "under" and *lingual* means "tongue." The pill dissolves and the med is absorbed quickly.

  Nitroglycerin is usually administered sublingually when the patient is having *angina* (chest pressure). The doctor writes this as *SL* or *under the tongue.*
- **Skin patch:** This route is also known as a *transdermal topical patch. Trans* means "across" and *dermal* refers to the skin, so this method involves administering the med across the skin with a patch. For example, the doctor can order Catapres (*kat*-uh-prez), which is used to treat high blood pressure, as either a pill or as a patch. Pain patches are a good example of skin-patch administration, too. Doctors usually write these orders in longhand.
- **Rectal:** Yes, some medications do go in there. Suppositories are a common example, which is why it pays to be regular! And a compounding pharmacist can make morphine suppositories for a cancer patient who cannot tolerate other delivery methods. Usually, the order says *PR*, meaning "per rectum."
- **Feeding tube:** Feeding tubes are very common, especially in hospitals, nursing homes, and rehabilitation units. When patients have trouble swallowing, they may have other problems in their gastrointestinal (GI) tract that require you to use a feeding tube. Some patients who are starting to eat still need the feeding tube for various reasons, including to receive meds. Jump to Chapters 9 and 18 for more details.

Medical professionals use various types of feeding tubes, from nasogastric (NG) tubes to percutaneous endoscopic gastrostomy (PEG) tubes, and you must know some of the workings of the particular feeding tube you need to use before you give a medication through it. The doctor usually writes *in the NG tube* or *via PEG tube*. If the doctor writes *PO*, you must call the doctor to clarify.

- **Inhalation**: You have to administer certain medications down the lungs. For example, patients with breathing problems, such as asthma or emphysema, use inhalers or nebulizers to administer drugs that help them breathe better.

  A *nebulizer* is a handy device that dispenses medication in mist form so that it can penetrate deep into the lungs. The most common medications ordered via a nebulizer are albuterol and ipratropium (Atrovent). A nebulizer machine is different from the inhalers commonly prescribed by doctors. For example, patients with asthma often carry a rescue inhaler — with albuterol (Proventil), for example — in their pocket to help them breathe. Nebulizers are used in hospitals when the person may not be strong enough to take in a deep breath, which is necessary for the inhalers to be effective. In many hospitals, respiratory therapists are responsible for dispensing these medications; however, in some settings, nurses administer nebulizer treatments. They can also be used at home, per the discretion of the prescribing physician.

Timing Is Everything: Knowing When and How Often to Give a Med

When do you medicate your patients? How often do you medicate them? The answers are based on time, of course, but you can't know when and how often to medicate your patients unless the doctor's orders are clear and unambiguous. The following sections take a quick look at some common time-related abbreviations as well as the 24-hour clock, both of which doctors use to make their prescriptions as clear as possible.

Medical abbreviations for time

Here are some time-related, generally accepted abbreviations — and their translations — that doctors often use on their medication orders:

- **BID:** To translate, *BID* means that you need to administer the medication twice a day. One caveat about this abbreviation is that many hospitals dispense meds at assigned times, usually 9 a.m. and 9 p.m. The doctor may not only order BID dosing, but may also specify the times the medication should be given (at 9 a.m. and 6 p.m., for example).

- **STAT**: As you're reading this abbreviation, you may be thinking to yourself: Is this a legit abbreviation or not? In fact, *STAT* is very legit. It means that you need to administer this medication NOW.

  Often with STAT orders, the doctor also talks to the nurse about the order and explains what may be going on with the patient. The patient's medical condition may have changed abruptly, prompting the STAT order.

  Some doctors write *ASAP*, meaning "as soon as possible" in place of STAT. Although this abbreviation is legitimate, it can be confusing and ambiguous. Do you give the medication now or later? An ASAP order requires the doctor to talk with you to explain the time frame in terms of ASAP.

  STAT comes from the Latin word *statim*, which means "immediately."

- **PRN:** Sometimes doctors schedule medications on an as-needed, or *PRN*, basis rather than around the clock. Examples of PRN orders include some pain medications, medications used to help with anxiety, and medications used to control blood pressure.

See the earlier section "Avoiding unacceptable abbreviations" for some totally unacceptable time-related abbreviations. The Joint Commission doesn't like them, and no good doctor should use them.

The 24-hour clock: Military time

If you live outside the United States, work in aviation, or serve in the military, you likely use a 24-hour clock rather than a 12-hour clock to tell time. The same is true for most hospitals and medical centers, so you definitely need to be familiar with military time. Sometimes this standard is called Coordinated Universal Time (UTC), which replaced Greenwich Mean Time (GMT). It's also sometimes called Zulu time. All these names refer to the 24-hour clock.

After midnight (0000), you start counting time from 0. The minute after midnight is 0001, and the minute after 0059 is 0100 (which you say as *one hundred hours*). After the noon hour (1200), the counting continues in the same way, so the minute after 1259 is 1300 (which you say as *thirteen hundred hours*). The last minute of the day is 2359.

Here are some more examples of what 12-hour time looks like in military time:

12-Hour Time	*Military Time*
3:00 p.m.	1500
6:00 p.m.	1800
9:00 p.m.	2100

This time notation is important in reading written medical orders and in dispensing medications. Every hospital has standard times when the nurses dispense medications unless the doc specifies different times, and the times are likely expressed in military time.

BID is usually designated as 0900 and 2100 (9 a.m. and 9 p.m.). If a doctor orders something TID, the most common times are before breakfast, lunch, and dinner unless the times are specified. Note that ordering something every eight hours is not the same as ordering as TID.

You may say, "I'm only a civilian!" Not to worry. A real pro easily adapts to hospital time. For the hours greater than 12, just subtract 12. For example, 1430 in military time is 2:30 p.m. in 12-hour time. Subtract 12 from 14 to get 2.

Individualized Dosing Modifications

All patients are different, especially in terms of their responses to medications, so don't be surprised when you see an order that has restrictions placed on when and how the medication should be given.

Restrictive parameters are very common, especially with certain groups of medications, like blood pressure medications, anxiety medications, and pain medications. For these meds, you often see restrictions based on patient blood pressure or pulse. For example, look at this order:

> labetalol 10 mg IV q6h hold if SBP < 110 or HR < 55

This order means that you should administer labetalol every 6 hours, measure the patient's blood pressure and heart rate before administering the medication, and hold the medication if the patient's systolic blood pressure is less than 110 mmHg or if the heart rate is less than 55 beats per minute (BPM). The doctor wrote the order this way because labetalol can slow the heart rate, and she wants you to take the pulse before administering the med.

You can also see restrictive parameters with sliding scale and insulin orders. For instance, you'd definitely need to hold a scheduled insulin dose if a patient's blood sugar is too low. As always, if you have any questions about the doctor's order, don't hesitate to call the doctor.

Verbal Orders: Make like a Parrot and Repeat Them to the Doctor

Sometimes the doctor has to give a medication order when he isn't there to physically write it. The doctor speaks to the nurse taking care of the assigned patient, and the nurse transcribes the doctor's order onto the physician order sheet. If the hospital has computerized order entry, the nurse enters the order into the system instead. Then the nurse dispenses the med.

The transcription process is efficient, and it could even save lives. But (as Boris Karloff said in the old horror movies) "it is fraught with danger." So take precautions!

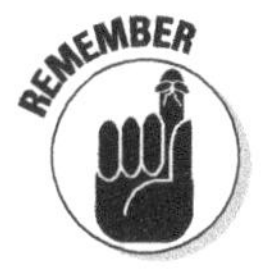

Before you write or electronically enter any medication order, repeat the order *verbatim* (as in "exactly" or "word for word") back to the doctor. Repeating med orders is especially important if the doctor is giving you more than one medication order verbally.

Be sure to repeat these items to the doctor:

- The name of the medication (If necessary, have the doctor spell out the name.)
- The dosage of the medication
- The route of administration
- The time(s) when the medication should be given, including frequency of dosing
- Any individualized dosing changes the doctor has made

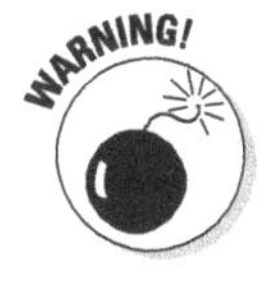

The biggest problem with verbal orders is that they run the risk of containing an error, with no reliable doctor-backed documentation (a paper trail) to substantiate them. To help minimize errors associated with verbal orders, the Joint Commission says that doctors should sign all verbal orders within 24 hours — or else!

As soon as the nurse transcribes the order, she often places a reminder on the patient's chart for the doctor to sign the verbal order. Different EMRs have different ways of reminding the doctor that orders need to be signed. So be sure to check with the hospital or med center where you work (or plan to work) to find out how to create a reminder that the doctor will see.

SODD: Same order, different day

SODD — which means "same order, different day" — is a made-up word that describes the questionable practice of continuing to administer a drug without thinking about whether it's still necessary to the patient's treatment and/or healing. It isn't a good practice to get into. Patients need protection against prolonged drug therapy.

Many hospitals have automatic stop orders on medications or fluid administration.

An *automatic stop order* is a policy to stop and review administering a med to a patient. Depending on the medical center, some medications need daily renewal orders by the physician. Hospitals have rules about how often doctors must renew medications.

For example, intravenous (IV) fluid orders often need to be renewed on a daily basis. Other medications, such as antibiotics, often need to be renewed after a few days, depending on the medication.

These rules are important because they allow (require, actually) the doctor to determine whether he should continue a certain medication. Sometimes the patient's condition changes, and the doctor needs to adjust the dosages accordingly.

Although verbal orders are problematic until they become written orders, you can work effectively with verbal orders by following these simple steps:

1. **Repeat the information provided by the doctor to the doctor when you get the verbal order.**
2. **Put a reminder on the patient's chart telling the doctor to sign the written order.**
3. **Stay alert for any unexpected patient reaction when you dispense the med.**

   If an unexpected reaction occurs, the order may have an error in it. Consult the doctor right away to find out what you need to do next.
4. **Recognize that your task isn't over until the verbal order becomes a written order.**

Real-Life Practice: Interpreting Orders

Table 5-4 shows you some examples of unambiguous, but compact, med orders. Spend some time looking over these orders and their translations, and notice which elements and abbreviations the doctor uses to make the orders clear and concise. To turn this exercise into a quiz, cover up the right column (the translations) and translate the orders in the left column on your own. Then compare your translations with the ones shown in the table.

Table 5-4 Interpreting Orders

Doctor's Order	*Translation*
Zestril 10 mg PO daily	Administer 10 milligrams of Zestril by mouth daily
Rocephin 1 gram IV q8h	Administer 1 gram of Rocephin intravenously every 8 hours.
Heparin 5,000 Units subq q8h	Administer 5,000 units of heparin subcutaneously every 8 hours.
Increase Vitamin D3 to 1,000 units PO daily	Increase Vitamin D3 (cholecalciferol) to 1,000 units by mouth daily.
Discontinue Hytrin. Start Norvasc 2.5 mg PO daily, hold if sbp < 110	Discontinue Hytrin. Begin administering 2.5 mg of Norvasc by mouth daily, but hold if the systolic blood pressure is less than 110.
Magnesium sulfate 8 mEq IV in 100 mL NS over 3 hrs	Administer magnesium sulfate 8 milliequivalents in a total of 100 milliliters of normal saline intravenously over 3 hours.
Lasix 80 mg IV q8h	Administer 80 mg of Lasix intravenously every 8 hours.
Dilaudid 2 mg IV q6h prn severe pain	Administer 2 milligrams of Dilaudid intravenously every 6 hours as needed for severe pain.
Kayexalate enema 30 g PR one dose STAT	Administer 30 grams of Kayexalate enema per rectum now!
1 L D5 ½ NS at 75 mL/hr	Administer 1,000 milliliters of dextrose 5% in one-half normal saline at a rate of 75 milliliters per hour.
1 L D5W with 75 mEq Na Bicarbonate at 125 mL/hr	Administer 1,000 milliliters of dextrose 5% in water with 75 milliequivalents of sodium bicarbonate at a rate of 125 milliliters per hour.
Demadex 60 mg PO, give daily at 0900 and 1800	Administer 60 mg of Demadex by mouth daily at 9 a.m. and 6 p.m.

Real-Life Practice: Evaluating a Script

Figure 5-2 shows a handwritten prescription for three meds — amlodipine, quinapril, and triamterene/hydrochlorothiazide (Dyazide). Is this prescription clear and concise, or not? List the items that the doctor should improve.

Here are the shortfalls in this prescription:

- The patient information is incomplete. (Unfortunately, this is common.)
- The date is funky. What does "12 -1 c 10" mean, anyway? Yes, it looks a little like it was written in December 2010, but who really knows?

- The numbers (5 mg, 40 mg, and 37.5/25) aren't too bad, except for the 5's.
- The mg's look more like g's or a squiggle.
- The first character in "PO" doesn't look at all like a "P."
- The line under each quantity (#100) is illegible, and what's QAU mean, anyway? Most likely, it's supposed to be "QAM," meaning "every a.m."
- The signature is impossible to read.

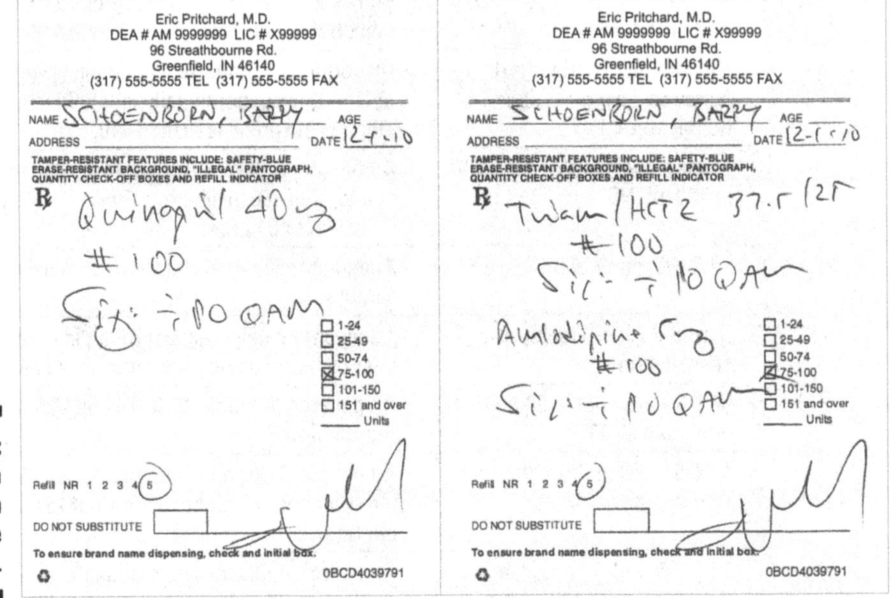

Eric Pritchard, M.D.
DEA # AM 9999999 LIC # X99999
96 Streathbourne Rd.
Greenfield, IN 46140
(317) 555-5555 TEL (317) 555-5555 FAX

NAME ______ AGE ____
ADDRESS ______ DATE ______

TAMPER-RESISTANT FEATURES INCLUDE: SAFETY-BLUE ERASE-RESISTANT BACKGROUND, "ILLEGAL" PANTOGRAPH, QUANTITY CHECK-OFF BOXES AND REFILL INDICATOR

℞

☐ 1-24
☐ 25-49
☐ 50-74
☒ 75-100
☐ 101-150
☐ 151 and over
____ Units

Refill NR 1 2 3 4 5

DO NOT SUBSTITUTE ☐

To ensure brand name dispensing, check and initial box.

0BCD4039791

Eric Pritchard, M.D.
DEA # AM 9999999 LIC # X99999
96 Streathbourne Rd.
Greenfield, IN 46140
(317) 555-5555 TEL (317) 555-5555 FAX

NAME ______ AGE ____
ADDRESS ______ DATE ______

TAMPER-RESISTANT FEATURES INCLUDE: SAFETY-BLUE ERASE-RESISTANT BACKGROUND, "ILLEGAL" PANTOGRAPH, QUANTITY CHECK-OFF BOXES AND REFILL INDICATOR

℞

☐ 1-24
☐ 25-49
☐ 50-74
☒ 75-100
☐ 101-150
☐ 151 and over
____ Units

Refill NR 1 2 3 4 5

DO NOT SUBSTITUTE ☐

To ensure brand name dispensing, check and initial box.

0BCD4039791

Figure 5-2: Handwritten prescription for three meds.

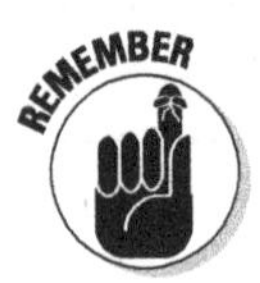

If a nurse has any difficulty reading or understanding a prescription, he should query the doctor. If an outpatient has trouble, she should ask the retail pharmacist about it. The pharmacist has two valuable tools: first, the knowledge of what typical dosing of a med should be; second, the skill to interpret the handwriting of local physicians. Then, if there's a problem, the patient should let the pharmacist contact the doctor, as she has better access.

The good news for the preceding example is that the patient understood the order and the mail-order pharmacy filled it correctly.

Chapter 6

Medication Labels and Patient Safety

In This Chapter

- Reviewing the components of a medication label
- Championing patient safety by being aware of possible medication-related problems
- Preventing medication errors by practicing the six "rights" of medication administration

The number-one concern of doctors and other medical professionals is promoting patient safety and preventing medical errors. Doing accurate medical dosage calculations is a vital part of patient care, but it's only one of several components in a total program of patient safety.

Successful healing and patient safety start with the medication label. In this chapter, you see all the components of medication labels and all the valuable information they provide you. You find out how to read and interpret drug labels correctly so that you can dispense the right drug to the right patient in the right way. You also discover what you can do to prevent and reduce the chances for medical error. Finally, you take a look at the six key factors you need to consider before you administer any medication.

Whether you're a parent giving medication to your ill son or daughter or a medical professional administering medication in a hospital or rehabilitation setting (or both, for that matter), you're in the trenches, so to speak. Accuracy — and, therefore, patient safety — very much rests with you.

Anatomy of a Medication Label

Like prescriptions, all medication labels contain essential elements that are important for you to know. (Take a look at Chapter 5 for details on the elements of a prescription.) As with the doctor's order, the medication label begins with a name, but it also includes several other components. This section discusses the label parts you need to identify and understand.

Brand and generic names

Every drug label includes a brand name, a generic name, or both. The difference between brand-name and generic medications is simple.

- **Brand name:** A brand-name drug is patented, and its name is trademarked. So don't be surprised to see a registered trademark (®) or trademark symbol (™) next to the drug name. The brand name is also called the *trade name* or the *proprietary name,* and it's usually the biggest word on the drug label. (The generic name is right underneath the brand name in smaller lettering. Having both the brand name and the generic name on the label minimizes confusion.)
- **Generic:** A *generic* drug is a med that has the same active ingredient as a brand-name drug but is produced without patent protection. Generic meds are almost always less expensive than their brand-name counterparts. The generic name appears alone on the drug label.

Figure 6-1 shows a label for donepezil HCI (Aricept), with both the brand and generic names.

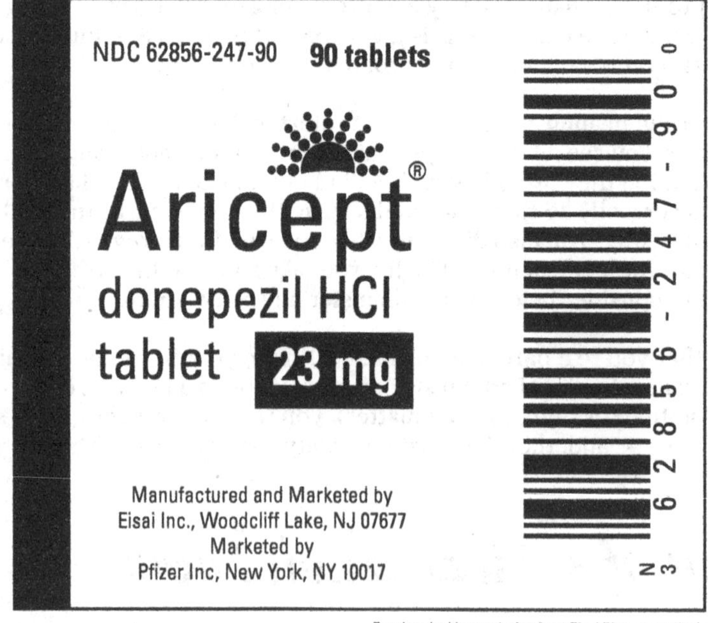

Figure 6-1: Label for donepezil HCI with brand name and generic name.

Reprinted with permission from Eisai Pharmaceuticals

Some people can't tolerate some generic medications. This intolerance may be due to the fillers in the formulation since the active ingredient is the same. In most cases, the generic form of a medication is often more affordable and may be covered under many prescription plans. If a patient finds, however, that he isn't tolerating the generic form of a medication, he must notify his doctor immediately. The patient may need to take the brand-name version or switch to another medication entirely.

Before giving any medication to a patient, ask the patient if she has had adverse reactions to any drug. If she has, be sure to ask whether it was the brand-name drug or the generic version.

Supply dosage strength or concentration

The *supply dosage strength* tells you how strong the medication you're administering is. For tablets and capsules, the most common unit of measurement is the milligram (mg). For example, hydrochlorothiazide (or HCTZ, for short) is a tablet commonly dosed at 12.5 mg daily. For liquids, the most common unit of measurement is milligrams per milliliters of solution (mg/mL). For example, you can dose amoxicillin, a commonly prescribed antibiotic, in liquid form at 250 mg/5 mL. This supply dosage means that the medication contains 250 mg of amoxicillin in every 5 mL of solution.

Medications can be tricky. You can dose some medications in either tablet form or liquid form. For example, amoxicillin comes as a 250 mg tablet or as a 250 mg capsule, but you can also dose the same strength in a 250 mg/5 mL liquid form. Many other meds, particularly antibiotics, are also available in both liquid and solid forms.

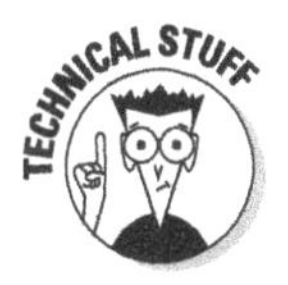

Doctors often prescribe medications in liquid form for infants and pediatric patients as well as elderly patients because that form may be easier for them to swallow. Depending on other medical conditions, a tablet may need to be crushed and administered in custard or applesauce. For example, patients who have suffered from a stroke may not be able to swallow liquids safely because they're at a higher risk of *aspiration*, which is when food and medication go into the lungs. Often, a doctor may order a swallowing evaluation to determine the safest way to orally administer a medication and provide nutrition.

Form

Every medication label includes the basic form of a drug. This form is typically *tablet, capsule, oral solution, suspension,* or *powder for reconstitution.* However, some forms of a medication denote the duration of action for that medication and aren't related to the med's physical structure. For those forms, look for abbreviations, such as *CD* (continuous dosing), *XR* (extended release), *XT* (extended release), and *SR* (sustained release), after the drug name. All these abbreviations indicate longer durations of action than their standard counterparts.

For example, diltiazem (Cardizem) is a commonly prescribed medication for high blood pressure and *atrial fibrillation* (an abnormal heart rhythm). It has many brand names, which all have different durations of action. For instance, the label for a 120 mg dose of diltiazem can include the following duration-of-action forms (*PO* means by mouth):

- Cardizem CD 120 mg PO daily
- Dilacor XR 120 mg PO daily
- Taztia XT 120 mg PO daily

Doctors dose many timed-release meds at a different frequency than their regular counterparts. For example, doctors often order Cardizem CD as a once-daily dose, whereas they order regular Cardizem as a twice-daily dose. Sometimes, the doc wants lower doses of the medication given three or four times a day to test its effect. For example, when treating atrial fibrillation, doctors may order 30 mg four times a day. If this dosing works, the doctor may then transition the order to a once-daily dose.

Route of administration

The *route of administration* is simply the way the patient takes the medication. If you have a medication that's a capsule or tablet, how you dose the med is self-evident — it's oral. The label usually doesn't declare this route of administration, but it always says *tablets* or *capsules*. One exception is nitroglycerin tablets, which should say *SL* (which means under the tongue).

If the medication you're dosing is a liquid (or a powder that will be reconstituted as a liquid), the label clarifies by saying *oral solution, for oral suspension, for intravenous or IV use only, for IV infusion only,* or *for IM, SC, or IV use.*

Total volume

All medication labels specify how much of the particular medication is present. For liquid formulations or intravenous medications, the label shows the total fluid volume of solution, usually in mL. For pills, the label shows the quantity of tabs or caps in the container.

For example, Figure 6-1 shows that the Amoxil will have a total volume of 100 mL when it's reconstituted.

Bar code

Every label for every medication that you'll ever administer includes a printed bar code (unless your job is dosing meds to people in a less modern culture). It's no surprise that, in many treatment settings, you also find a bar code on every patient's wristband. Together, the two bar codes help confirm that the correct med is being given to the correct patient.

Medication bar codes have really improved patient care and patient safety because they provide you a quick and easy way to double-check that you're administering the right meds to the right patients. Before you administer any medication, you're required to scan the bar code on the medication and the patient's bar code. The rule is: No Bar Code Match, No Medicine!

Although every medication has a bar code, not every healthcare setting uses patient IDs with bar codes. For example, long-term-care facilities without a bar code system use a patient picture ID system. In that case, the nurse uses the patient number and picture ID to identify the patient and then checks the order to be sure it's for the correct patient.

National Drug Code number

The *National Drug Code number,* or NDC, is a 10- or 11-digit, 3-segment number. It appears on every medication label and identifies the vendor, generic entity, strength, dosage form, and package size for the given med. It often appears right under the bar code.

Directions for reconstituting

Some drugs come in powder form, even though you have to administer them intravenously or by injection. In those cases, you find directions for reconstituting the medication on the label. For example, reconstituting directions for a drug like 1.2 g tobramycin say to constitute to 40 mg/mL with 30 mL of sterile water for IV use.

NF or USP quality assurance

Every medication you administer must be safe, of good quality, pure, and potent. When you see NF or USP on the label, you know the medication is okay to give to your patients. In case you're curious, *NF* stands for National Formulary and *USP* stands for United States Pharmacopeia. The two organizations are now merged. USP establishes standards for medicines. Manufacturers and regulatory agencies use the standards to guarantee that drugs have the right identification, purity, and strength.

Manufacturer's name and lot number

If you're wondering who made the wonderful medication you're about to administer, check the label. The name of the manufacturer should appear on every drug label.

The manufacturer's *lot number* (sometimes called a *control number*) also appears on every drug label. Every batch of a particular drug has its own lot number. In the event that the manufacturer must recall a med, the hospital uses the lot number to determine which batch needs to be returned.

Combination medications

If a med is made up of more than one substance, the label will clearly say so. For example, atorvastatin/amlodipine (Caduet) is a combination of atorvastatin (Lipitor — when uncombined, a drug used to treat high cholesterol) and amlodipine (Norvasc — when uncombined, an antihypertensive medication). Diovan HCT, a common antihypertensive medication, is a combination of hydrochlorothiazide (HCTZ) and valsartan.

Controlled substance classifications

As a medical professional, you may have to administer controlled substances. What exactly is a *controlled substance?* It's any medication whose dispensation and administration is regulated by the U.S. Drug Enforcement Administration (DEA). The DEA classifies controlled substances into five different schedules (I, II, III, IV, and V) based on the med's potential for abuse, its use as an accepted medical treatment, and its potential for drug dependence.

The schedules of controlled substances include street drugs, such as once-legal heroin, and prescription drugs, such as oxycodone (OxyContin). They also include plant/fungus forms, such as psilocybin, peyote, marijuana, opium blossoms, and coca leaves. (For more information, refer to the DEA's Web site on controlled substances: `www.deadiversion.usdoj.gov/schedules/index.html`.)

Find out if the drug you're administering is a controlled substance by looking for a big *C* on the label; the classification schedule of the controlled substance appears in Roman numeral form next to or within the *C*.

Expiration date

Every medication label has an expiration date. Never administer a medication that's expired because it may not be effective or safe to take. For outpatients, if the expired medication is a sample given by a doctor's office, discard it. If you're working in a hospital and find an expired med, notify the pharmacist and return it.

Label alerts and FDA drug alerts

Many medication labels, both in hospitals and in retail pharmacies, include simple label alerts. For instance, a label may explain storage conditions for the drug ("Store below 25 degrees C, 77 degrees F," for example), or it may explain when the medicine shouldn't be used ("Do not use if precipitated," for example). A drug from a retail pharmacy may explain when to take the medicine ("Take with food," for example).

The label may include other instructions as well. For example, for some oral solutions or IV medications, the label says that you must shake the medication before you dispense it.

If you find a discrepancy between the label and the doctor's order, don't dispense the medication until you consult with the doctor about the discrepancy. Go with your gut: If it doesn't make sense, don't dispense!

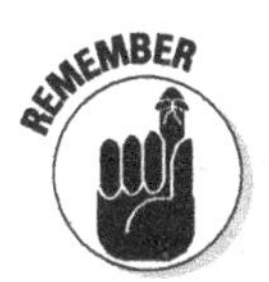

If there's ever a problem with a med's safety, the Food and Drug Administration (FDA) issues an alert. Although the FDA's alerts don't appear on the drug labels, you can receive them automatically on some smartphone apps or consult the Internet. You can also get specific alert information directly from the FDA. For more information about drug alerts, refer to `www.drugs.com/fda_alerts.html`.

Highlighting the Four Big Patient Safety Concerns

As a healthcare worker, you must be aware of the four big patient safety concerns that can (at a minimum) affect the effectiveness of medications. The maximum effect of these concerns, unfortunately, may be a threat to the patient's life. These four concerns are

- Medication allergies
- Adverse drug reactions
- Drug-drug interactions
- Herbal medications and nutritional supplements

Checking for medication allergies

A *medication allergic reaction* is an unexpected or unintended side effect. The nature and degree of the allergic reaction can vary from a simple skin rash to anaphylactic shock (which is life threatening).

Any med can cause an allergic reaction. However, common allergies you're likely to see on patients' charts include allergies to penicillins (like amoxicillin), cephalosporins (like Keflex or Rocephin), sulfa medications like trimethoprim-sulfamethoxazole (Bactrim), and nonsteroidal anti-inflammatory drugs (NSAIDs).

Before you administer any drug, ask the patient if he has any medication allergies. Then double-check the information recorded on the medication reconciliation form (MRF) and the doctor's initial admission note. You can also see that info on the doctor's initial history and physical form. (*Medication reconciliation* is the process of comparing a patient's medication orders to all the medications the patient has been taking at home. See Chapter 7 for more details.)

Finally, always triple-check your own documentation to make sure you've listed any pertinent medication allergies. List the nature of the allergy if that information isn't present. You'd be surprised how often errors occur in the transcriptions of medications from one form to the other.

If the patient doesn't have any medication allergies, simply note this by using the abbreviation *NKDA,* which stands for "No Known Drug Allergies."

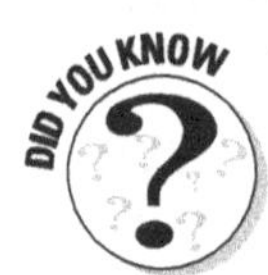

In certain situations, knowing that a patient has an allergy to one medication can prevent the doc from prescribing a medication from a similar drug class. Why? Because it could produce the same symptoms. *Cross-reactivity* is when one class of medications may be so similar to another class that a person might be at risk for similar allergic reaction. One significant example is the cross-reactivity between penicillins and cephalosporins, which are both antibiotics.

Suppose you're asked to administer cephalexin (Keflex) 500 mg PO BID. You check for medication allergies and find out that your patient is allergic to penicillin. Although the patient has no history of allergies to cephalexin, a cephalosporin, you remember that cross-reactivity can occur between these two classes of antibiotics. In other words, if the patient had an allergic reaction to penicillin, there's a small chance that she'll have a reaction to cephalosporins just because she had a reaction to penicillin. Because these two classes of antibiotics are so commonly administered, the prescribing physician must be aware of the patient's prior drug allergies. Call the doctor to clarify the order before administering the medication if you notice possible cross-reactivity.

Asking about adverse drug reactions

As you do your initial patient assessment, you ask about medication allergies (see the preceding section). Patients often give you lists that include pain medications like codeine or dextropropoxyphene (Darvocet).

However, if a patient tells you about a pain medication (or any other med, for that matter) and says that it causes "stomach upset" or "nausea," be aware that this type of reaction doesn't necessarily constitute a drug allergy. Instead, it likely represents an *adverse drug reaction* (or ADR). The patient doesn't develop an allergy to the medication; he develops a side effect because of the medication. ADRs are medication effects that are not caused by an allergic reaction.

Most common ADRs affect the gastrointestinal (GI) system and include nausea, dry heaves, vomiting, constipation, diarrhea, and stomach upset. Some medications lead to very unique reactions in certain people; you can find these reactions in the PDR (Physician's Desk Reference). Labetalol, for example, has a unique side effect of causing the scalp to tingle. Other drugs may cause some people to have drug reactions that aren't listed anywhere.

Some medications cause *expected drug reactions.* For example, a class of medications called *beta blockers* can slow the heart rate and lower the blood pressure. These bodily effects are expected medication reactions. In contrast, if someone who's taking a beta blocker develops nausea or diarrhea, she's experiencing an adverse drug reaction.

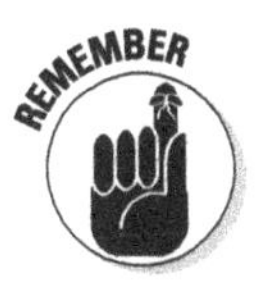

The important thing is to be able to differentiate between allergic reactions and adverse drug reactions.

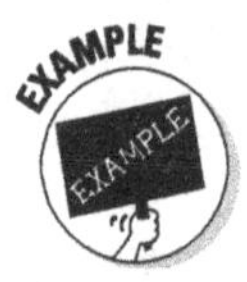

You're asked to administer hydromorphone (Dilaudid) 2 mg IV every four hours as needed for pain to a person with metastatic cancer. (You're on the oncology floor of a hospital, and the patient is in incredible pain.) You check the patient's allergy list and notice that hydromorphone is listed as an allergy. You question the patient and find out that he had taken hydromorphone and that it caused significant constipation. You take note that constipation is *not* a true medication allergy; it's what a drug reference calls a *common reaction.*

You call the doctor, explain the nature of the patient's drug reaction as well as the intractable pain. The doctor orders a bowel regimen to prevent constipation so that your patient can receive hydromorphone.

Dealing with drug-drug interactions

The average person takes more than four medications to treat more than one chronic condition. The older a person is, the more likely he is to be on more meds to treat more chronic conditions, such as hypertension, diabetes, heart disease, and emphysema, just to name a few.

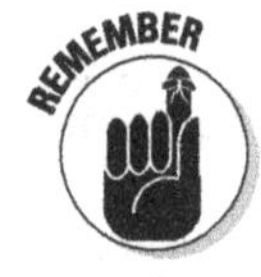

The more medications a person is taking, the higher the chance of a significant drug-drug interaction.

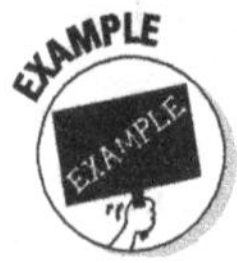

You're administering amiodarone 200 mg PO daily to a patient with atrial fibrillation. You look at the patient's list of meds and note that he's also taking warfarin (Coumadin). Three days later, he develops a GI bleed. The doctor asks you to do a PT/INR check, using a ProTime coagulation tester, STAT. (*PT/INR* stands for International Normalized Ratio, based on prothrombin time; it's a measure of how quickly blood clots. INRs above 5.0 are bad.) The INR is 7.0.

What happened? The amiodarone interfered with the metabolism of the Coumadin, causing the INR to increase dramatically. There's a direct drug interaction between amiodarone and Coumadin.

You're asked to administer sertraline (Zoloft) 50 mg daily to a patient for depression. The patient has a history of a cardiac arrhythmia and is taking propafenone (Rythmol) 100 mg daily.

What could possibly happen? Bad stuff (to use the medical term). The setraline could interfere with the metabolism of the propafenone and cause a life-threatening heart arrhythmia. Call the doctor for order clarification.

A valuable resource for patient safety

The Institute for Safe Medication Practices (ISMP, for short) is a nonprofit organization dedicated to preventing medical errors and promoting medication safety. It's a certified patient safety organization and has many education programs and safety tools designed to help medical professionals practice safe medicine. For more information, visit their Web site at www.ismp.org.

Dealing with a mix of herbal and traditional

Ask about any herbal medications or nutritional supplements that the patient may be taking. These substances aren't inherently bad, but they can potentially interact with prescription meds.

For example, St. John's Wort, a common herbal medication used for its antidepressant properties, can interact with many medications, including some antibiotics and blood thinners like warfarin. The interaction can change the way the body handles the prescription meds. The change, which is known as *drug metabolism,* can result in toxication or detoxication and may increase the risk of significant medication reactions.

If the patient is using herbals or other supplements, advise the doctor and get clarification for any drug order.

Reviewing the Six "Rights" of Medication Administration

You're probably familiar with many different kinds of rights — human rights, the Bill of Rights, and Miranda rights, just to name a few. These rights are legal or moral claims. But another common definition of *right* is to do things the correct way, in conformity with a principle or a standard. That's the kind of right we're talking about in this section.

To ensure patient safety, nurses and other medical professionals are expected to adhere to the Six Rights of Medication Administration, which guide them in administering meds the right way. Nursing schools everywhere teach these six rights, although some hospitals incorporate additional rights into their daily practices, and there are now as many as eight rights. The Six Rights are

- Right patient
- Right medication
- Right dose
- Right time
- Right route
- Right documentation

To prevent medication errors and to keep your patients safe, you must know and practice these rights.

Right patient

Give the medication to the right patient. You may think it would be impossible to give a med to the wrong patient, but such events occur every day. A medication error can happen if the hospital doesn't have patient bar code identification or if the nurse fails to scan it. In a manual system, a medication error can occur if the nurse fails to check the patient's number, name, or picture on a wristband.

Every hospital patient wears a plastic wristband that contains several patient identifiers, including her name, her medical record number (also known as the hospital number), and (in EMR systems) a bar code. See Chapter 5 for more details.

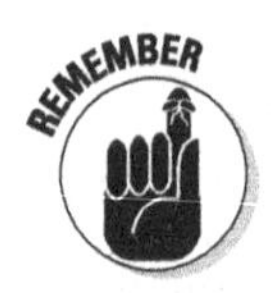

Make sure the patient in front of you is the one who is supposed to receive the medication you're administering. Scan the bar code, and always check at least two different patient identifiers before giving a medication to a patient. In a system without bar codes, check the patient name, patient number, and photo ID.

Right medication

Make sure the medication you're giving to the patient matches the doctor's order. A med can easily get mixed up because the doctor's handwriting on the prescription is illegible, and hospital pharmacies have been known to make mistakes, too. When in doubt about whether a med matches the written prescription, confirm before administering the med.

Too many Rich Snyders

In school, Rich Snyder, one of this book's authors, was one of several children with the same name. There was a Richard Snyder, a Richard Snider, and a Richard Schneider. Co-author Rich often found himself just a few steps away from having an identity crisis. When his frustrated and confused teacher wanted to call on him in class, she would sometimes point or just yell "You!" During recess (and later in life), Rich gained the unique nickname Snyder-Man!

But wait, the story gets better. Later in life, as a medical resident in training, another physician had the exact same name, right down to the middle initial.

What's the moral of this story? The concept of confusing similar names doesn't just apply to medication names; it also applies to people's names. Imagine the confusion that could develop if there were two Rich Snyders in the hospital as patients at the same time. If you ask Barry, the other author of this book, one Rich is more than enough.

Take the same care when you transcribe an order, especially a verbal order. Note that many medication names sound similar and resemble each other in spelling (visit Chapter 5 for more on confusing similar names). Double- and triple-check the name of the medication to avoid any confusion. If anything's unclear, confirm it.

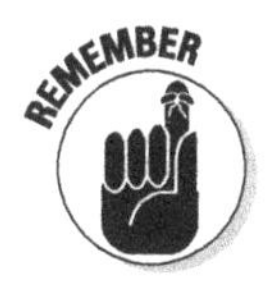

Before you administer the medication, look at the label. Make sure that all aspects of the label match the doctor's order, beginning with the name of the medication. Then double-check that the strength, time, and route of administration also match the doctor's order (see the next three sections for more on these rights).

Apply your knowledge of medicine and your common sense as you review the medication label to make sure the med matches the diagnosis. You must give the medication for the right reason in the right situation. For example, if the order calls for digoxin and the patient doesn't have a diagnosis of atrial fibrillation or congestive heart failure, you need to figure out why you're dispensing that particular med. Call the doctor for clarification.

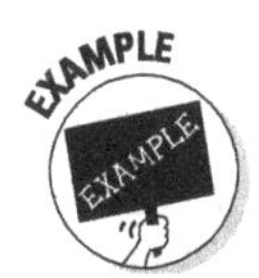

You're instructed to give aspirin 81 mg PO daily. You check the patient's chart and see that he was admitted to the hospital with a bleeding ulcer. Red flag! He's getting aspirin, which has stomach bleeding as a possible side effect. Do the right thing and question the doctor about the order.

You're asked to administer terazosin (Hytrin), a treatment for an enlarged prostate, 2 mg at night to a patient. But the patient has a history of high blood pressure. There are no *restrictive parameters* (patient conditions requiring modified dosing, such as if BP is too high, BP is too low, HR is too high, HR is too low, and so forth) noted on the order. You do a vital signs assessment on the patient and discover that his systolic blood pressure is 95 mmHg, which is close to the textbook definition of hypotension (systolic less than 90 mmHg). And you know that terazosin can lower the systolic BP even more. In this case, you hold the medication and call the doctor for clarification.

Right dose

Administer the correct dose. Seems simple, doesn't it? Yet you must check the dose very carefully to verify that the dose you're about to give is the dose the doctor ordered.

For tablets and capsules, verifying the right dose means accurately comparing the doctor's order to the medication label. You shouldn't find any discrepancies; if you do, call the doctor for clarification. Look at various places in the patient chart where the medication order has been transcribed — it should match word for word with the doctor's order and the medication label. Of course, you may need to calculate the number of tabs or caps to give.

For injections and intravenous administration, verifying the right dose starts with comparing the doctor's order to the label on the med. You may then need to calculate the exact amount to inject. When medicating intravenously, you may also have to calculate the flow rate and time.

Right time

Check the time the medication should be given with the time you're actually giving the med to make sure the times match. The order is transcribed onto the Medical Administration Record (MAR), and you find the correct time of administration there. If the times don't match, you may be administering the med at the wrong time. Note that sometimes the doc orders a schedule that doesn't fit in with standard hospital policy, and you must use the doctor-ordered times. Check out Chapter 7 for more about proper medical documentation.

Right route

Determine and confirm the route of administration. Check the doctor's order and the medication label to make sure you can administer the medication as ordered.

If you're dosing a liquid medication, verify whether you're supposed to administer it orally, by injection, or intravenously. Check the doctor's order and the medication label.

Right documentation

After you administer any medication, document that you did so. Record the date and the time on the patient's medical administration record — the MAR (see Chapter 7) — and add your initials for each medication you administer.

Two more rights for patients

Some hospitals train their nurses to adhere to two additional medication administration rights. These rights aren't about doing the right dosing; they're about providing patients with the right information and medication options.

Right to know about the med

Patients have the right to be informed of any medication administered to them, including the reason for the medication to be administered as well as possible side effects of the medication. Patients also have the right to refuse any medication. Certain medications, including chemotherapy, require written permission to be given because of their toxic side effects.

The medications that a doctor orders to treat the patient's condition are tailored to that condition (for example, an antibiotic to treat a pneumonia). In situations where the prognosis of the patient is grim, the doc always has a conversation with the family and patient concerning the overall plan of care and options for treatment.

Recognize that a doctor orders the patient's meds because she believes them to be correct for effecting a cure or providing palliative care. The doctor has an obligation, based in state law, hospital policy, and/or personal ethics, to inform the patient about the medications she dispenses.

Realize that the patient may ask you what medication he's getting, the reason for its being prescribed, and its intended purpose. Don't let the queries surprise you; as doctors and other healthcare professionals increasingly believe, patients must be active participants in their healing. The Internet helps people to be better informed, but some patients remain poorly informed.

Either way, you need to be prepared to deal with queries from patients and their families about medications. Patients and families are concerned, of course, with the likely effects of medications. Also, in this time of skyrocketing medical costs, they want to get a sense of the costs of various medications.

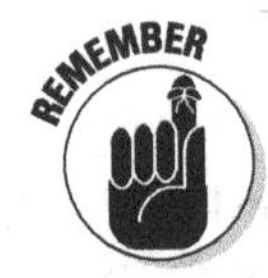

It may be inappropriate (because of the scope of your education and/or hospital policy) for you to discuss drug therapy directly with the patient. In such cases, inform the doctor that she should discuss her assessment with the patient. The common sense assumption is that the physician is responsible for ordering the drugs and is most capable of discussing them with the patient.

Right to refuse the med

This book isn't about medical ethics, but you need to be aware that controversies exist about a patient's right to refuse medication — or treatment, for that matter. The issue originally centered around the administration of psychotropic drugs by psychiatrists and the treatment of involuntary patients, such as prisoners.

In 1990, the Florida Supreme Court recognized that a patient has the inherent right to make choices about medical treatment. A competent patient, said the court, has the constitutional right to refuse treatment.

Hospital policies about dealing with a patient who refuses to take a medication may vary. Be sure to ask about the policy at the institution where you plan to work. Generally, to avoid a sticky situation down the road, inform the doctor right away if your patient refuses to take a prescribed med.

Chapter 7

Proper Medical Documentation and Dispensation

In This Chapter

- Familiarizing yourself with the Medication Reconciliation Form and the Medication Administration Record
- Delivering meds using a pneumatic tube system
- Dispensing meds with the Pyxis system
- Practicing medical documentation and dispensation with some real-life problems

Forms, forms, and more forms! As a medical professional, sometimes you may feel like all you do is fill out forms. Just when you're done with one form, you find that you have to fill out yet another one. You may feel a bit overwhelmed with too many forms and too little time, but proper documentation is very important to patient care. Good medical record keeping is essential to reducing medical errors and improving the care and safety of patients (see Chapter 6 for more on patient safety).

You'll become familiar with many different forms over the course of your career, and all of them are important. But the one form that stands out above the rest is the Medication Administration Record (MAR). This form is so important that we dedicate a whole section to it. Whatever you do, make sure you document correctly on this form and don't mar your MAR!

The other important form you need to know about is the Medication Reconciliation Form (MRF). The MRF, coupled with the physician's orders, forms the basis of the MAR. In this chapter, we introduce you to the MRF and the MAR, and we provide some examples and practice that simulate using these forms in the real world. We also discuss proper dispensation of controlled substances and explain what documentation you need to provide to stay out of trouble.

The Medication Reconciliation Form — Essential for Patient Care

The *Medication Reconciliation Form* (MRF) lists the medications a person is taking at home when she is admitted to the hospital. It's called a *reconciliation* form because it does more than just list the patient's home meds. For the admitting physician, it provides a system of checks and balances he can use to make sure the patient's home medications match up with the newly prescribed hospital medications.

The medication reconciliation process typically has the following steps:

1. **An RN/LPN/LVN takes inventory of the patient's home medication regimen when the patient is admitted to the hospital.**

   This list includes prescription drugs, over-the-counter meds, herbal supplements, patches, inhalers, eye/ear/nose drops, and vitamins. The MRF also has space to include medication allergies and adverse drug reactions, or ADRs (see Chapter 6 for more details).

2. **The nurse writes the list of meds on a preprinted paper form or enters the list into a computer terminal.**

   For each med, the nurse identifies the drug, dosage, frequency, and last time taken. According to Rich (one of the authors), some hospitals write out each medication by hand, but many others use electronic entry.

3. **The doctor studies the patient's home medication list and reconciles it by deciding whether each med should be continued or discontinued while the patient is in the hospital.**

   Next to each medication on the MRF are boxes that say Continue or Discontinue. The doc checks the appropriate box. Alternately, the doctor may circle the preprinted letters *C* and *DC*.

   For example, if a patient's MRF shows that he's taking furosemide (Lasix) 40 mg PO bid (orally, twice a day), and if he's admitted to the hospital for a CHF (coronary heart failure) exacerbation, then the admitting doctor may order that the furosemide be administered intravenously. In that case, the admitting physician would check the box next to Discontinue for the home dose of furosemide.

4. **The doctor finalizes the medication orders, and a list is generated.**

   This list becomes the basis of the MAR (see the next section).

Figure 7-1 shows an example of a printed MRF.

GENERAL HOSPITAL CARVER, KY

HOME MEDICATION RECONCILIATION FORM

USE BALL POINT PEN (PRESS FIRMLY) **Meds Sent Home** **Meds Stored In Pharmacy**
If additional space is needed, please use a 2nd copy of Home Medication Reconciliation Form.
PATIENT PHARMACY: **PHONE:**
Information about medications prior to admission obtained from:
Patient ***Medication List*** ***Other***

Date	Medication / Herbal Supplement / Dose / Route / Frequency / Indication	Last Dose		Admission Meds	
		Date	Time	Cont.	Stop

THE ABOVE HOME MEDICATIONS HAVE BEEN REVIEWED BY: (Continue medications ✓'d above during Inpatient/Outpatient Admission)
INDICATE IF ADDITIONAL FORMS — OF ________
Signature of Person taking history ________ *Date: ________*
Physician ________
Signature ________ *Date ________*

Figure 7-1: A sample Medication Reconciliation Form.

The doctor must review and update the patient's medication list each time the patient is transferred to a different level (usually meaning a transfer to a different medical-surgical floor). For example, if the patient's condition worsens and she goes into a critical state (and is transferred to the ICU), the most current medication list is printed, and the doc reconciles the current medication regimen with the most recent change in the patient's condition.

After a patient gets out of surgery, recovers, and is to be brought back to the medical-surgical floor, the doctor must reconcile the medication list again. For example, if the patient is to be NPO (nothing by mouth), the doc needs to change the route of administration for many meds (or hold some medications) until the patient is able to take them orally again.

When a patient is to be discharged, expect to see a Discharge MRF, containing only the medications that the patient can take at home.

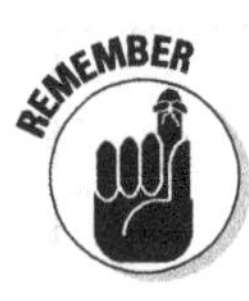

The important point to remember is that reconciling medications doesn't just happen once; it can happen multiple times during a patient's hospitalization. You need to be aware of all updates being made to the MRF (and subsequent inpatient medication lists) because changing the MRF affects the MAR, and the MAR needs to be up to date with the doctor's orders at all times (see the next section for details on the MAR).

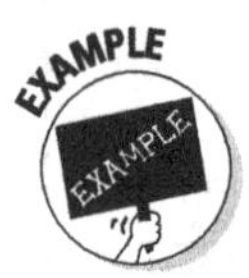

You're taking care of a patient who has just been admitted for accelerated hypertension. The patient was taking a clonidine (Catapres TTS-2) transdermal patch at home. You note that the doctor's orders call for clonidine 0.3 mg PO tid (three times daily). Is this order okay?

To find out, follow these steps:

1. **Do some research.**

   You check a drug reference and see that Catapres TTS-2 is a seven-day patch that should provide 0.2 mg/day of the medication.

2. **Inspect the MRF.**

   You look at the MRF and see that the patch was discontinued (per the doctor's order). The patient will start taking a higher dosage in pill form while in the hospital.

The order looks good. The old med was discontinued, and the new med will start in a different form with a higher dosage.

The Medication Administration Record — Don't Mar Your MAR!

The *Medication Administration Record* (MAR) is simply a record of the medications you give to a patient. These include both routine meds (given on a schedule) and prn meds (given as needed).

Two key points to keep in mind about the MAR are

- **Proper documentation (known as "right documentation") is a patient right.** Obviously, you and your team need to know what meds the patient received (and how much and when). The MAR is essential both for patient safety and for confirmation that the patient is getting the prescribed drugs.
- **The MAR is a legal document.** The MAR requires noting everything from side effects to the location of injections. The MAR can reveal a lot in liability lawsuits, so accuracy rules. As Patricia Iyer, Barbara Levin, and Mary Ann Shea point out in *Medical Legal Aspects of Medical Records,* the MAR is a very important element in an attorney's review of medication-related records.

The MAR is made up of transcribed medication orders. Whether you fill it in manually or get help from a computerized system, the potential for error always exists. Your mantra must be "Check, double-check, and check again."

Knowing where to find the MAR

Where do you find a patient's MAR? It depends on the setup of the hospital where you work or may work.

- If the facility doesn't have an electronic medical record (EMR) system (see Chapter 5), much of the documentation must be done by hand. The MAR is sometimes kept in the patient's chart, but, in most hospitals, it's kept in a ring binder. Either way, it must be in a place where you have easy access to it.
- If the hospital has an EMR system, the MAR is part of the patient's computerized record. Just pull up the patient's electronic record to find the MAR.
- In many healthcare facilities, nurses have portable computers with computer-based EMRs. They can input all the patient's information, including the MAR, on the portable computer.

Understanding what's in the MAR

Don't lose your MAR-bles worrying about what's in the MAR. Every MAR contains the same main components, which we cover in the following sections. The form may look different at different facilities, but the basic information is the same. Figure 7-2 shows an example of a very simple MAR.

Pausing for patient identification

The patient name, patient identification number, and date appear somewhere on the MAR. Like a physician's order form (see Chapter 5 for details) or an MRF, the information may be stamped at the top or the bottom of the page. In other instances, you may need to put a patient sticker, complete with this ID information, on the MAR form. Check and double-check the patient ID — you don't want to give the wrong patient the wrong medications!

Listing allergies and ADRs

Allergies (usually in reference to drug allergies) and adverse drug reactions (ADRs) must appear in a prominent place on the MAR, often at the top of the page. The allergy-specific info needs to include the names of the medications causing the allergies and the nature of the allergies. Noting an adverse drug reaction versus a true allergic reaction can mean a huge difference in the treatment of a patient.

Medication Administration Record (MAR)

MO/YR:	Start/Stop Date		Facility Name																															
Medication		Hour	1	2	3	4	5	6	7	8	9	10	11	12	13	14	15	16	17	18	19	20	21	22	23	24	25	26	27	28	29	30	31	
	Start																																	
	Stop																																	
	Start																																	
	Stop																																	
	Start																																	
	Stop																																	
	Start																																	
	Stop																																	
	Start																																	
	Stop																																	
	Start																																	
	Stop																																	

Diagnosis:

DIET (Special instructions, e.g. Texture, Bite Size, Positions, etc.)

Comments

Allergies:

Physician Name

Physician Number

A. Put initials in appropriate box when medication is given.
B. Circle initials when not given.
C. State reason for refusal/omission on back of form.
D. PRN Medications: Reason given and results must be noted on back of form.
E. Legend: *S* = School; *H* = Home visit; *W* = Work; *P* = Program

NAME:

Record #

Date of Birth:

Sex:

Figure 7-2: A typical MAR.

Mapping out the medications

Expect to see all the details of each prescription in the medications section of the MAR (see Chapter 6 for a lot more details on medication labels).

- **Drug name:** The drug names listed on the MAR must match the MRF exactly and include all the drugs the doc checked to be continued in the hospital as well as any new drugs the doc prescribed. Expect to see the generic name, but know that many computer-based systems list both the generic name and the brand name. The MAR also shows the med's type (for example, long acting, sustained release, and so on).

- **Dosage:** The medication's dosage strength and amount must be clear on the MAR, and they should match the doctor's orders and the MRF exactly. If the doctor changes the medication or the dosage, the medication is crossed out or discontinued from the current form, if an EMR is used. The new medication or dosage is then placed in the updated MAR.

- **Route of administration:** The route of administration is an important element on the MAR because you need to dispense the meds correctly. Also, you need to be able to find this info fast if the medication is not on the hospital formulary, if the prescribed form of the medication isn't available, or if the doctor needs to change a dosage.

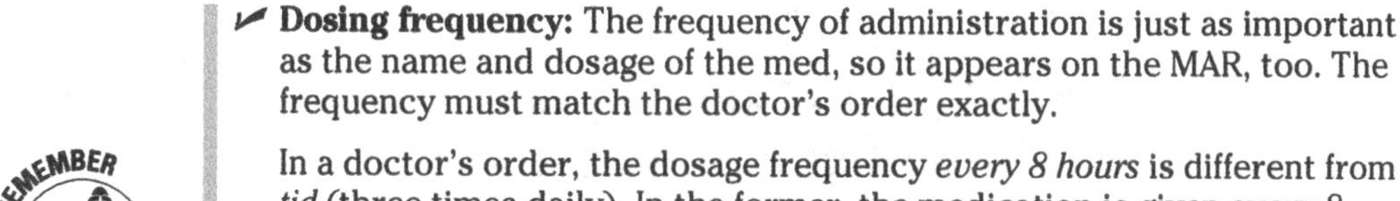

- **Dosing frequency:** The frequency of administration is just as important as the name and dosage of the med, so it appears on the MAR, too. The frequency must match the doctor's order exactly.

  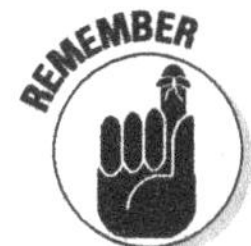

  In a doctor's order, the dosage frequency *every 8 hours* is different from *tid* (three times daily). In the former, the medication is given every 8 hours (for example, 5 a.m., 1 p.m., and 9 p.m.). In the latter, it can be given three times a day, not always in 8-hour intervals.

  You may encounter a *PRN MAR,* a supplemental form that lists only the meds prescribed prn (take as needed).

- **Dates and timing for the medication:** The MAR includes when the doctor ordered each medication started and when each med should be stopped. Many hospitals place an automatic stop order on meds that doctors don't specify stop times or stop dates for as part of hospital policy; these stop orders depend on the medication.

Staying up to date with a daily chart

A large part of the MAR is a daily chart, which often has a range of 31 days. Expect to see all the details of *each* dosing of the meds on the MAR, including the time (in military time) that the med was given and a place for the administering nurse's initials.

Calling all doctors: Physician information

The MAR includes the prescribing physician's contact information in case a question arises concerning the medication order. Because more than one doctor can be taking care of a patient, you may find yourself calling several doctors about different medication orders.

Marking your spot: Nurse's initials

After you give any medication, put a slash through the time, or if you administer prn, write in the time and then slash through the time. Add your initials to show that you administered the medication. This is an important step, and you can't forget to do it.

Surveying other sections

MARs vary from hospital to hospital. For example, you may see a prn section, codes for where in the body you gave an injection, or codes for *refused, asleep,* or *NPO* (nothing by mouth).

Making changes

If the patient's status changes and the doctor orders a new medication, you must document what the new medication is, why it's being given, and all the other med details we cover in the section "Mapping out the medications."

Getting a handle on other forms and documentation

Here are some of the other forms and documents, besides the MRF and MAR, that you find in your patients' charts:

- **Physician History and Physical:** This form, also called an *H&P*, is the initial form the doctor uses to record necessary information when a patient is admitted to the hospital.

  The History section consists of all the information relevant to the patient's admission. It includes the patient's chief complaint and history before admission to the hospital, the patient's past medical and surgical history, and a detailed review of the patient's home medication regimen, including allergies and medically relevant family and social history.

  The Physical section consists of a detailed physical examination, including vital signs, laboratory results, and pertinent radiological studies. The final part of the H&P form is the Assessment and Plan, where the admitting physician lists the admission diagnoses and her plan of treatment.

- **Nursing Assessment and Care Plan:** The nurse does a comprehensive assessment when a patient is first admitted to the hospital. She does a review of the patient's history, as well as a physical examination and medication review. The nurse also formulates a plan of care for the patient. This plan of care includes instructions concerning patient care as well as goals for the patient to achieve during the hospitalization.

- **Physician Progress Note:** This document is where the physician documents the daily progress of the patient as it relates to the admission diagnosis. Think of it as a mini H&P. The Physician Progress Note documents the patient's past 24 hours in the hospital, the vital signs, any pertinent physical exam findings, a list of lab and radiological studies, and an assessment and plan for further treatment. Depending on your hospital system, this note can be handwritten or charted electronically.

- **Nursing Daily Note:** Like the doc, the nurse also takes daily progress notes. These notes can be handwritten or electronically charted.

- **Notes by other caregivers:** Other caregivers, including a dietician, a physical therapist, an occupational therapist, and a case manager, may see the patient while he's in the hospital. Each caregiver has a section in the patient's chart where she documents her findings.

- **Discharge Form:** This comprehensive instruction sheet includes instructions to the patient, the outpatient physician the patient is to see for follow-up, any follow-up lab tests the patient needs to have done, and a printout of the patient's in-hospital medication regimen — with a review of the medication reconciliation form to see what has changed. A Discharge MRF describes what the patient's home medications are to be.

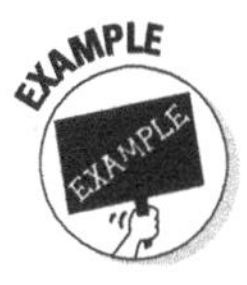

A patient is receiving furosemide (Lasix) IV. On your rounds, you note that he's significantly short of breath. What do you do?

Follow these steps:

1. **Record the vitals, and call the doctor.**

   The physician comes up to see the patient and ascertains that the patient is in CHF. He orders furosemide 80 mg IV times 1 dose now. The doctor should write the order, including the date and time, on the physician order form, or order it electronically if the medical center has an EMR.

2. **Administer the ordered dose of furosemide.**
3. **Document the change on the patient's MAR.**

   Document why this dose was given, and note the change in the patient's condition. Include the date and time of the event. Sign and include your credentials.

If you transcribe any medication from the physician's order sheet, don't forget to sign that sheet as well. Again, include the date, time, and your credentials.

Reviewing Medication Dispensation

Depending on the medication being administered, you may already have the medication in your medication drawer. If you don't, you have to get the med from the pharmacy or use a Pyxis system.

Tubing up the meds

Many hospitals have a very efficient way of getting medications from the pharmacy to the medical-surgical floor — the *pneumatic tube system.*

Pharmacies can "tube" many medications, like antibiotics and continuous infusions, directly to the medical-surgical floor, which is especially handy in critical care units.

Note: Although tube systems are efficient and quick, they aren't right for all medications. For example, glass vials and other medications may exceed the weight or size limits of the pneumatic tube; they must be brought to the floor directly.

Using the Pyxis to give narcs

You need to follow a special procedure when administering narcotics or other controlled substances (often referred to as *narcs*). Many medical-surgical floors use a special type of medication dispensing machine for narcs, a common one being the Pyxis.

The Pyxis MedStation is a branded product from Cardinal Health. It provides a secure place for hospitals to store the narcs that you'll dispense to patients. A Pyxis machine uses bar codes to ensure that medications being administered are the right dose for the right patient. To access the Pyxis, you need a username and password (kind of like signing in to access your e-mail).

After you administer a narc and note it on your patient's MAR, you must also sign the delivery sheet, which is then reconciled with a Pyxis activity report.

The use of narcs is monitored closely, and some hospitals use *inventory sheets* to monitor the use of such medications. An inventory sheet keeps a running count of all the medications in stock compared to the number of meds that have been used.

That being said, most hospital centers use an electronic tracking system, which means you don't have to fill out an inventory sheet because the medication usage is tracked electronically. You do, however, have to count and record the amount of narcotic left after each usage. The pharmacy department double-checks this amount to make sure there's no discrepancy.

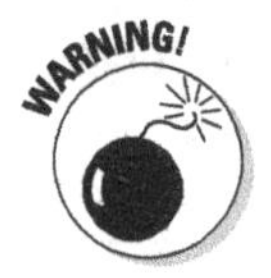

Government and hospitals are very paranoid about "losing count" of controlled substances. If a miscount can't be reconciled and no one takes responsibility for it, supervisors and the director of nursing will get involved, and you'll have to deal with write-ups and other negative consequences.

Real-Life Practice: Administering a Narcotic

You're ordered to administer hydromorphone (Dilaudid) 2 mg IV prn (as needed) for pain. You administer the medication. How would you document that you administered it?

Follow these steps:

1. **Withdraw the hydromorphone from the medication dispensing machine.**

   Hydromorphone is a Schedule II controlled substance. If your hospital has a Pyxis system, use your username and password to withdraw the medication. Your username serves as your electronic signature.

   If your hospital doesn't have a Pyxis system, record how much of the med you withdrew on a special drug inventory sheet, designed specifically for controlled substances.

2. **Administer the hydromorphone.**
3. **Record the controlled substance transaction.**

   Sign the delivery sheet, which will later be reconciled with a Pyxis activity report, or (in a manual system) manual inventory reports. More commonly, the controlled substance transaction is recorded electronically, with a running count being maintained, as we describe in the preceding section.

4. **Document the administration on the patient's MAR.**

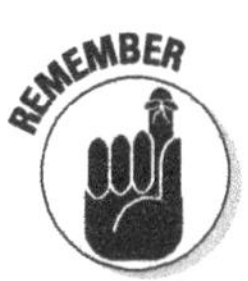

When you're working with controlled substances, if you don't administer all the medication in the syringe, you need another nurse to watch you dispose of the extra medication. In addition, you must record the discarded amount in the Pyxis as wasted.

Real-Life Practice: Checking Vitals and Administering Fluids

You're taking vital signs on a patient with pneumonia and record that her blood pressure is low, with a systolic BP (the upper number) of 80 mmHg. The patient is *mentating* (exhibiting normal brain function) well and otherwise feels fine. What do you do? How do you record this situation?

Follow these steps:

1. **Call the doctor.**

   The doctor orders you to give a fluid bolus of normal saline 500 mL IV "wide open" over a half-hour. The doctor asks you to call him back after the infusion with another set of vital signs.

2. **Administer the fluid bolus.**

   See Chapter 11 for details on intravenous dosing and administration.

3. **Record the bolus on the MAR.**

4. **Check the patient's vital signs.**

   The blood pressure is still the same.

5. **Call the doctor back with updated vital signs.**

   The doctor orders the patient to be transferred to the intensive care unit.

6. **Print a new, updated patient medication list.**

   This is the form the doctor reviews to determine which of the current medications to continue or discontinue and which new medications to add to the physician order form.

7. **Record the events.**

   On a Nursing Progress Note, you record that the fluid order is different from the fluid order given on admission because of the patient's change in status (that is, her low blood pressure).

Chapter 8

Mastering Calculation Methods for Dosing Meds

In This Chapter

- Looking at the general rules for all dosage calculations
- Examining three distinct calculation methods
- Practicing some real-life dosing math using different calculation methods

Calculating dosages is an everyday task if you're a nurse or other health-care provider. Correct dosing is important in every medical setting, but especially in critical care units, pediatric units, and obstetrics units. Your goal is to do calculations accurately and with minimum effort.

In this chapter, we show you a general approach to doing all dosing calculations and then focus on the details of each of the three calculation methods: formula, ratio-proportion, and dimensional analysis. Then you get to try your hand at a handful of sample dosing problems, most of which we show you how to do using all three methods.

Taking a General Approach to Dosage Calculations

Some dosage calculations look difficult, but they're not. After all, inside every "hard" problem is an easy problem (or maybe a couple of them) just waiting to get out. This section shows you a general approach that you can take for all dosing problems. It helps you figure out how to break the doctor's order down and how to use the right calculation method to determine the right dosage to give the patient.

Knowing some basic mathematical principles

Every dosage calculation involves some sort of arithmetic, whether it's addition, subtraction, multiplication (usually of fractions), or division, and many calculations also involve algebra. (See Chapter 2 for more details on arithmetic basics.)

Three equations for three methods

Medical dosing calculations amount to the following three algebraic equations.

Formula method:

$$x = \frac{a}{b} \times c$$

Ratio-proportion method:

$$\frac{a}{b} = \frac{c}{d}$$

Dimensional analysis method:

$$x = \frac{a}{b} \times \frac{b}{c} \times \frac{c}{d} \times \frac{d}{e} \times \frac{e}{f}$$

See the sections "Focusing on the Formula Method," "Relying on the Ratio-Proportion Method," and "Dosing with the Dimensional Analysis Method" for more information.

Improper fractions

When you do dosing math, you can make life easier by expressing whole numbers as improper fractions. For example:

$$12 = \frac{12}{1}$$

Unity

When the numerator and denominator of a common fraction are the same, you have *unity*. Any number divided by itself is equal to 1. The same is true for units. For example:

$$\frac{12}{12} = 1 \quad \frac{\text{mg}}{\text{mg}} = 1 \quad \frac{\text{tablets}}{\text{tablets}} = 1$$

Canceling out units

When the numerator and denominator of a common fraction share a unit, you can "cancel out" that unit because they're equal to 1 (see the preceding section).

For example, to calculate how many mg are in twelve 50 mg tablets, set up and solve the following equation:

$$x = \frac{12\text{ tablet}}{1} \times \frac{50\text{ mg}}{1\text{ tablet}}$$

$$x = \frac{12\ \cancel{\text{tablet}} \times 50\text{ mg}}{1 \times 1\ \cancel{\text{tablet}}}$$

$$x = \frac{600\text{ mg}}{1} = 600\text{ mg}$$

This is an easy example of multiplying fractions and canceling out units. Because the tablet unit appears in both the numerator and the denominator, you can eliminate it.

Commutativity

You can freely rearrange addition and multiplication terms in a mathematical expression because of a property of math called *commutativity*. Essentially, it means that for addition and multiplication:

$$a + b = b + a$$

$$a \times b = b \times a$$

For example, you can rearrange the elements from the example in the section "Canceling out units" like so:

$$x = \frac{12\text{ tablet}}{1} \times \frac{50\text{ mg}}{1\text{ tablet}}$$

$$x = \frac{50\text{ mg} \times 12\text{ tablet}}{1 \times 1\text{ tablet}}$$

$$x = \frac{50\text{ mg} \times 12}{1 \times 1} \times \frac{\cancel{\text{tablet}}}{\cancel{\text{tablet}}}$$

$$x = 600\text{ mg}$$

The equation and the result are the same as the ones from the preceding section. Twelve tablets contain a total of 600 mg.

Conversion factors

A *conversion factor* is a simple equation that expresses equivalent amounts in differing units. Generally, memorizing conversion factors is easy to do, and when you know some conversion factors, all you have to do to convert units is use simple multiplication or division. For example:

1 kg = 2.2 lb

lb = kg ÷ 2.2

kg = lb × 2.2

The general rule is

desired unit = given unit × conversion factor

See Chapter 4 for more details.

Following the process

Doing a dosage calculation takes a few simple steps. Follow the procedure we outline in this section, but recognize that some calculations don't require all the steps. As you work through these calculation steps, consider this sample dosing problem:

> You're instructed to administer heparin via a weight-based regimen. First, you're required to give an 80 unit/kg bolus and then to start an infusion at 18 unit/kg/hr (units per kilogram of patient body weight per hour). The heparin comes as 25,000 units in 500 mL of 0.9% NS. The patient weighs 220 pounds. What's the flow rate in mL/hr?

1. **Think about the dose.**

   Get a grip on what the final dose would look like. Are you dosing units, mg, or mL? Is patient weight a factor? Is time a factor, as it is with flow rates?

   For instance, in the sample order, you know you have to do an IV infusion, which involves a flow rate, commonly expressed in mL/hr. A single mL must contain the right number of units for the patient's body weight, of course, but your final answer needs to be a flow rate.

2. **Break the order into separate steps.**

   The process of doing a dosage calculation may have multiple steps. Identify them, and separate them. For example, when you examine the preceding sample problem, you see that you have to work through two dosing steps: The bolus is one calculation and the infusion is another.

3. **Convert units to match the order.**

The units provided in a doctor's order have to match the units you use in your calculations. Be prepared to convert units (see Chapter 4 for details).

4. **Use one of the three calculation methods (formula method, ratio-proportion method, or dimensional analysis method) to calculate the dosage.**

   Set up the equation, plug in the values, and determine the dosage.

5. **Double-check your answer to make sure it's reasonable.**

   As always, your number-one goal is patient safety, so you must exercise caution in all your dosage calculations. The med you dose has to be a likely amount. If it isn't, review your math. If the math is right, you may need to question the doctor's order.

   If an answer looks "way off," the chances are excellent that you've inverted one of the equation's terms or used an incorrect conversion factor. For example, prevention of myocardial infarction calls for a dose of 1 aspirin 80 to 325 mg every day. If calculating a dose gives you an answer of 8,000 mg every day (100 children's tablets/day!), you can feel pretty sure you made a mistake somewhere. When you find and correct the error, you'll probably come up with a reasonable answer.

Some calculations are so simple that you don't have to do any steps. For example, if the order is 5 mg of warfarin (Coumadin) PO qday (orally, once a day), then you don't have to do any calculation. Warfarin comes in 5 mg tablets, and the patient should take 1 tablet/day. We'd really be stretching things if we asked you to calculate how many mg are in a 5 mg tablet.

Watch out for orders specifying *gr.* Errors in dosing by grain (gr) rather than gram (g) will "mess you up," as we say in professional doctor talk. Grains are an artifact in the U.S. Pharmacopeia, and they surely make too high a contribution to overdosing and underdosing situations.

Using the right tools

Calculations are easy to do when you use the right tools. Make sure you know or have handy the following (see Chapter 4 for a whole lot more details):

- **Metric system equivalents:** Metric equivalents like 1,000 mcg = 1 mg, 1,000 mg = 1 g, and 1,000 g = 1 kg will become second nature to you.
- **Metric-to-U.S. equivalents:** You'll come to know the relationships between metric units and U.S. customary units (including household units) like the back of your hand. For example, you know that 5 mL = 1 tsp, 3 tsp = 1 Tbsp, and, of course 1 kg = 2.2 lb.
- **Conversion factors:** You don't have to memorize some conversions, such as mmol to mEq (millimoles to milliequivalents), which is used in

electrolyte therapy, but be aware that such units and such conversions exist. You may never be intensely involved with electrolyte therapy, but you can bet you'll be tested on this subject in your classes.

- **Helpful tools:** You can use pencil and paper, a hand calculator, a spreadsheet, a smartphone app, or an online calculator to help you do calculations.

Focusing on the Formula Method

The *formula method* of dosing calculations is simple and straightforward. In fact, some nurses make it their first choice in dosing calculations because of its simplicity. Generally speaking, the formula method is the fastest way to calculate the dosing of tablets and capsules, but it's less useful in complex calculations. The structure is

$$D\ (\text{dose}) = \frac{O\ (\text{ordered})}{H\ (\text{have})} \times Q\ (\text{quantity})$$

Here's what the variables represent in this general formula:

- **D (dose):** The dose you will give
- **O (ordered):** The dose ordered by the doc
- **H (have, or on hand):** The dose on the medication label per unit on the medication label
- **Q (quantity):** The unit on the label that contains an amount of the dose (for tablets and capsules, this number is always 1)

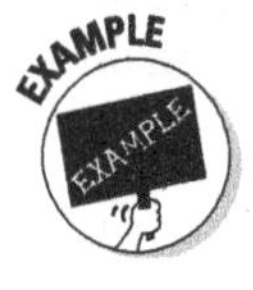

The doctor orders you to give 6 mg diazepam (Valium), and you have 2 mg tablets on hand. How many tablets do you give?

To find out, use the formula method and follow these steps:

1. **Set up the following equation:**

$$D\ (\text{dose}) = \frac{O\ (\text{ordered})}{H\ (\text{have})} \times Q\ (\text{quantity})$$

$$D\ \text{tablet} = \frac{6\ \text{mg}\ (\text{ordered})}{2\ \text{mg}\ (\text{have})} \times 1\ \text{tablet}$$

2. **Multiply and solve.**

$$D = \frac{6\ \cancel{mg}}{2\ \cancel{mg}} \times 1 \text{ tablet}$$

$$D = 3 \text{ tablets}$$

The mg units cancel out, and you're left with tablets. Give three 2 mg tablets to make up a dose of 6 mg.

You're ordered to dose 200 mg of a liquid suspension orally. The strength of the supplied medication is 125 mg/5 mL. How much do you give?

To answer this question, use the formula method and follow these steps:

1. **Set up the following equation:**

$$D \text{ mL} = \frac{200 \text{ mg (ordered)}}{125 \text{ mg (have)}} \times 5 \text{ mL (quantity)}$$

2. **Multiply and solve.**

$$D = \frac{200\ \cancel{mg}}{125\ \cancel{mg}} \times 5 \text{ mL}$$

$$D = \frac{200 \times 5 \text{ mL}}{125}$$

$$D = 8 \text{ mL}$$

The mg units cancel out, and you're left with mL. Provide 8 mL orally.

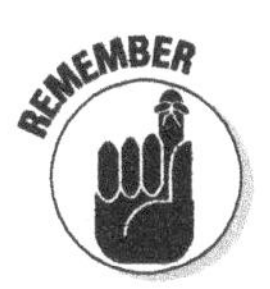

When you have to convert units, you can often use a simple conversion factor that resembles the formula method for calculating medications. We mention conversion factors in the section "Knowing some basic mathematical principles" and discuss unit conversions in detail in Chapter 4.

For example, to convert 1 g to mg, set up the following equation:

desired unit = given unit × conversion factor

$$N \text{ (new unit)} = a\ (\cancel{\text{old unit}}) \times \frac{b \text{ (new unit)}}{c\ (\cancel{\text{old unit}})}$$

$$\text{mg} = \cancel{g} \times \frac{1{,}000 \text{ mg}}{1\ \cancel{g}}$$

This is just a complicated way of saying that 1,000 mg = 1 g. It looks a little like the formula method and a little like the dimensional analysis method (which we discuss later in this chapter).

Relying on the Ratio-Proportion Method

A *proportion* is a relationship between four quantities. The first divided by the second equals the third divided by the fourth, as the following equation shows:

$$\frac{a}{b} = \frac{c}{d}$$

You say this equation as "*a* is to *b* as *c* is to *d*." When you know three of the variables, you can solve for the fourth variable.

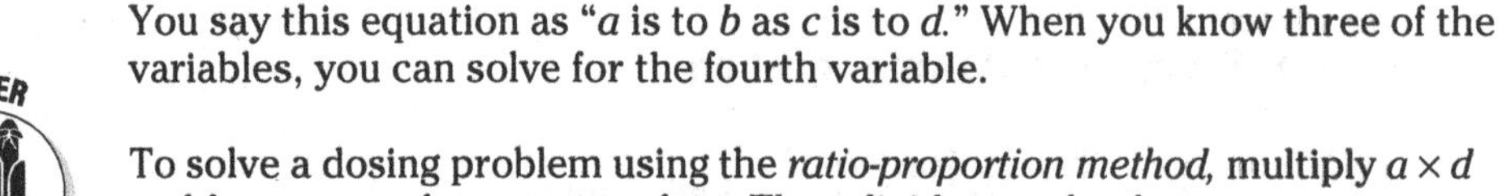

To solve a dosing problem using the *ratio-proportion method,* multiply $a \times d$ and $b \times c$ to get the cross-product. Then divide to solve for x.

Note: A *ratio* is commonly understood to be the relationship between two quantities, and it doesn't change. For example, a med that has 100 mg/mL contains that much medicine in that much volume, no matter how much or little of it you dispense.

Some proportions are obvious. For example, if there are 8 slices in 1 pie, how many slices are in 2 pies? This one's easy (as pie). There are 16 slices in 2 pies.

Here's the structure for solving a ratio-proportion dosing problem, using the pie example:

$$\frac{\text{known equivalent}}{\text{known equivalent}} = \frac{\text{known equivalent}}{\text{desired equivalent}}$$

$$\frac{1 \text{ pie}}{8 \text{ slices}} = \frac{2 \text{ pie}}{x \text{ slices}}$$

$$x = 2 \times 8$$

$$x = 16$$

The answer is 16 slices.

You can also flip the right side upside down, like so:

$$\frac{\text{known equivalent}}{\text{known equivalent}} = \frac{\text{desired equivalent}}{\text{known equivalent}}$$

$$\frac{8 \text{ slices}}{1 \text{ pie}} = \frac{x \text{ slices}}{2 \text{ pie}}$$

$$2 \times 8 = x$$

$$16 = x$$

The answer is 16 slices.

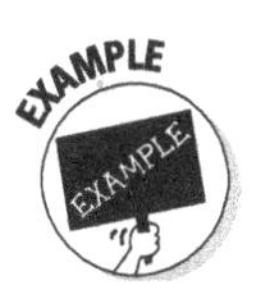

You're ordered to infuse magnesium sulfate 2 g. You have a solution of 40 g in 1 L (1,000 mL). What volume will deliver 2 g?

To solve this problem, use the ratio-proportion method and follow these steps:

1. **Set up the following proportion:**

$$\frac{\text{known equivalent}}{\text{known equivalent}} = \frac{\text{known equivalent}}{\text{desired equivalent}}$$

$$\frac{40 \text{ g}}{1{,}000 \text{ mL}} = \frac{2 \text{ g}}{x \text{ mL}}$$

2. **Cross-multiply and solve.**

$$40x = 2{,}000$$

$$x = 50$$

The answer is 50 mL.

Dosing with the Dimensional Analysis Method

Dimensional analysis is a calculation method that puts all the elements in a dosing calculation together into a single equation. The elements can include conversion factors as well as med-specific ratios. The structure is

$$\text{Dose} = \frac{\text{factor}}{\text{factor}} \times \frac{\text{factor}}{\text{factor}} \times \frac{\text{factor}}{\text{factor}} \times \frac{\text{factor}}{\text{factor}} \times \frac{\text{factor}}{\text{factor}} \times \frac{\text{factor}}{\text{factor}} \times \frac{\text{factor}}{\text{factor}}$$

For example, to calculate the number of seconds in a day, set up the related ratios, as follows:

$$x \text{ sec/day} = \frac{60 \text{ sec}}{1 \cancel{\text{min}}} \times \frac{60 \cancel{\text{min}}}{1 \cancel{\text{hr}}} \times \frac{24 \cancel{\text{hr}}}{1 \text{ day}}$$

$$x \text{ sec/day} = \frac{60 \times 60 \times 24 \text{ sec}}{1 \text{ day}}$$

$$x \text{ sec/day} = \frac{86,400}{1}$$

$$x \text{ sec/day} = 86,400$$

When you multiply, the min and hr units cancel out, leaving only the sec and day units. The answer is 86,400 sec/day.

You're administering a med in syrup form at a dose of 600 mg every 12 hr. It comes in a strength of 100 mg/5 mL. What's the equivalent dose in tablespoons (Tbsp) per day?

To solve this problem, you need to know a few basic conversion factors (see Chapter 4 for details). With those factors in hand, you can use dimensional analysis by following these steps:

1. **Set up the following equation:**

$$\text{Dose} = \frac{\text{factor}}{\text{factor}} \times \frac{\text{factor}}{\text{factor}} \times \frac{\text{factor}}{\text{factor}} \times \frac{\text{factor}}{\text{factor}}$$

$$x \text{ Tbsp/day} = \frac{600 \cancel{\text{mg}}}{12 \cancel{\text{hr}}} \times \frac{24 \cancel{\text{hr}}}{1 \text{ day}} \times \frac{5 \cancel{\text{mL}}}{100 \cancel{\text{mg}}} \times \frac{1 \text{ Tbsp}}{15 \cancel{\text{mL}}}$$

2. **Multiply and solve.**

$$x \text{ Tbsp/day} = \frac{600 \times 24 \times 5 \times 1}{12 \times 1 \times 100 \times 15}$$

$$x \text{ Tbsp/day} = \frac{72,000}{18,000}$$

$$x \text{ Tbsp/day} = 4$$

The various units cancel out, leaving Tbsp and day. The answer is 4 Tbsp/day.

Real-Life Practice: Using Various Methods for Common Dosage Calculations

Most of the following examples demonstrate how to solve the same problem by using the three different calculation methods we cover earlier in this chapter.

For some problems, one or more of the methods may not be appropriate, as they may be too complicated a way to get the desired result. We always recommend using the simplest method as your first approach to doing a dosing calculation.

Determining total flushes

During your shift, you gave a patient 0.75 L, 300 mL, and 500 mL flushes. What is the total amount you gave, in L?

To solve this simple problem, just use a conversion factor so all your units are the same and then do some basic addition. Follow these steps:

1. **Use the conversion factor 1 L = 1,000 mL to convert mL to L.**

   L = mL ÷ 1,000

   L = 300 mL ÷ 1,000 = 0.3 L

   L = 500 mL ÷ 1,000 = 0.5 L

2. **Add the three flush volumes together.**

   x = 0.75 L + 0.3 L + 0.5 L

   x = 1.55 L

   You gave the patient a total of 1.55 L of flushes on your shift.

Figuring out how many amoxicillin tablets to administer

You're asked to administer 2 grams (2,000 mg) of amoxicillin times 1 dose to a patient before a dental procedure. The only amoxicillin you have available is in 250 mg tablets. How many tablets do you need to give?

To solve this problem, you can use any of the three calculation methods we cover earlier in this chapter. However, the formula method is the simplest and fastest method. The ratio-proportion method is almost as simple. (***Note:*** Tablet dosing isn't a very good use of the dimensional analysis method, but we show you how to use it here anyway.)

Formula method:

1. **Set up the following equation:**

$$D \text{ tablet} = \frac{2{,}000 \text{ mg (ordered)}}{250 \text{ mg (have)}} \times 1 \text{ tablet (quantity)}$$

2. **Divide and solve.**

$$D = \frac{2{,}000 \cancel{\text{mg}}}{250 \cancel{\text{mg}}} \times \text{tablet}$$

$$D = \frac{2{,}000}{250} \text{tablet}$$

$$D = 8 \text{ tablet}$$

Give 8 tablets (250 mg each) to make up a dose of 2,000 mg.

Ratio-proportion method:

1. **Set up the following proportion:**

$$\frac{250 \text{ mg}}{1 \text{ tablet}} = \frac{2{,}000 \text{ mg}}{x \text{ tablet}}$$

2. **Cross-multiply and solve.**

$250x = 2{,}000$

$x = 8$

The answer is 8 tablets.

Dimensional analysis method:

1. **Set up the following equation:**

$$x \text{ tablet/dose} = \frac{1 \text{ tablet}}{250 \cancel{\text{mg}}} \times \frac{2{,}000 \cancel{\text{mg}}}{1 \text{ dose}}$$

2. **Divide and solve.**

$$x \text{ tablet/dose} = \frac{2{,}000}{250}$$

$$x \text{ tablet/dose} = 8$$

The mg cancel out. The answer is 8 tablets for 1 dose.

Giving a potassium chloride piggyback

A patient needs potassium chloride (KCl) 25 mEq IV piggyback (meaning you need to stop the main infusion while you introduce the KCl). The potassium chloride is labeled 10 mL = 40 mEq. How many mL should you put in the line?

Use any one of the three calculation methods we discuss earlier in the chapter to solve this problem. Ratio-proportion provides the clearest picture of the calculation.

Formula method:

1. **Set up the following equation:**

$$D\text{ mL} = \frac{25\text{ mEq (ordered)}}{40\text{ mEq (have)}} \times 10\text{ mL (quantity)}$$

2. **Multiply and solve.**

$$D\text{ mL} = \frac{25\ \cancel{\text{mEq}}}{40\ \cancel{\text{mEq}}} \times 10\text{ mL}$$

$$D\text{ mL} = 6.25\text{ mL}$$

The answer is 6.25 mL.

Ratio-proportion method:

1. **Set up the following proportion:**

$$\frac{40\text{ mEq}}{10\text{ mL}} = \frac{25\text{ mEq}}{x\text{ mL}}$$

2. **Cross-multiply and solve.**

$40x = 250$

$x = 6.25$

The answer is 6.25 mL.

Dimensional analysis method:

1. **Set up the following equation:**

$$x\text{ mL/dose} = \frac{25\ \cancel{\text{mEq}}}{1\text{ dose}} \times \frac{10\text{ mL}}{40\ \cancel{\text{mEq}}}$$

2. **Divide and solve.**

$$x \text{ mL/dose} = \frac{250}{40}$$

$$x \text{ mL/dose} = 6.25$$

The mEq cancel out. The answer is 6.25 mL.

Figuring the dose and total volume of an antibiotic

A doctor's order reads to administer the antibiotic cefpodoxime (Vantin) 200 mg PO q12h (orally, every 12 hours) for 5 five days. It's available as an oral suspension at 50 mg/5 mL. How many mL do you give for each dose? What's the total volume to be administered over 5 days?

This problem has two parts. To find out how many mL you give per dose, you can use any of the three calculation methods we cover in this chapter. To determine the total volume to be administered over 5 days, though, the best method to use is dimensional analysis, as you see at the end of this section.

Formula method:

1. **Set up the following equation:**

$$D \text{ mL} = \frac{200 \text{ mg (ordered)}}{50 \text{ mg (have)}} \times 5 \text{ mL (quantity)}$$

2. **Multiply and solve.**

$$D \text{ mL} = \frac{200 \cancel{\text{mg}}}{50 \cancel{\text{mg}}} \times 5 \text{ mL}$$

$$D \text{ mL} = 20 \text{ mL}$$

The answer is 20 mL/dose.

Ratio-proportion method:

1. **Set up the following proportion:**

$$\frac{50 \text{ mg}}{5 \text{ mL}} = \frac{200 \text{ mg}}{x \text{ mL}}$$

2. **Cross-multiply and solve.**

$$50x = 1{,}000$$

$$x = 20$$

The answer is 20 mL/dose.

Dimensional analysis method:

1. **Set up the following equation:**

$$x \text{ mL/dose} = \frac{200 \cancel{\text{mg}}}{1 \text{ dose}} \times \frac{5 \text{ mL}}{50 \cancel{\text{mg}}}$$

2. **Multiply and solve.**

$$x \text{ mL/dose} = \frac{1{,}000}{50}$$

$$x \text{ mL/dose} = 20$$

The mg cancel out. The answer is 20 mL/dose.

Finding total volume with the dimensional analysis method:

1. **Using the volume/dose (20 mL) that you calculated in the previous sections, set up the following equation:**

$$x = \frac{20 \text{ mL}}{1 \cancel{\text{dose}}} \times \frac{1 \cancel{\text{dose}}}{12 \cancel{\text{hr}}} \times \frac{24 \cancel{\text{hr}}}{1 \cancel{\text{day}}} \times \frac{5 \cancel{\text{day}}}{1}$$

2. **Multiply and solve.**

$$x = \frac{20 \times 1 \times 24 \times 5}{1 \times 12 \times 1 \times 1}$$

$$x = \frac{2{,}400}{12}$$

$$x = 200$$

All the units except mL cancel out. You give a total of 200 mL over 5 days.

Administering furosemide in mL

You're asked to administer furosemide (Lasix) 40 mg IV to a patient in congestive heart failure. The furosemide is available in a concentration of 10 mg/mL. How many mL do you administer?

To solve this problem, use any one of the three calculation methods we cover in this chapter. They are equally good and equally fast.

Formula method:

1. **Set up the following equation:**

$$D\text{ mL} = \frac{40\text{ mg (ordered)}}{10\text{ mg (have)}} \times 1\text{ mL}$$

2. **Multiply and solve.**

$$D\text{ mL} = \frac{40\,\cancel{\text{mg}}\text{ (ordered)}}{10\,\cancel{\text{mg}}\text{ (have)}} \times 1\text{ mL}$$

$$D\text{ mL} = 4\text{ mL}$$

The answer is 4 mL.

Ratio-proportion method:

1. **Set up the following proportion:**

$$\frac{10\text{ mg}}{1\text{ mL}} = \frac{40\text{ mg}}{x\text{ mL}}$$

2. **Cross-multiply and solve.**

$$10x = 40$$

$$x = 4$$

The answer is 4 mL.

Dimensional analysis method:

1. **Set up the following equation:**

$$x\text{ mL/dose} = \frac{40\,\cancel{\text{mg}}}{1\text{ dose}} \times \frac{1\text{ mL}}{10\,\cancel{\text{mg}}}$$

2. **Divide and solve.**

$$x \text{ mL/dose} = \frac{40}{10}$$

$$x \text{ mL/dose} = 4$$

The mg cancel out. The answer is 4 mL.

Figuring the dosage of phenobarbital

You must administer phenobarbital gr ii (2 gr) PO to a child. The label on the vial reads 160 mg/5 mL. How many mL of phenobarbital do you give?

You can use any one of the three calculation methods we cover in this chapter to solve this problem. But if you use either the formula method or the ratio-proportion method, be aware that you must set up two separate equations: one to convert gr to mg and one to determine the required mL. Regardless of which method you use, you have to look up the conversion factor for going from gr to mg (1 gr = 64.79891 mg, which you can round up to 1 gr = 65 mg).

Formula method:

1. **Use the conversion factor 1 gr = 65 mg to convert from gr to mg.**

$$\text{mg} = \text{gr} \times 65$$
$$x = 2 \times 65$$
$$x = 130$$

The answer is 130 mg. The order for 2 gr means giving 130 mg of phenobarbital.

2. **Set up the following equation to determine the required mL:**

$$D \text{ mL} = \frac{130 \text{ mg (ordered)}}{160 \text{ mg (have)}} \times 5 \text{ mL (quantity)}$$

3. **Multiply and solve.**

$$D \text{ mL} = \frac{130 \cancel{\text{mg}}}{160 \cancel{\text{mg}}} \times 5 \text{ mL}$$

$$D \text{ mL} = 4.06 \text{ mL}$$

The answer 4.06 mL, which you can round down to 4 mL.

Ratio-proportion method:

1. **Set up the following proportion to convert from gr to mg:**

   $$\frac{1\text{ gr}}{65\text{ mg}} = \frac{2\text{ gr}}{x\text{ mg}}$$

2. **Cross-multiply and solve.**

   $$x = 2 \times 65$$
   $$x = 130$$

3. **Set up the following proportion to convert from mg to mL:**

   $$\frac{160\text{ mg}}{5\text{ mL}} = \frac{130\text{ mg}}{x\text{ mL}}$$

4. **Cross-multiply and solve.**

   $$160x = 5 \times 130$$
   $$x = 4.06$$

   The answer is 4.06 mL, which you can round down to 4 mL.

Dimensional analysis method:

1. **Set up the following equation:**

   $$x\text{ mL/dose} = \frac{2\text{ }\cancel{\text{gr}}}{1\text{ dose}} \times \frac{65\text{ }\cancel{\text{mg}}}{1\text{ }\cancel{\text{gr}}} \times \frac{5\text{ mL}}{160\text{ }\cancel{\text{mg}}}$$

2. **Multiply and solve.**

   $$x\text{ mL/dose} = \frac{650}{160}$$

   $$x\text{ mL/dose} = 4.06$$

   The mg and gr cancel out, leaving mL/dose. The answer is 4.06 mL, which you can round down to 4 mL.

Part III

Calculations for Different Routes of Administration

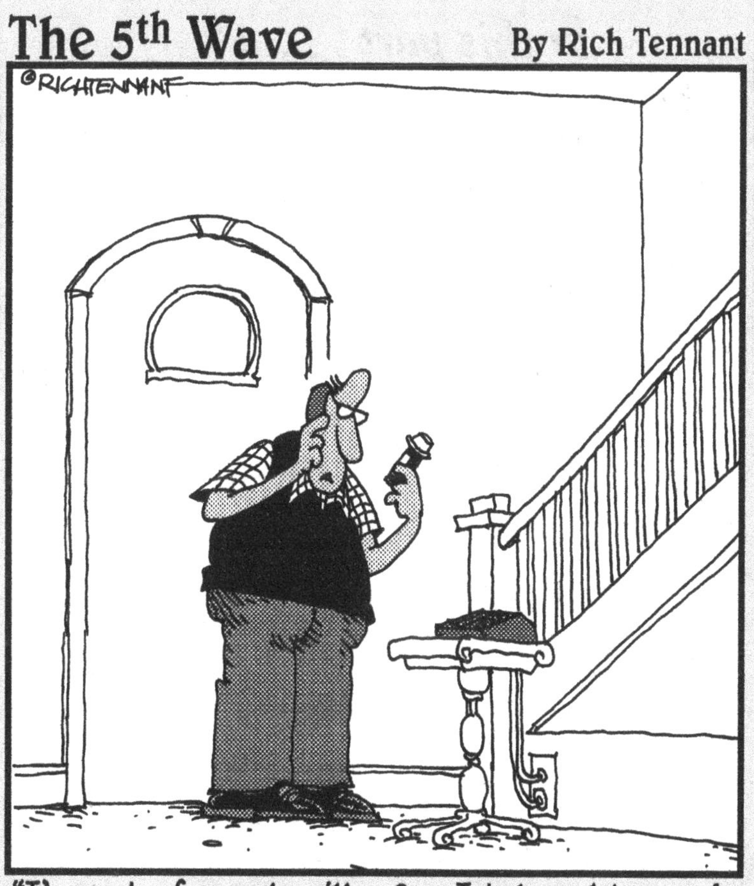

"I'm out of purple pills. Can I take 1 blue and 1 red instead?"

In this part . . .

Part III shows you how to do dosing calculations for the different routes of administration. Chapter 9 covers calculations for oral dosing (tablets, capsules, and liquids). Chapter 10 makes dosing for parenteral administration (injections) easy. Take a look at how to do intravenous dosing in Chapter 11 and how to reconstitute meds in Chapter 12. The math is pretty simple after you practice it.

Chapter 9

Oral Calculations: Tablets, Capsules, and Liquids

In This Chapter

- Reading oral medication labels carefully
- Working through dosing calculations for tablets, capsules, and liquids
- Converting from one drug form to another
- Being extra cautious when administering meds through a feeding tube
- Putting your oral calculation skills to the test with some practice problems

As a healthcare professional, you'll encounter many ways to administer a medication. But the all-time most popular route of administration is oral (via tablets, capsules, and liquids) because it's the most convenient, effective, and economical way to dose a patient.

In this chapter, we show you how to calculate and administer oral meds. We start by taking a quick look at the drug label. Then we introduce you to the fundamentals of dosing — the key is to avoid errors — and show you how to do dosing calculations. Because flexibility is an important part of dosing calculations, we also show you how to go from one medication form to another (oral to intravenous, for example) and give you tips about how to administer through a feeding tube. Finally, we offer a couple of practice problems to get you rolling with real-life oral calculations.

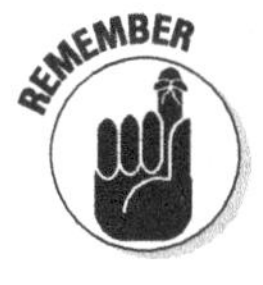

When you calculate or dose medications, patient care and patient safety come first. The first part of safety lies in understanding the medication label. If you don't read the label and check it thrice, then you're being naughty rather than nice. The second part of safety is in calculating accurately and rechecking your work. (See Chapter 6 for a ton more details about medication labels and patient safety.)

Checking Out the Label

Have you ever looked over a man or woman at a party, in speed dating, or at a church social? If you have, then you know what "checking out" someone means. You pay attention to every nuance, every detail — the way a person walks, acts, and talks. Nothing of importance escapes you. But just the same, what you see isn't always what you get.

Fortunately, medical labels aren't like people; what you see *is* what you get. (If people had labels like meds do, dating would be a lot easier.)

When you're dosing oral meds, you must check the label carefully. Because you're in a position of assigned responsibility for any medication errors, you must pay attention to every detail, including the following. (To see a lot more about labels, take a trip to Chapter 6.)

- **Name:** The name identifies the medication, of course. You may see the brand name or the generic name. A great label has both names on it to eliminate any confusion. For example, the med clonazepam is called Klonopin in the United States, as shown in Figure 9-1, but it's also called Ravotril in Chile and Rivotril or Rivatril in other places.

  Two entirely different medications can have two very similar names. For example, Cerebyx and Celebrex look similar, but they are by no means the same. Celebrex is used to treat arthritis, pain, and colon/rectal polyps, while Cerebyx is an epileptic seizure treatment.

- **Dosage strength:** The label shows the strength of the med, which is important because the wrong strength won't be effective (and may not be safe) for the patient. For example, the ACE inhibitor quinapril (Accupril) comes in 5 mg, 10 mg, 20 mg, and 40 mg tablets.
- **Dosage units:** Expect to see the dosing units expressed as mg for tablets, mg/mL or mEq/mL for liquids, and units for penicillin. (Turn to Chapter 4 for details on units of measurement and their abbreviations.)
- **Description:** The label for tablets and capsules includes a description of what the drug looks like. For example, the label for Darvocet-N 100 includes this description: "Film-coated orange oblong tablet. Front: 5112V." Such descriptions can be invaluable in identifying and verifying medications.
- **Warnings:** Expect to see warnings about possible side effects and other important considerations the patient needs to know. Both retail and hospital pharmacies use warnings when the patient will be self-dispensing the med. The warnings are usually printed in bold letters. Examples include "MAY CAUSE DIZZINESS" and "DO NOT DRINK ALCOHOLIC BEVERAGES." (Of course, you won't see warnings if you're using an ADC — an automated dispensing cabinet. The warnings are available on package inserts and in drug references).

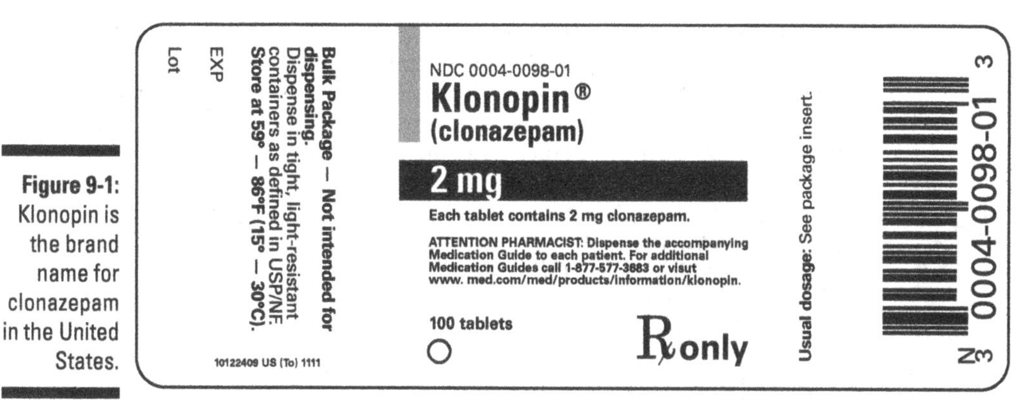

Figure 9-1: Klonopin is the brand name for clonazepam in the United States.

Reprinted with permission from Roche Pharmaceuticals

Examining and Dosing Tablets

A tablet is a pressed form of medication, and it's usually taken orally. Tablets have both active ingredients and *excipients,* which are the inactive ingredients, like binders and disintegrating agents.

Almost all tablets are round, oval, or capsule-shaped, and many of them have coatings that help the patient swallow them. Tablets come in different colors, which help you identify them. Tablets almost always have clear, easy-to-read letters printed on them to make identifying them even easier.

The best thing about tablets is that you administer an accurate dosage every time because the medications the doctor prescribes usually come in the exact dosages ordered. However, sometimes you may need to administer multiple tablets to achieve the correct dosage as ordered by the doctor. Read on to find out more about dosing and administering tablets.

Everybody calls tablets *pills,* but that term is technically incorrect. The word *pill* comes from the Bad Old Days, when an apothecary mixed the ingredients in a mortar, added an excipient like glucose syrup, and rolled the stuff into little balls using his fingers or maybe a new-fangled pill-rolling machine. Today's "pills" are no longer rolled by hand, so the correct term for them is *tablets.*

Splitting scored tablets

If you see a groove down the tablet's center (the *score line*), you're allowed to break it in half. The score line indicates the exact center of the tablet.

If, on the other hand, the doctor's order says to administer half a tablet to a patient but the tablet isn't scored, don't halve it. Call the doctor or pharmacist to find out if there's an acceptable substitute, such as a lower-dosage tablet, a tablet scored to provide the correct dosage when split, a capsule, a liquid, or maybe another medication entirely.

Sometimes those nasty little buggers are hard to split in two. If you have a hard time splitting the tablet using a sharp knife and a cutting board, use the recommended method — a *pill splitter.* A pill splitter is a handy-dandy device that lets you split a tab in two with ease. Figure 9-2 shows a pill splitter.

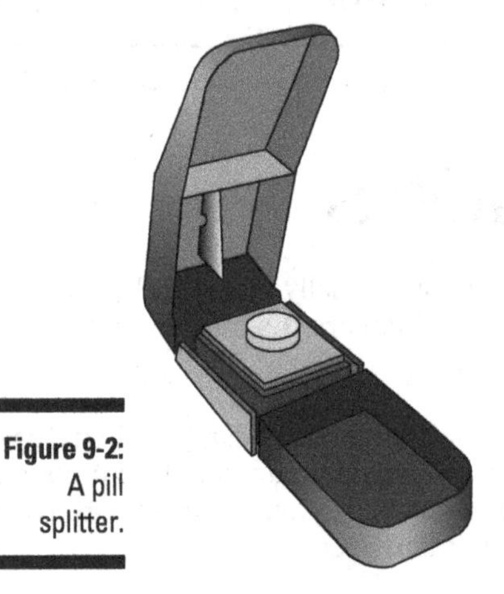

Figure 9-2: A pill splitter.

Needing to crush — The tablet, not the person

To crush or not to crush? That is the question. Generally, it's not a good idea to crush tablets because crushing may change the way the body absorbs the med.

The ideal alternative to crushing is using a liquid form of the medication. But if the patient has a feeding tube and a liquid form of the prescribed medication isn't available, you must consult with the doctor to find out whether you can crush the tablet. When administering a crushed tablet through a feeding tube, you must mix the med very well with about 15 mL of water.

When a patient must take a tablet PO (orally by mouth) but has trouble swallowing, the doctor may permit you to mix a crushed tablet with applesauce, pudding, or yogurt. To crush tablets, you can use a *pill crusher,* which is just a handheld device that allows you to crush tablets easily. Pill crushers are available in both institutional and retail versions.

On the other hand, some meds, like nitroglycerin, go directly under the patient's tongue when he has an angina (chest pain) episode, so you don't need to crush these meds before administering them. Other tablets have a chewable form, so you don't need to crush them either.

Giving timed-release tablets

Some meds have a timed-release feature. A *timed-release medication* delivers the dose gradually instead of releasing (or dumping) the active ingredient all at once. One example is diltiazem ER (Cardizem CD, Dilacor XR, and Taztia XT), which is a calcium channel blocker used to treat high blood pressure and some abnormal rhythms of the heart (also referred to as *arrhythmias*). Nifedipine (Procardia XL) is another calcium channel blocker; it's used to treat hypertension.

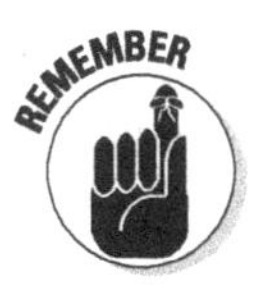

You know you're working with a timed-release med because the label says so. Don't try to split such tablets in half. They aren't scored, and with good reason; they work effectively only as whole tablets. Don't crush them, either.

Protecting the tummy with coated tablets

Many people suffer from stomach problems, such as *gastritis* (inflammation of the stomach lining), peptic ulcer disease (PUD), and *dyspepsia* (a kind of symptom complex consisting of nausea and an upset stomach). For that matter, many people find that common aspirin upsets their stomachs. To avoid causing stomach problems, the doctor may prescribe enteric-coated medications.

An *enteric coating* is a coating that causes a tablet to dissolve in the small intestine rather than the stomach, thus, eliminating any painful stomach side effects.

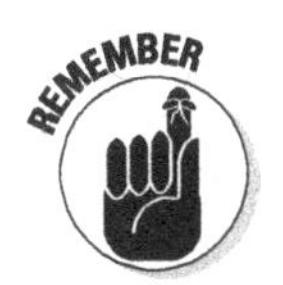

Don't crush an enteric-coated tablet, or you'll defeat its purpose.

Dosing tablets

Tablets are the most widely used form of oral medication. Tablets are effective because of their reliable medicine content, durability, and convenience. Tablets are useful both in a hospital setting and in the patient's home. This section shows you how to dose them.

Basic milligram (mg) calculations

The vast majority of tablets have specified mg dosages (for example, 1 mg, 5 mg, 100 mg, and 500 mg). A few drugs are specified in grains (see the next section). Lastly, a very small number of drugs are specified in units (for example, alpha-tocopherol, commonly known as vitamin E). This section deals with tablets specified in mg.

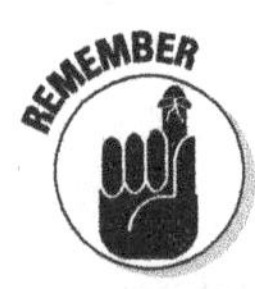

You can use more than one calculation method (ratio-proportion, formula, or dimensional analysis) to do tablet calculations. But as the following examples show, one method is usually better suited for solving a particular problem. See Chapter 8 for more about these calculation methods.

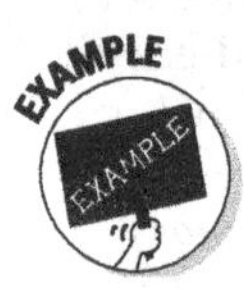

You must administer 750 mg of ciprofloxacin every 12 hours (two times a day) for 7 days. The medication is available only in 250 mg doses. First, how many tablets do you need to give in each dose? Second, how many total tablets do you need?

To solve this problem, use the ratio-proportion method and the dimensional analysis method. Follow these steps:

1. **Set up the following ratio-proportion equation to find out how many tablets you must give each day:**

   $$\frac{\text{known equivalent}}{\text{known equivalent}} = \frac{\text{known equivalent}}{\text{desired equivalent}}$$

   $$\frac{250 \text{ mg}}{1 \text{ tab}} = \frac{750 \text{ mg}}{x \text{ tab}}$$

2. **Cross-multiply and solve.**

   $250x = 750$

   $x = 3$

   You must give the patient 3 tablets per dose.

3. **Set up the following dimensional analysis equation to determine how many total tablets you need.**

   The dimensional analysis method has the advantage of presenting all the terms in one equation.

   $$\text{desired units} = \frac{\text{unit factor}}{\text{unit factor}} \times \frac{\text{unit factor}}{\text{unit factor}} \times \frac{\text{unit factor}}{\text{unit factor}}$$

   $$x \text{ tabs/week} = \frac{3 \text{ tabs}}{1 \text{ dose}} \times \frac{2 \text{ doses}}{1 \text{ day}} \times \frac{7 \text{ days}}{1 \text{ week}}$$

4. **Multiply and solve.**

$$x \text{ tabs/week} = \frac{3 \times 2 \times 7}{1 \times 1 \times 1}$$

$$x \text{ tabs/week} = 3 \times 2 \times 7$$

$$x \text{ tabs/week} = 42$$

The units cancel out. The patient needs 42 tablets total.

You have to give a total of 2.4 g of ibuprofen (Motrin) daily to a patient with bad arthritis. The tablet strength is 200 mg. How many tabs should you give each day?

Use dimensional analysis to find out. Dimensional analysis has the advantage of presenting all the terms clearly in a single equation:

1. **Set up the following equation:**

$$x \text{ tabs/day} = \frac{1 \text{ tab}}{200 \text{ mg}} \times \frac{1{,}000 \text{ mg}}{1 \text{ g}} \times \frac{2.4 \text{ g}}{1 \text{ day}}$$

2. **Multiply and solve.**

$$x \text{ tabs/day} = \frac{1 \times 1{,}000 \times 2.4}{200 \times 1 \times 1}$$

$$x \text{ tabs/day} = \frac{2{,}400}{200}$$

$$x \text{ tabs/day} = 12$$

The units cancel out. The patient needs 12 tablets daily.

You're asked to give labetalol 150 mg twice a day to treat high blood pressure. The medication is dosed at 300 mg. How would you administer this medication?

Use the formula method to find out, as it's the simplest method of calculation:

1. **Set up the following equation:**

$$x \text{ (amount)} = \frac{d \text{ (desired)}}{h \text{ (have)}}$$

$$x = \frac{150 \cancel{\text{mg}}}{300 \cancel{\text{mg}}}$$

2. **Divide and solve.**

$$x = \frac{150}{300}$$

$$x = \frac{1}{2}$$

You administer ½ tablet of labetalol twice a day.

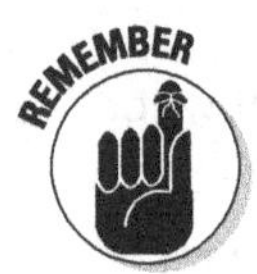

Be sure to check the medication to see whether it's scored. Lucky for you, it is, so you can split each tablet in two to get the correct dose. (Yay! Score one for your side!)

Going against the grain

The *grain* is the basic unit of the traditional English *apothecaries' system* of weights (the outdated system that uses scruples, drams, and ounces as its units).

Weight by grain can be a pain — a pain in the butt to calculate, that is. Fortunately for everyone, the grain isn't used very often in the medical field today. However, it's still a measurement you need to be familiar with. (Take it with a grain of salt, and head out to Chapter 4 for more on systems of measurement.) As far as dosing calculations go, here's what you need to know:

7,000 grains = 1 avoirdupois pound

15,432.3584 grains = 1 kilogram

15.4323584 grains = 1 gram

1 grain = 65 milligrams

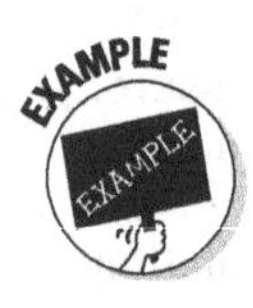

You must give thyroid tablets at a dose of 1¼ gr daily. How do you dose this in mg?

Follow these steps to find out:

1. **Convert the fractional dosage into a mixed decimal fraction.**

$$1\frac{1}{4} = 1 + \frac{1}{4} = 1 + 0.25 = 1.25$$

2. **Use dimensional analysis to set up the following equation to convert grains to mg:**

$$x \text{ mg/day} = \frac{1 \cancel{g}}{15.4 \cancel{gr}} \times \frac{1{,}000 \text{ mg}}{1 \cancel{g}} \times \frac{1.25 \cancel{gr}}{1 \text{ day}}$$

3. **Multiply and solve.**

$$x \text{ mg/day} = \frac{1 \times 1{,}000 \times 1.25}{15.4 \times 1 \times 1}$$

$$x \text{ mg/day} = \frac{1{,}250}{15.4}$$

$$x \text{ mg/day} = 81 \text{ mg/day}$$

The units cancel out. The patient needs 81 mg daily.

Be doubly cautious as you work through this problem. First, don't confuse the abbreviation for grain (gr) with the abbreviation for gram (g). Second, when you convert between different systems of units, recheck your calculations. They can be tricky.

Considering the Colorful Capsule in Medical Dosing

How many different kinds of capsules can you think of? Well, there's a space capsule, which is useful for holding astronauts. There's a time capsule, the kind you put a bunch of stuff in and bury for a hundred years or so. Then there's the medication capsule. Notice the trend here? In every *case,* the capsule is a *case* that holds something.

The following sections take a closer look at the different types of medication capsules and show you how to do dosing calculations for them.

Shelling out for a capsule

In the medical world, a *capsule* is a small case (usually made of gelatin) that contains a dose of medication. The patient swallows it whole. The two types of capsules are

- **Hard shell:** This capsule usually holds powder or little pellets (technically known as *spheroids*).
- **Soft gel:** This capsule usually holds an oil-like substance, such as fish oil or vitamin E.

The shells of both types of capsules are made of gelatin so they can dissolve after ingestion. Like M&Ms, capsule shells won't melt in your hand. But unlike M&Ms, they won't melt in your mouth, either. Capsules dissolve in the patient's GI tract.

Don't try to split a capsule. For it to be effective for the patient, the capsule must remain intact until it reaches the patient's GI tract.

A *spansule* is a capsule that releases one or more drugs over time.

Calculating dosages for capsules

In many ways, the dosage calculations for capsules are similar to those for tablets. The main exception is that capsules aren't scored, so you can't give them in divided doses.

You're instructed to give mycophenolic acid (CellCept) to a patient who has had a recent kidney transplant. She is taking 2 g/day in two divided doses. The only capsules available are 250 mg. How many capsules does the patient need to take each day?

Use dimensional analysis and follow these steps to find out (see Chapter 8 for details on this calculation method). The dimensional analysis method has the advantage of expressing all terms of the calculation in one equation.

Getting the capsule down

Sometimes the patient can't swallow a capsule, so be prepared to change forms, if necessary. Find out if the prescribed drug comes in a liquid form, and ask the doctor if you can use it as a substitute.

But what if the med isn't available as a liquid? With a doctor's order, you can mix the medication into a small amount of applesauce to help the patient swallow it. In this case, a spoonful of sugar doesn't help the medicine go down, but a spoonful of applesauce does! Consider using custard and other puddings for the same purpose.

1. **Set up the following equation:**

$$x \text{ capsule/day} = \frac{1 \text{ capsule}}{250 \cancel{\text{mg}}} \times \frac{1{,}000 \cancel{\text{mg}}}{1 \cancel{\text{g}}} \times \frac{2 \cancel{\text{g}}}{1 \text{ day}}$$

2. **Multiply and solve.**

$$x \text{ capsule/day} = \frac{1 \times 1{,}000 \times 2}{250 \times 1 \times 1}$$

$$x \text{ capsule/day} = \frac{2{,}000}{250}$$

$$x \text{ capsule/day} = 8$$

The units cancel out. The patient needs a total of 8 capsules/day in two doses of 4 capsules.

Looking at Liquids and Knowing How to Dose Them

Meds in liquid form have several advantages over their solid counterparts (tablets and capsules). For example, they eliminate pill-swallowing problems, and they're easy to introduce through a feeding tube.

Keep reading to find out about the different types of liquid meds doctors can prescribe as well as the steps you need to take to do liquid dosing calculations.

Surveying the different types of liquids

The term *liquid* is very generic and doesn't tell you much about what kind of med you're dealing with, other than the fact that it's not solid, of course. The two most common types of liquids that docs and other medical professionals use for liquid med formulations are

- **Suspension:** A *liquid suspension* is a formulation in which the drug is in the solution but not completely dissolved in it.

  When you administer any medication in a liquid suspension, you need to shake it up to make sure you get just the right amount of medication with each dose. So treat your suspensions as you would martinis, and shake (or stir) them up!

- **Elixir:** An *elixir* is a solution that serves as a medium for a medication to be ingested and absorbed. The medicine is completely dissolved in it. Elixirs are very popular with infants and young children.

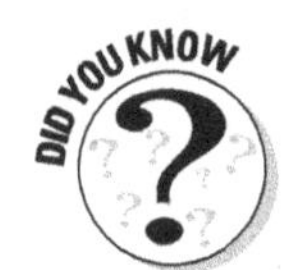

The *elixir of life* is also called the *elixir of immortality*. If you drink it, you'll live forever. Many people in many cultures have tried to create it, but so far, nobody (as far as we know) has succeeded. If you'd like a natural alternative, search for the Fountain of Youth.

The following liquid-associated terms are less common but prevalent enough that you need to be familiar with them:

- **Solution:** Broadly speaking, most liquid meds are solutions. In a *solution*, a medication (called the *solute*) is dissolved in a liquid (called the *solvent*). Even normal saline (0.9% NS) is a solution. An elixir is a solution, too, but a suspension isn't.
- **Emulsion:** An *emulsion* contains two or more unblendable liquids, and you need to shake any emulsion before using it. This term is more common with meds you apply topically.
- **Syrup:** A *syrup* is a medication dissolved in a sugar and water mixture.
- **Tincture:** A *tincture* is an extract of plant material in alcohol. You may see the word in the world of flower essences and other alternate therapies.

Dosing liquid meds

In medical dosage calculations for liquid formulations, you typically calculate the strength of a medication per mL of solution and then figure out how many mL to administer. As part of your calculations, you may need to convert between different measurement systems (for example, from the apothecaries' system to metric or from metric to the U.S. customary system; see Chapter 4 for more details).

Note: Professionally, you work mostly with the metric system. But at home, everybody (including doctors, nurses, and patients) clings to elements of different systems, such as the U.S. customary system, household system, or apothecaries' system. For example, you may have to dose liquid medications in ounces, teaspoons, and tablespoons in addition to milliliters.

You must administer a dose of ciprofloxacin (Cipro) in liquid form because the patient doesn't tolerate the tablet form. You have to give the patient 0.75 g of ciprofloxacin, and it's available in a liquid suspension of 500 mg/5 mL. How many mL do you give for each dose?

In calculations with liquids, the ratio-proportion method and the dimensional analysis method work equally well. The ratio-proportion method allows you to solve a problem one step at a time and shows a clear relationship between terms of the equation. Dimensional analysis lets you see the connection between all the terms you're using in one equation (check out Chapter 8 for details on calculation methods).

To use dimensional analysis to solve this problem, follow these steps:

1. **Set up the following equation:**

$$x \text{ mL} = \frac{5 \text{ mL}}{500 \cancel{\text{mg}}} \times \frac{1{,}000 \cancel{\text{mg}}}{1 \cancel{\text{g}}} \times \frac{0.75 \cancel{\text{g}}}{1}$$

2. **Multiply and solve.**

$$x \text{ mL} = \frac{5 \times 1{,}000 \times 0.75}{500 \times 1 \times 1}$$

$$x \text{ mL} = \frac{3{,}750}{500}$$

$$x \text{ mL} = 7.5$$

The units cancel out. The patient needs a total of 7.5 mL for each dose.

To solve the problem using the ratio-proportion method, follow these steps:

1. **Convert 0.75 g to mg by multiplying by 1,000.**

   $0.75 \text{ g} \times 1{,}000 = 750 \text{ mg}$

   Remember that to go from g to mg, all you have to do is move the decimal point three places to the right. (See Chapter 4 for more details on converting units.)

2. **Set up the following proportion:**

$$\frac{500 \text{ mg}}{5 \text{ mL}} = \frac{750 \text{ mg}}{x \text{ mL}}$$

3. **Cross-multiply and solve.**

   $500x = 3{,}750$

   $x = 7.5$

   You administer 7.5 mL for each dose.

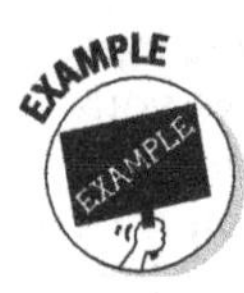

You're instructed to dose sodium citrate (Bicitra) to your patient at a dose of 30 mL PO BID (by mouth, twice a day). If the standard dosing of oral sodium citrate is 500 mg/5 mL of solution, then how many grams are you administering with each dose?

To find out, use the ratio-proportion method and follow these steps:

1. **Set up the following proportion:**

   $$\frac{500 \text{ mg}}{5 \text{ mL}} = \frac{x \text{ mg}}{30 \text{ mL}}$$

2. **Cross-multiply and solve.**

   $5x = 15{,}000$

   $x = 3{,}000$

   The answer is 3,000 mg.

3. **Convert milligrams to grams by dividing by 1,000.**

   $3{,}000 \text{ mg} \div 1{,}000 = 3 \text{ g}$

   The answer is 3 grams. (See Chapter 4 for more details on converting units.)

Nurses say sodium citrate tastes terrible. You can water it down with a better-tasting liquid or simply tell the patient to "knock it back" like a shot of tequila.

A doctor's order tells you to give thiamine to a patient at a dose of 5 mg daily in two divided doses. The elixir form is available in the strength 250 mcg/5 mL. How much thiamine, in mL, should you give the patient?

To find out, use the ratio-proportion method and follow these steps:

1. **Convert micrograms to milligrams by dividing by 1,000.**

   $250 \text{ mcg} \div 1{,}000 = 0.25 \text{ mg}$

   The answer is 0.25 mg, meaning that the elixir's concentration is 0.25 mg/5 mL. (See Chapter 4 for details on converting units.)

2. **Set up the following proportion:**

   $$\frac{0.25 \text{ mg}}{5 \text{ mL}} = \frac{5 \text{ mg}}{x \text{ mL}}$$

3. **Cross-multiply and solve.**

   $0.25x = 25$

   $x = 100$

   The answer is 100 mL. Because you dose two times daily, you must administer 50 mL in each dose.

You have to give cephalexin (Keflex) at 250 mg twice a day. It's available in a suspension form of 100 mg/mL. How many teaspoons is this?

Use a combination of the ratio-proportion method and dimensional analysis to solve this problem. Follow these steps:

1. **Set up the following proportion to calculate how many mL you need:**

   $$\frac{100 \text{ mg}}{1 \text{ mL}} = \frac{250 \text{ mg}}{x \text{ mL}}$$

2. **Cross-multiply and solve.**

   $100x = 250$

   $x = 2.5$

   The answer is 2.5 mL, meaning that each dose of 250 mg cephalexin requires 2.5 mL of solution.

3. **Use dimensional analysis to set up the following equation:**

   $$x \text{ tsp} = \frac{1 \text{ tsp}}{5 \cancel{\text{mL}}} \times \frac{2.5 \cancel{\text{mL}}}{1}$$

   If you're not sure how many mL are in a teaspoon, turn to Chapter 4; there you see that 1 teaspoon is equivalent to 5 mL.

4. **Divide and solve.**

   $$x \text{ tsp} = \frac{1 \times 2.5}{5 \times 1}$$

   $$x \text{ tsp} = \frac{2.5}{5}$$

   $$x \text{ tsp} = 0.5$$

   You give one-half of a teaspoon (0.5 tsp) twice a day.

Converting from One Form of a Med to Another

Be prepared to be flexible as you do your medical dosage calculations. For example, when a person's admitted to the hospital, it's not uncommon for his doctor to change a medication that he's been taking in tablet or capsule form to one in intravenous form. As the patient's condition stabilizes, the doctor may switch the medication back from intravenous to oral. (The doctor may also order medications to be injected while the patient is in the hospital. Check out Chapter 10 for more info on how to calculate dosages for injection.)

The following sections show you how to convert from intravenous to oral dosing and from oral to oral dosing. (For more details on intravenous dosing, turn to Chapter 11.)

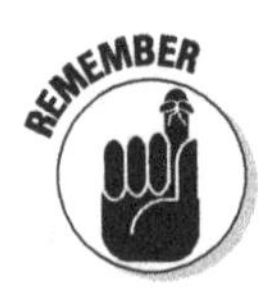

You can use several different resources to figure out the equivalent doses of many medications. The most convenient resources are printed drug reference guides, such as the Physicians' Desk Reference; online references, such as `www.rxlist.com`; and smartphone apps, such as Epocrates. However, if you have any questions at all, call the pharmacist or the prescribing doctor. (***Note:*** We include equivalent doses for the examples in this section to help you get started.)

Going from intravenous to oral (and back again)

For many medications — like the antibiotic levofloxacin (Levaquin), for example — converting between oral and intravenous dosing is one-to-one. But for other commonly prescribed meds, like diuretics and thyroid hormone, the intravenous dose may not match the oral dose. The examples in this section show you how to switch between the two drug forms with ease.

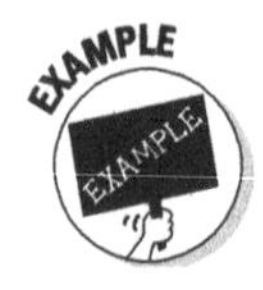

Mr. Smith has been receiving furosemide (Lasix) 40 mg IV BID. If you were to switch him to an equivalent oral (PO) dose, what would it be?

The answer to this problem is easy to calculate because dosing 1 mg of furosemide intravenously is equivalent to dosing 2 mg PO. So the equivalent oral dose of 40 mg IV BID is 80 mg PO BID (40 mg × 2 = 80 mg).

Obviously, the problem works the other way, too. If Mr. Smith had been receiving furosemide 80 mg PO BID and you were to switch him to an equivalent IV dose, what would it be? To solve this problem, all you have to do is work backward: If dosing 2 mg PO is equivalent to dosing 1 mg IV, the equivalent dose of 80 mg PO BID is 40 mg IV BID.

You're instructed to administer levothyroxine (Synthroid) at a dose of 100 mcg PO daily. The condition of your patient has changed, and the doctor has written an order that your patient be NPO (nothing by mouth). The physician's order states to administer levothyroxine at a dose of 50 mcg IV, which is one-half of the prescribed oral dose.

The intravenous form of levothyroxine comes as a 500 mcg vial, and when reconstituted with 5 mL of normal saline, it has a concentration of 100 mcg/mL. How many mL of this solution do you administer? (See Chapter 12 for more information about the reconstitution of solutions.)

Use the ratio-proportion method to find out:

1. **Set up the following proportion:**

   $$\frac{100\text{ mcg}}{1\text{ mL}} = \frac{50\text{ mcg}}{x\text{ mL}}$$

2. **Cross-multiply and solve.**

   $$100x = 50$$

   $$x = 0.5$$

   You administer 0.5 mL intravenously.

Converting between meds with the same purpose

Sometimes you have to convert between two oral meds with the same therapeutic function, particularly if a medication isn't on the hospital formulary. (A *formulary* is the inventory of medicines in a hospital.)

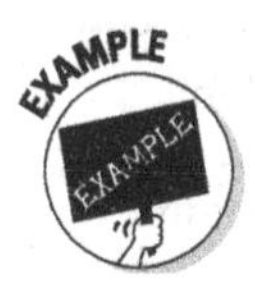

You're asked to give bumetanide (Bumex) 2 mg PO BID. You find out from the patient that he had an adverse drug reaction to bumetanide but has tolerated furosemide (Lasix) well in the past. You call the prescribing physician, and she instructs you to give an equivalent dose of oral furosemide. How many mg do you administer for each dose?

The conversion from bumetanide to furosemide is 1 to 40, meaning that 1 mg of bumetanide is equivalent to 40 mg of furosemide. Use the ratio-proportion method to find out how many mg of furosemide you need to administer. Just follow these steps:

1. **Set up the following proportion:**

   $$\frac{1 \text{ mg bumetanide}}{40 \text{ mg furosemide}} = \frac{2 \text{ mg bumetanide}}{x \text{ mg furosemide}}$$

2. **Cross-multiply and solve.**

   $x = 2 \times 40$

   $x = 80$

   You give 80 mg furosemide PO BID.

Administering to the Patient with a Feeding Tube

You may have to calculate and administer a medication through a feeding tube. Before you even start calculating, though, make sure you do the following:

- **Verify that the prescribed med is safe to administer through a feeding tube.** Don't assume that because you can give a med orally that it's safe to give through a feeding tube. Coated medications and timed-release capsules, for example, don't work well in feeding tubes. Find out if there's a liquid form of the medication that will go down the tube better, and ask the doctor if you can administer it.

  If a liquid formulation isn't available, call the doctor or pharmacist to find out if there's a form of the medication you can crush. Then mix the crushed med with at least 15 mL of water before putting it through the tube.

- **Ask the doctor or pharmacist if the medication you're about to administer interferes with tube feedings.** If it does, the doc may instruct you to stop the tube feeding before you administer the medication and restart it after you're done. Just be sure to flush the feeding tube before and after you give the medication. If you're administering a liquid medication that is very thick, you may need to dilute it with more water (30–60 mL, depending on the medication). You don't want an *occluded* (blocked) feeding tube. If you find that the tube is occluded, call the doctor for further instruction.

If you have any questions about administering a medication through a feeding tube, call the doctor.

A *PEG tube* is a percutaneous endoscopic gastrostomy tube. It goes into a patient's stomach through the abdominal wall as a means of feeding her. The doc places the tube with the help of an endoscope. An *NG* tube (nasogastric feeding tube) is a tube that's passed through the patient's *nares* (nostril).

Real-Life Practice: Doxycycline, the Infection Fighter

You have to give a patient doxycycline 100 mg PO every 12 hours for 21 days. It's available in a liquid suspension at a dose of 25 mg/5 mL. How many mL do you give with each dose, and how many mL do you need for all 21 days?

Use a combination of the ratio-proportion method and dimensional analysis to solve this problem. Ratio-proportion is a compact method of finding the mL/dose, and dimensional analysis is the best way to calculate the total of multi-day doses. Follow these steps:

1. **Use the ratio-proportion method to set up the following proportion:**

   $$\frac{25\text{ mg}}{5\text{ mL}} = \frac{100\text{ mg}}{x\text{ ml}}$$

2. **Cross-multiply and solve.**

   $25x = 500$

   $x = 20$

   You administer 20 mL for each dose of doxycycline.

3. **Use dimensional analysis to set up the following equation:**

$$x \text{ mL} = \frac{20 \text{ mL}}{1 \cancel{\text{dose}}} \times \frac{2 \cancel{\text{dose}}}{1 \cancel{\text{day}}} \times \frac{21 \cancel{\text{day}}}{1}$$

4. **Multiply and solve**

$$x \text{ mL} = \frac{20 \times 2 \times 21}{1 \times 1 \times 1}$$

$$x \text{ mL} = \frac{840}{1}$$

$$x \text{ mL} = 840$$

The day and dose units cancel out. The patient needs a total of 840 mL for the three-week period.

You can use different dosing calculation methods to solve a dosing problem (see Chapter 8 for details on the three main methods). Find which calculation method works best for you, and stick with it (although you should be familiar with all three).

Real-Life Practice: In Need of Potassium

You're instructed to administer metronidazole 750 mg extended release (available as Flagyl ER) via a PEG tube daily. Before you administer or calculate anything, what's wrong with this order?

Here's what's wrong. You realize that you can't give the extended release form of metronidazole through a PEG tube. When you call the pharmacy, you find out there's no liquid formulation of the medication but there is a tablet form. So you do the following:

1. **Speak with the doctor, who reorders the medication at 250 mg every 8 hours.**
2. **Crush the medication and mix the crushed tablet in 15 mL of water.**
3. **Administer the med via the PEG tube.**
4. **Administer the med again 8 hours later and then again 8 hours later.**
5. **Flush the PEG tube with 30 mL of water before and after administering the medication.**

The dosing you do for this example is mathematically simple. The key component to dosing this patient correctly is to notice the problem and get it fixed.

You get a call from the lab 30 minutes later because your patient's potassium is very low! You're instructed to give a potassium solution that comes in an oral form at a dose of 20 mEq/15 mL. The doctor orders you to give 60 mEq via PEG now and then to administer another 30 mEq 4 hours later. How many mL will you administer total for the two doses?

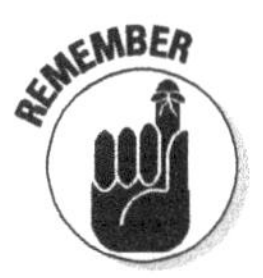

Most oral dosing situations deal with milligrams or grams, but when you're doing oral replacement of electrolytes, particularly potassium, you see milliequivalents (mEq) a lot. Take a look at Chapter 18 for more on feeding and electrolytes.

To find out how many total mL you need to administer, first use the ratio-proportion method to calculate the mL for each dose individually. Then add them together. Follow these steps:

1. **Set up the following proportion for the first dose:**

   $$\frac{20 \text{ mEq}}{15 \text{ mL}} = \frac{60 \text{ mEq}}{x \text{ mL}}$$

2. **Cross-multiply and solve.**

   $20x = 900$

   $x = 45$

   The answer is 45 mL for the first dose of potassium.

3. **Set up the following proportion for the second dose:**

   $$\frac{20 \text{ mEq}}{15 \text{ mL}} = \frac{30 \text{ mEq}}{x \text{ mL}}$$

4. **Cross-multiply and solve.**

   $20x = 450$

   $x = 22.5$

   The answer is 22.5 mL for the second dose of potassium.

5. **Add the two doses together.**

   45 mL + 22.5 mL = 67.5 mL

   The cumulative total dose is 67.5 mL.

Chapter 10

Parenteral Injections and Calculations

In This Chapter

- Getting familiar with the syringe
- Knowing what to look for on medication labels for meds administered parenterally
- Looking at the different parenteral injections and doing basic dosing calculations for them
- Putting your skills to the test with some real-life practice problems

This chapter's all about medications that you administer parenterally (pair-*en*-ter-il-ly). The word *parenteral* comes from the Greek *para,* meaning "beside," and *enteron,* meaning "intestine," so it makes sense that the parenteral route of administration bypasses the intestines. By contrast, *enteral* medications (which you administer orally and which include capsules, tablets, and oral liquids) are absorbed in the body through the stomach and small intestine (see Chapter 9 for details).

Commonly, you administer medications parenterally by injecting them directly into a vein (*intravenous*), a muscle (*intramuscular*), the fatty tissue beneath the skin (*subcutaneous*), or a very superficial layer under the skin (*intradermal).* Less commonly, but still important, you may administer an injection into the abdominal cavity (*intraperitoneal),* the heart (*intracardiac),* or the artery (*intraarterial).*

Doctors prescribe parenterally administered medications when the patient's body needs to absorb the meds faster than oral administration allows. The absorption rate of parenteral injections varies widely, but all the injection methods are faster than their enteral counterparts.

Intravenous administration (through the vein) is such a big topic that we cover it alone in Chapter 11. This chapter focuses on the basics of what you need to know to calculate injections. It also offers plenty of information about syringes, medication labels, and the different types of injections you may have to administer.

Packing a Syringe — It's Essential to be Equipped

To administer a medication parenterally via an injection, you need a syringe. A *syringe* is a simple piston pump made up of a plunger that fits tightly in a tube. This section covers the basics about syringes and shows you how to use them.

Anatomy of a syringe

All syringes have the following five parts:

- **Barrel:** The *barrel* (also called the *tube*) is a cylinder made of plastic, glass, or (less commonly) metal.

  The base of the barrel has a flange, which lets you hold the barrel with two fingers while you press on the plunger with your thumb. (Think of the flange as a ring or a pair of arms running perpendicular to the barrel.)

  A syringe is *calibrated,* meaning that it has numbers and lines that show measurement values — typically mL or insulin units. These numbers and lines appear on the side of the barrel.

- **Plunger:** The *plunger* is a piston that moves inside the barrel. It has a tight-fitting rubber head inside the barrel and a flange for pushing on.
- **Hub:** The *hub* (also called the *needle adapter*) is a plastic or aluminum adapter that fits a needle to the barrel.
- **Needle:** The *needle* is a hollow stainless steel tube. The needle has a bevel to help it pierce the patient's skin. Depending on how deep the injection (or fluid extraction) needs to be, the needle's orifice can be thinner or wider and the needle's length can be shorter or longer. (*Needle stick* is the official term for an accidental piercing wound caused by a needle.)

  The *bevel* refers to the sharp, angled opening at the end of the needle. If you can *see* the bevel, then it's "up." Whether you do an injection with the bevel up or down depends on the type of injection you're doing. The majority of the time (as with subcutaneous injections), you'll likely be instructed to administer an injection with the bevel up.

- **Cap:** The syringe has a protective cap on top of the needle. The cap is there for your safety. To prevent accidental needle sticks, never cap your needle before discarding it. Discard it? Yes! Disposable syringes are common in medical practice.

Who invented the syringe?

The idea of the syringe goes back to the ninth century BCE, but credit for inventing the modern hypodermic syringe belongs to Alexander Wood, a Scots physician, in 1853. However, the Irish disagree, saying that Francis Rynd invented the hollow needle in 1845. Still others give credit to Charles Pravaz, a French surgeon, for inventing the first practical syringe, which used Rynd's needle.

The terms *syringe* and *hypodermic needle* are used interchangeably, but actually the hypodermic needle is just the little stainless steel part at the end. Medical professionals also commonly call syringes *sharps*.

Syringes come with different capacities to handle different injection tasks. Figure 10-1 shows the four most common syringes with capacities of 1 mL, 3 mL, 5 mL, and 100 units (for insulin).

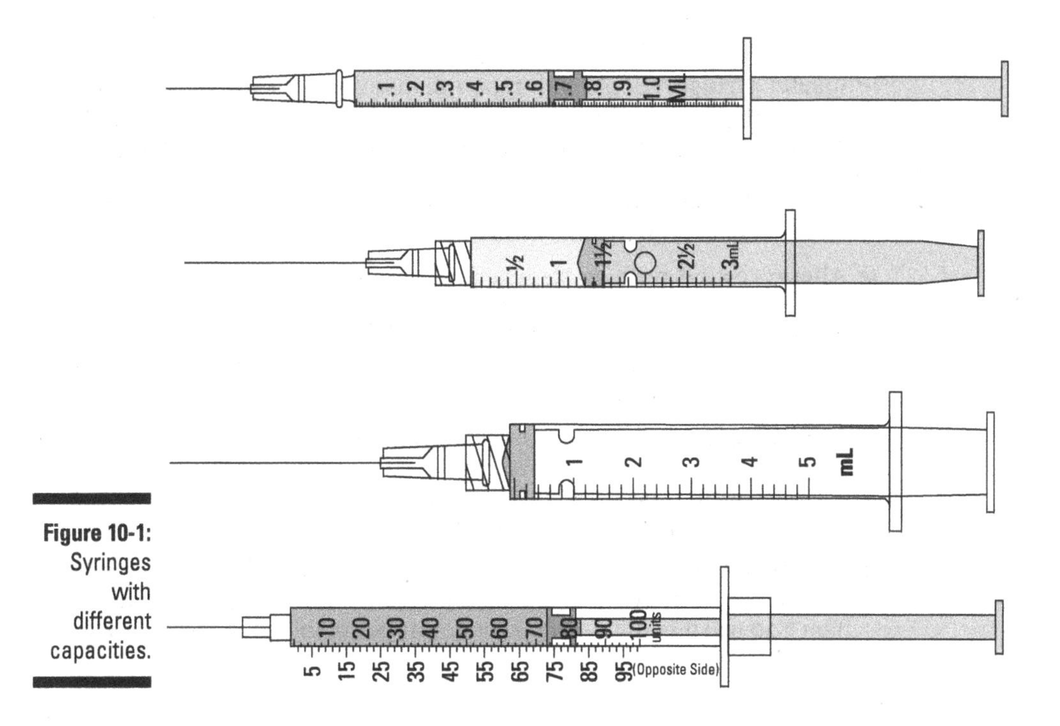

Figure 10-1: Syringes with different capacities.

Surveying several syringe types

Syringes come in quite a few varieties. The syringe you use depends on the parenteral route of administration ordered — usually IM ("muscle shot"), ID ("intradermal"), or subcut ("subcutaneous"). The most common syringes used in medicine are

- **Standard syringe:** The standard syringe is an empty syringe made of plastic and meant to be thrown out after one use. You draw up the medication from either a vial or an *ampule* (a small glass vessel that holds the solution to be injected).
- **Prefilled syringe:** Prefilled syringes are already filled with the medication when you get them from the pharmacist, making them more accurate than standard fill-them-yourself syringes. Consider what happens when you have to draw up medication from a vial or ampule. Sometimes you draw up more medication than needed.
- **Safety syringe:** Many newer syringes are safety syringes. They have built-in safety devices that help prevent accidental needle sticks. For example, the needles may be retractable after use, or the syringes may have snap covers over the needles.
- **Insulin syringe:** People with type 1 diabetes inject themselves several times a day with an insulin syringe. The special needle on an insulin syringe is made specifically for subcutaneous injection; it tends to be shorter and thinner (meaning it has a higher gauge, as we discuss in the nearby sidebar "Sizing up syringes") than a standard needle. The barrel of an insulin syringe is marked in units, not mL.
- **Allergy-testing syringe:** Medical professionals use this narrow, small syringe to administer intradermal injections to test for potential allergic responses. If you work in an allergist's office, or if you or a loved one has significant allergy problems, you've probably seen allergic skin testing done by means of intradermal injections.
- **Oral syringe:** You're probably reading this and going, "Say what?" A syringe that you put in your mouth? Well, this is the exception to the injection. It's a syringe with no needle. You use this type of syringe to administer liquid medicine to infants, children, and adults who have difficulty swallowing.
- **Tuberculin syringe:** Despite what its name suggests, you use a tuberculin syringe for more than just intradermal testing for TB (tuberculosis). You also use it to administer different types of injections intradermally.

Every medical professional undergoes the infamous *PPD* test (also known as the Purified Protein Derivative or tuberculin skin test) every year. A medical professional injects PPD extract into the dermal layer, forming a *wheal* (a small swelling on the skin). The wheal should go away in a few hours, but you need to have a medical professional look at the site in 48 to 72 hours. Depending on the size of the wheal after 72 hours, you may require further testing.

Sizing up syringes

When it comes to syringes, one size doesn't fit all. You can classify syringe size by capacity, needle thickness or diameter *(gauge)*, and needle length.

- **Capacity:** Syringe capacity refers to how much liquid it can hold. Syringes are sized in mL or units and come in many sizes, ranging from as small as 0.5 mL to as big as 100 mL. You can tell a syringe's capacity by looking at its packaging. For example, if the packaging says *3 mL*, the syringe can hold up to 3 mL of fluid. (Note that 1 cc, or cubic centimeter, is the same as 1 mL.) The smaller sizes, usually 1 mL or less, are the most precise. You can also see the capacity on the barrel of the syringe. Medical professionals use larger-volume syringes to administer liquid medication and also to irrigate wounds.
- **Needle thickness and length:** Look at a syringe's packaging: You see a number, followed by a *G* and another number. The first number indicates the gauge of the needle. Basically, the higher the number, the thinner the needle. So a 22-gauge needle is thinner than a 14-gauge needle. The second number indicates the length of the needle. For example, a 22 G ½ needle has a gauge of 22 and a length of ½ inch.

  There are several systems for gauging needles, including the Stubs Needle Gauge and the French Catheter Scale. Needles in common medical use range from 7 gauge (the largest) to 34 gauge (the smallest). You can see the dimensions of needles at `www.worldlingo.com/ma/enwiki/en/Needle_gauge_comparison_chart`, which also has links to explanations of the origins of the two gauging systems.

The choice of needle gauge and needle length depend, of course, on the type of injection you're administering. The standard needle to use for IM (intramuscular) injections is a 19- or 21-gauge needle. The choice usually depends on what your facility has available. In terms of needle length, use a 1-inch needle for a very thin person, and consider using a 2-inch needle for a heavy person.

Medical professionals commonly use 21-gauge needles to draw blood for testing purposes. But they typically use 16-gauge or 18-gauge needles for blood donation because they're wide enough to allow red blood cells to pass through the needle without rupturing.

Using the right syringe to inject a med

Calculating a dose accurately is a major part of dosing correctly, but you must also deliver the dose accurately. (See the section "Practicing Parenteral Dosing Calculations" for details on calculating doses.) After you determine the volume of a dose to inject, you must pick the correct syringe and then draw the medication into it.

When you're ready to choose which syringe to use to administer a certain med, keep the following tips in mind:

- For medication doses that are less than 0.5 mL, use a 1-mL syringe.
- For doses that are more than 1.0 mL, use a 3-mL syringe.
- For doses between 0.5 mL and 1.0 mL, choose either a 1-mL or a 3-mL syringe.

You're asked to give an injection of ketorolac (Toradol) 10 mg IM (intramuscularly) for pain. Ketorolac is available in injection form at 15 mg/mL. The dose is 0.67 mL. Which type of syringe should you use?

To select the correct syringe, let the volume to be dosed be your guide. Use a tuberculin syringe with 1 mL (sometimes marked "1 cc") capacity. It has graduations of 0.01 mL (or cc) on the barrel, so you can dispense 0.67 mL accurately.

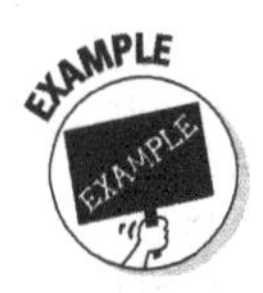

You have to give 10 mg morphine sulfate PRN for pain. (*PRN* or *prn* means "as needed." It's the abbreviation for *pro re nata*, Latin for "in the circumstances.") The correct dose is contained in 1 mL of solution. Which syringe should you use?

Again, let the volume to be dosed be your guide when choosing the right syringe. Use either a 1-mL syringe or a 3-mL syringe.

Getting the med into the syringe

After you pick the right syringe to use for a given injection, you need to know how to get the medication into the syringe. Meds that you have to inject via syringes come in several different containers. The two main med containers are

- **Vial:** A *vial* is a container you put the needle into to draw up a medication; you can use a vial more than once. A vial can have different types of coverings — a rubber stopper and metal cap, a cork seal, or some other type of stopper. *Screw vials* have coverings that are screwed on.

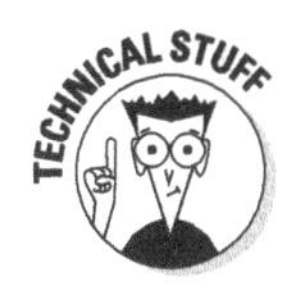

To draw medication into a syringe from a vial, draw back the plunger to a position equal to the amount of medication you'll inject, inject the air into the vial, and withdraw the correct amount of medication into the syringe.

In case you're curious, a Vacutainer (a brand name) is the type of vacuum-filled vial used in blood draws.

- **Ampule**: An *ampule* is a glass container that you have to break open to get to the medication inside it. You use it only once. You need to use a filter needle to draw medication from an ampule to avoid drawing glass up into the syringe.

Look at Figure 10-2 to get a better idea of the differences between different medication containers. Figure 10-2a shows examples of a vial, Figure 10-2b shows examples of an ampule, and Figure 10-2c shows a Vacutainer.

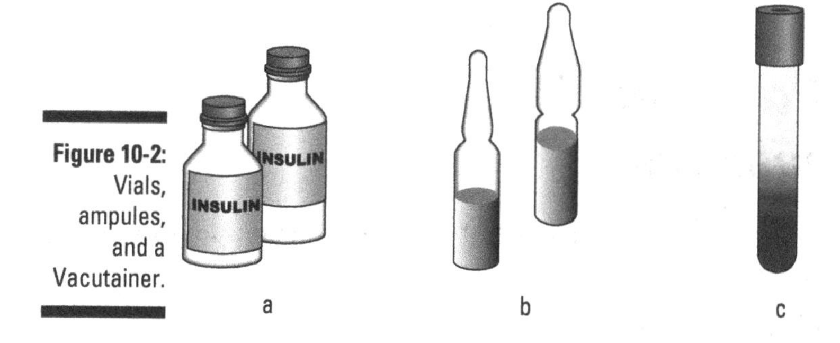

Figure 10-2: Vials, ampules, and a Vacutainer.

Looking At the Label and Following Hospital Protocols

When you examine a drug label before administering a medication parenterally, focus on the medication strength (typically in mg/mL). It's the key number you need for determining the right volume to administer. You also see the following on the label:

- Brand name
- Generic name
- Vial capacity
- Route of administration, such as "Injection USP"
- Warnings, such as "For IM use only," "Not for intravenous use," or "Do not use if precipitated"

For more information on medication labels, go to Chapter 6.

If you're working in a hospital setting, the hospital protocols concerning parenterally administered drugs are important, too. For example, for labetalol, the protocols may read something like the following:

- This drug is to be administered only in critical care areas where patient is on a cardiac monitor.
- Labetalol may be given by 2 methods: repeated IV bolus or continuous infusion. If administered as a continuous infusion, it must be administered on an infusion pump using a safety software program.

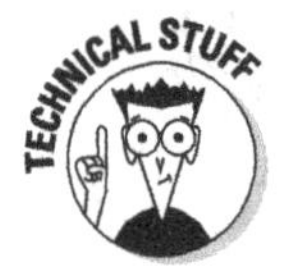

A *bolus* or *IV push* is a single dose. In IV therapy, you connect a syringe to an access port in the IV setup and push the injection in. For *continuous infusion,* by contrast, an Alaris infusion pump uses a software program called *Guardrails* to set safety limits for dosing. See Chapter 11 for more details.

Practicing Parenteral Dosing Calculations

This section shows you how to do medical dosing calculations for three of the four types of parenteral injections:

- **Subcutaneous:** Under the skin
- **Intradermal:** Into the dermal layer
- **Intramuscular:** Into the muscle

Note: Intravenous injections (those made into the vein) are also parenteral injections, but they differ substantially from injections made using a syringe. See Chapter 11 for a complete discussion about the intravenous route of administration.

The calculation of volumes to inject is essentially the same for each of the preceding three injection types. The formula method and the ratio-proportion method work well, although we authors often favor the ratio-proportion method because the terms are so clearly presented.

Which of the different types of parenteral injections is absorbed the fastest? Intravenous (IV) injections have the fastest effect, followed by intramuscular (IM) injections. In third place is the subcutaneous (subq) injection. Coming in last place is the intradermal (ID) injection.

Subcutaneous dosing: Getting under the skin

When you administer a med subcutaneously, you're injecting it into the area of fatty tissue under the skin. (Not surprisingly, the word *subcutaneous* means "under the skin.") This area consists of fat and connective tissue loaded with vessels and nerves. Doctors prescribe many medications that must be given in this manner.

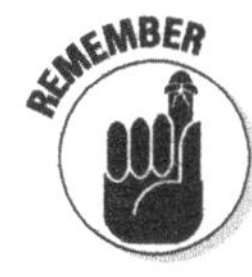

When you give a subcutaneous injection, keep these important points in mind:

- **Pick the right site for injection.** Common injection sites include the abdominal wall (common for heparin and insulin injections), the outer part of the upper arms, the thigh area, and the lower back. Be sure to inspect the area before injecting; you don't want to inject into scar tissue, bruised tissue, or a site that has been used recently.
- **Always alternate injection sites.** The site of the last injection isn't a good place for the next injection.
- **Use the right needle.** Because you're injecting into the fatty tissue below the skin, you need to use a shorter needle. A needle that's ½ inch to ⅝ inch long with a gauge of 25 to 30 is usually sufficient to administer a medication subcutaneously.
- **Be aware of how the medication is packaged.** Is it in a vial or an ampule? If it's in an ampule, you need to "break the neck" of the ampule to get the medication.
- **Inject at the correct angle.** Pinch a small aspect of skin between your thumb and forefinger, and insert the needle at a 45-degree angle into the skin fold. Don't change your angle or go deeper than the skin fold. There! You're done!
- **Know whether or not you need to apply gentle pressure to the injection site.** Whether you should apply pressure after injection depends on the medication you're injecting. For any kind of blood-thinning medication, don't apply pressure after injection.
- **Discard your waste.** Put the needle in an approved needle disposal (or "sharps") container.

You're asked to administer epoetin alfa (Procrit) 10,000 units subcut (subcutaneously) for a person with anemia. Epoetin alfa is available in 20,000 units/mL, and it comes in a glass vial with a rubber top that doesn't need to be broken. How many mL do you administer?

You can use either the formula method or the ratio-proportion method to solve this problem. (For details on both calculation methods, turn to Chapter 8.)

Follow these steps to use the formula method:

1. **Set up the following equation:**

$$x\ (\text{amount}) = \frac{d\ (\text{desired})}{h\ (\text{have})} \times q\ (\text{conversion factor})$$

$$x\ \text{mL} = \frac{10{,}000\ \text{units}}{20{,}000\ \text{units}} \times 1\ \text{mL}$$

2. **Divide and solve.**

$$x\ \text{mL} = \frac{10{,}000}{20{,}000}$$

$$x\ \text{mL} = 0.5$$

You administer 0.5 mL of epoetin alfa subcutaneously.

Follow these steps to use the ratio-proportion method:

1. **Set up the following proportion:**

$$\frac{\text{known equivalent}}{\text{known equivalent}} = \frac{\text{known equivalent}}{\text{desired equivalent}}$$

$$\frac{20{,}000\ \text{units}}{1\ \text{mL}} = \frac{10{,}000\ \text{units}}{x\ \text{mL}}$$

2. **Cross-multiply and solve.**

$$20{,}000x = 10{,}000$$

$$x = 0.5$$

The answer is 0.5 mL of epoetin alfa.

You're instructed to administer fondaparinux (Arixtra) for the treatment of deep venous thrombosis (DVT) at a dose of 7.5 mg subcutaneously daily. The solution available is 5 mg/0.4 mL. How many mL do you administer?

You talk to the pharmacist and he confirms that dosing fondaparinux is weight dependent. Fortunately, the prescribed dose is correct because the patient weighs 70 kg.

To find out how many mL you need to administer, use the ratio-proportion method and follow these steps:

1. **Set up the following proportion:**

   $$\frac{5 \text{ mg}}{0.4 \text{ mL}} = \frac{7.5 \text{ mg}}{x \text{ mL}}$$

2. **Cross-multiply and solve.**

   $$5x = 3$$

   $$x = 0.6$$

   You need to administer 0.6 mL of fondaparinux subcutaneously.

Intradermal dosing: Feeling the wheal

Unlike the subcutaneous injection (which goes *under* the skin), an intradermal injection sends the medication you're administering right *into* the dermal layer of the skin.

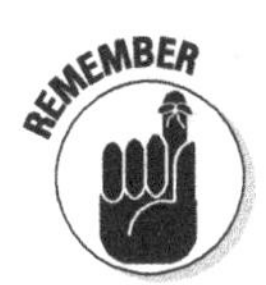

When you give an intradermal injection, keep these important points in mind:

- **Always alternate injection sites.** The site of the last injection isn't a good place for the next injection.
- **Pick the right site of injection.** Use the inner aspect of the forearm. (An *aspect* is a part of a surface facing in any direction.) The person's arm should be relaxed and the elbow in a flexed position.
- **Use the right needle and syringe.** The most common needle used for intradermal injection is 26 gauge. Lengths vary but are generally ½ inch or smaller. As for the type of syringe, you typically use a tuberculin syringe or 1-mL syringe.
- **Inject at the correct angle.** Hold the needle at 15 degrees.

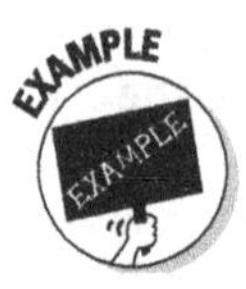

You're instructed to administer calcitonin to a patient diagnosed with hypercalcemia. It's available as a solution at 200 IU/mL in 2 mL vials (*IU* stands for International Units). You're to administer 4 IU/kg of patient weight every 12 hours subcutaneously. The patient weighs 80 kg. Before you proceed with the subcutaneous injection, however, you're instructed to give a test dose of calcitonin intradermally. The test dose is usually prepared by the pharmacy. It may come diluted to 10 IU/mL. You take 0.05 mL. How many units are in the 0.05 mL quantity of the intradermal test dose? And how much calcitonin do you need to administer subcutaneously?

To find out how many units are in the test dose, use the ratio-proportion method and follow these steps:

1. **Set up the following proportion:**

   $$\frac{1 \text{ mL}}{10 \text{ units}} = \frac{0.05 \text{ mL}}{x \text{ units}}$$

2. **Cross-multiply and solve.**

   $x = 0.05 \times 10$

   $x = 0.5$

   The answer is 0.5 units.

Now you're ready to make the test solution. Take 0.05 mL of solution and dilute with 0.9% normal saline to make 1 mL of solution. Mix well and waste 0.9 mL so that you have 0.1 mL to inject. Inject 0.1 mL over the inferior aspect of the forearm, and examine the injection site after 15 minutes. If no wheal is present, it's safe to administer the calcitonin subcutaneously.

To determine how many mL of calcitonin to administer per dose, use a simple formula and the patient's weight to find out how many IU to administer. Then convert IU to mL using the ratio-proportion method. Follow these steps:

1. **Use the following formula to determine how many IU to administer, based on patient weight.**

   $4 \text{ IU/kg} \times 80 \text{ kg} = 320 \text{ IU}$ for each injection

   You're going to administer 320 IU every 12 hours.

2. **Set up the following proportion to convert IU into mL:**

   $$\frac{200 \text{ units}}{1 \text{ mL}} = \frac{320 \text{ units}}{x \text{ mL}}$$

3. **Cross-multiply and solve.**

   $200x = 320$

   $x = 1.6$

   The answer is 1.6 mL. Administer 1.6 mL of calcitonin every 12 hours.

Intramuscular dosing: Going straight for the muscle

Sometimes you have to administer intramuscular (IM) injections. You may be in a situation where you're having difficulty getting intravenous access, and the need for the med (such as an antibiotic) is urgent.

Unfortunately, IM injections aren't fun for you or the patient. Because they go into the muscle below the subcutaneous layer, the needle used must be thicker and longer to ensure that the medicine gets injected into the proper tissue.

When you give an intramuscular injection, remember these important points:

- **Pick the right site of injection.** The best places to give an IM injection are the vastus lateralis muscle (thigh), ventrogluteal and dorsogluteal muscles (outer hip area), and deltoid muscle (upper arm).
- **Use the right needle.** Typically, 20- or 22-gauge needles that are 1 to 1½ inches long are appropriate for this type of injection. For a patient who's thin, with very little fatty tissue, you can use a 1-inch-long needle; for a heavier person, you may need to use a 1 ½-inch-long needle.
- **Hold the syringe the right way.** Hold the syringe in the hand you write with, like you would hold a pen or pencil. Then move your thumb to the plunger.
- **Inject at the correct angle.** Rather than the 45- and 15-degree angles you use for subcutaneous and intradermal injections, inject at a 90-degree angle for IM injections.
- **Do an IM injection only when you have no other choice.** They can be uncomfortable.

You're asked to give an injection of ketorolac (Toradol) 10 mg IM for pain. It's available in injection form at 15 mg/mL. How many mL do you give?

To find out, you can use either the formula method or the ratio-proportion method. (For details on both calculation methods, turn to Chapter 8.) Follow these steps to use the formula method:

1. **Set up the following equation:**

$$x = \frac{10 \text{ mg/mL}}{15 \text{ mg/mL}} \times 1 \text{ mL}$$

2. **Divide and solve.**

$$x = \frac{10}{15} \times 1$$

$$x = 0.67$$

The answer is 0.67 mL.

Follow these steps to use the ratio-proportion method:

1. **Set up the following proportion:**

$$\frac{15 \text{ mg}}{1 \text{ mL}} = \frac{10 \text{ mg}}{x \text{ mL}}$$

2. **Cross-multiply and solve.**

$$15x = 10$$

$$x = 0.67$$

The answer is 0.67 mL.

You're ordered to administer clindamycin IM now — one dose of 300 mg until you can obtain intravenous access. Clindamycin comes in a premixed container at 150 mg/mL. How many mL do you give?

To find out, use the ratio-proportion method and follow these steps:

1. **Set up the following proportion:**

$$\frac{150 \text{ mg}}{1 \text{ mL}} = \frac{300 \text{ mg}}{x \text{ mL}}$$

2. **Cross-multiply and solve.**

$$150x = 300$$
$$x = 2$$

You must administer 2 mL IM.

Real-Life Practice: Dosing an IM Med

You're ordered to administer 1 dose of penicillin G 2.4 million units IM. The medication is available in 600,000 units/mL. How many mL do you administer?

To solve this problem, use the ratio-proportion method and follow these steps:

1. **Set up the following proportion:**

$$\frac{600{,}000 \text{ units}}{1 \text{ mL}} = \frac{2{,}400{,}000 \text{ units}}{x \text{ mL}}$$

2. **Cross-multiply and solve.**

$$600{,}000x = 2{,}400{,}000$$
$$x = 4$$

You administer 4 mL intramuscularly.

Real-Life Practice: Dosing a Subcutaneous Med

You have to administer octreotide 150 mcg subq every 8 hours. It's available in a concentration of 0.2 mg/mL. How many mL do you need to administer?

To find out, use the ratio-proportion method and follow these steps:

1. **Use the conversion factor 1,000 mcg = 1 mg to convert from mg/mL to mcg/mL.**

   0.2 mg/mL × 1,000 mcg/1 mg = 200 mcg/mL

2. **Set up the following proportion to see how many mL you need to administer:**

   $$\frac{200 \text{ mcg}}{1 \text{ mL}} = \frac{150 \text{ mcg}}{x \text{ mL}}$$

3. **Cross-multiply and solve.**

   $200x = 150$

   $x = 0.75$

   You need to inject 0.75 mL subcutaneously every 8 hours.

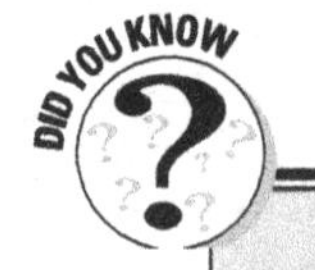

What else is a syringe good for?

Syringes have many uses outside of healthcare for humans. Here are just a few:

- Technicians may use a syringe to apply laboratory grease to lubricate ground glass joints and stopcocks.
- Animal-care technicians sometimes use a large syringe without a needle to feed small baby mammals during artificial rearing.
- You can use syringes in your home kitchen. Use a turkey syringe (a "marinade injector syringe") to improve the flavor of meat by injecting juices into it. You can also use a syringe to inject vodka into oranges, pineapples, grapes, kiwis, and strawberries.
- Hippy Sippy was an outrageous and controversial candy introduced in the late 1960s. It was a toy syringe that contained small multicolored candy pellets. The intent was to mimic drug use in the hippie culture. The maker took it off the market right away.

Chapter 11

The IV League: Intravenous Dosing and Calculations

In This Chapter

- Calculating flow rates, infusion times, and drip rates for intravenous fluids
- Getting to know the IV system and how to use it
- Administering IV fluids manually versus automatically
- Performing dosing calculations for intravenous infusions with some practice problems

One of the most common tasks you do as a medical professional is to administer fluids and medications intravenously (IV). *Intravenous therapy* is the route of administration during which you put a substance into a vein; it's the fastest way to get a liquid into a patient. (In case you're wondering where the term comes from, *intra* is Latin for "into" and *venous* comes from the Latin word *vena,* which means "vein.") The substances that you infuse during IV therapy vary widely and include medications, fluids, nutrition, blood, and blood products.

In this chapter, we introduce you to the practice of administering meds intravenously and show you how to do the dosing calculations for IV infusions. Keep in mind that we focus on the type of IV dosing you'd see and do on a general medical-surgical floor in a hospital. Take a look at Chapter 18 for information about calculating and dosing life-sustaining medications for very ill patients.

Note: If you're not comfortable with calculating how many mL of a medication you should give to deliver the right mg dose, turn to Chapter 10 for everything you need to know about doing dosing calculations for non-IV parenteral injections. If you're already comfortable with such calculations, stay right here!

Infusion 101: Calculating Flow Rates, Infusion Times, and Drip Rates

When you start an IV, you're starting an *infusion* (the process of introducing a liquid into a vein). Unlike an injection, which you administer all at one time, you give an infusion at a certain rate over time. You usually calculate the exact rate, based on the total time and the amount of medication specified in the doctor's order. An intravenous infusion is either continuous or intermittent.

- A *continuous* infusion lasts for 24 hours or more. Doctors can order many IV fluids and medications to run continuously. For example, heparin and insulin are likely to be infused over 24 hours.
- An *intermittent* infusion is one that you administer over a defined period of time (for example, 30 minutes, 1 hour, or 4 hours). Doctors order many intravenous meds, like antibiotics and electrolytes, to be administered as intermittent infusions.

Doctors or other medical professionals write orders for intravenous fluids in a variety of ways, but most of them require you to calculate a flow rate, an infusion time, or a drip rate. The following sections show you how to do all three.

Going with the flow: Calculating the flow rate

The *flow rate* (often called *infusion rate*) is the rate the doctor orders you to give an intravenous infusion in mL/hr. In many cases, the doctor writes exactly what she wants the flow rate to be, so it's a given. For example, a common intravenous fluid order is 1 L (1,000 mL) of 0.9% NaCl (called NS or normal saline) at 80 mL/hr. The flow rate of 80 mL/hr is a given.

Other times, though, you must calculate the flow rate. For example, flow rate isn't a given if the doc orders you to give a quantity of fluid over several hours. In this case, you need to calculate the flow rate in mL/hr.

You also have to calculate the flow rate if the order specifies g or mg rather than mL. To determine the flow rate for such orders, first calculate mg/mL; then figure out the flow rate in mL/hr.

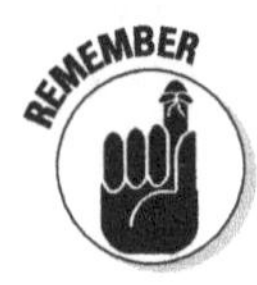

A simple formula for calculating flow rate is

flow rate (mL/hr) = total volume ÷ designated time

The doctor gives an order first to administer an IV fluid infusion of 500 mL over 2 hours and then to administer another 1 L (1,000 mL) over 5 hours. What are the flow rates in mL/hr?

To find out, use the ratio-proportion method and the flow rate formula (see Chapter 8 for details on the ratio-proportion method and other calculation methods). Follow these steps:

1. **Set up the following proportion to calculate the first flow rate to administer 500 mL over 2 hours:**

   $$\frac{\text{known equivalent}}{\text{known equivalent}} = \frac{\text{known equivalent}}{\text{desired equivalent}}$$

   $$\frac{2\text{ hr}}{500\text{ mL}} = \frac{1\text{ hr}}{x\text{ mL}}$$

2. **Cross-multiply and solve.**

   $2x = 500$

   $x = 250$

   Your initial fluid infusion is 250 mL/hr for 2 hours.

3. **Use the flow rate formula to figure out the flow rate for the second infusion of 1 L (1,000 mL) over 5 hours.**

   flow rate (mL/hr) = total volume ÷ designated time

   flow rate (mL/hr) = 1,000 mL ÷ 5 hr

   flow rate (mL/hr) = 200 mL/hr

   After 2 hours of infusing at 250 mL/hr, you decrease the intravenous flow rate to 200 mL/hr for another 5 hours. (The calculation is similar if you have to figure out flow rates for infusions of less than 1 hr.)

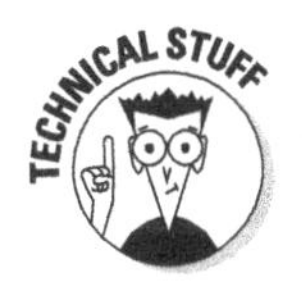

You have to change the IV bag after 4 to 5 hours. In a modern hospital, the IV equipment alerts you when the bag is ready to be changed. But if you're working in a field hospital in a developing country, you need to know how to manage the equipment manually. See the section "Going with gravity: Manual IV systems" for more details.

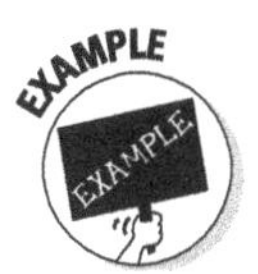

The doctor's order says to give a 0.9% NaCl (NS) fluid infusion 250 mL IV over 30 minutes. After 30 minutes, give the other 750 mL (the remainder of a 1 L bag) over the next 10 hours. What are the respective flow rates?

To solve this problem, follow these steps:

1. **Convert the time for the first infusion from minutes to hours.**

   desired unit = given unit × conversion factor

   $$x = 30\text{ min} \times \frac{1\text{ hr}}{60\text{ min}}$$

   $$x = \frac{30}{60}\text{ hr}$$

   $$x = 0.5\text{ hr}$$

   See Chapter 4 for a whole lot more on converting units.

2. **Use the flow rate formula to calculate the first flow rate to administer 250 mL over 30 minutes.**

   flow rate (mL/hr) = 250 mL ÷ 0.5 hr

   flow rate (mL/hr) = 500 mL/hr

   The initial flow rate is 500 mL/hr.

3. **Use the flow rate formula to calculate the second flow rate to administer 750 mL over 10 hours.**

   flow rate (mL/hr) = 750 mL ÷ 10 hr

   flow rate (mL/hr) = 75 mL/hr

   After infusing for 30 minutes at a rate of 500 mL/hr, you have to adjust the flow rate to be 75 mL/hr for 10 hours.

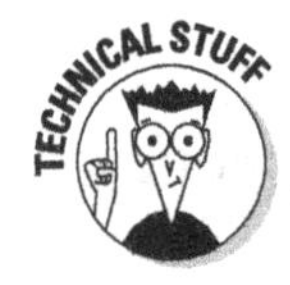

The initial infusion is called a *fluid bolus* (from the Latin, meaning "ball"). Normal saline is better at raising the patient's blood pressure than many other fluids.

So how do you set the flow rate or adjust it? The most common way is to use an *electronic infusion pump,* which lets you program the pump at a certain rate. See the section "Getting pumped up" for more details.

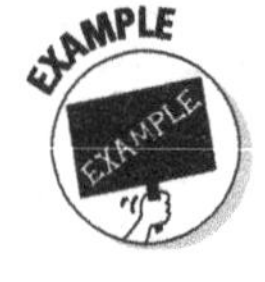

You're instructed to give the antibiotic levofloxacin (Levaquin) 750 mg in 150 mL D5W (5% dextrose in water) over 90 minutes. What's the flow rate?

To find out, follow these steps:

1. **Determine the quantity of mL containing 750 mg.**

   This quantity is a given; there are 750 mg in 150 mL.

2. **Convert minutes to hours.**

$$x = 90\ \text{min} \times \frac{1\ \text{hr}}{60\ \text{min}}$$

$$x = \frac{90}{60}\ \text{hr}$$

$$x = 1.5\ \text{hr}$$

3. **Use the flow rate formula to calculate the flow rate.**

   flow rate (mL/hr) = 150 mL ÷ 1.5 hr

   flow rate (mL/hr) = 100 mL/hr

   The flow rate is 100 mL/hr.

Timing is everything: Calculating the infusion time

The *infusion time* is the flip side of the flow rate. When you know the volume of fluid you need to administer in mL and the flow rate in mL/hr, the remaining factor to figure out is the time interval.

For continuous infusions lasting more than 24 hours, the physician gives all the parameters in his order. For example, look at the following order:

D5W 1,000 mL at 60 mL/hr

This order is understood to be a continuous IV infusion that will last more than 24 hours. More commonly, your job is to calculate infusion times for shorter intermittent time intervals.

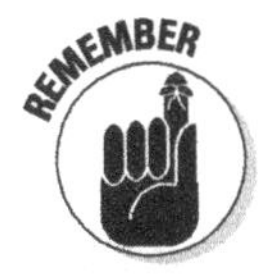

A simple formula for calculating infusion time is

infusion time (hr) = total volume (mL) ÷ flow rate (mL/hr)

You're instructed to administer 0.45% NaCl (called one-half normal saline or ½ NS) 1,000 mL at 60 mL/hr. What's the infusion time?

To solve this problem, all you have to do is use the infusion time formula, like so:

infusion time (hr) = total volume (mL) ÷ flow rate (mL/hr)

infusion time (hr) = 1,000 mL ÷ 60 mL/hr

infusion time (hr) = 16.67 hr

The infusion time is 16.67 hr, or 16 hours and 40 minutes.

IV drips and drops: Using the drop factor to calculate drip rate

When you're administering an IV by gravity without an infusion pump, you need to use the drip rate rather than the flow rate for your dosing calculations (see the sections "Going with gravity: Manual IV systems" and "Getting pumped up: Automated IV systems" for details on gravity versus pump). The *drip rate* is a measurement of flow in drops per minute (gtt/min), not mL/hr. For calculations involving drip rate, you also need to be familiar with the *drop factor,* a measurement of the IV tubing set's carrying capacity in gtt/mL.

Note: Medical professionals don't use drip rates very often because of the widespread use of infusion pumps, but you need to be prepared for anything. Although the drip rate math isn't hard and the principles are important, with the advent of the electronic infusion pump, most of the time you're just going to program in the flow rate.

IV tubing sets have drop factors that are preset by the manufacturer. The two types of tubing sets are

- **Macrodrip (larger gtt/mL):** Macrodrip tubing sets usually have drop factors of 10, 15, or 20 gtt/mL. Adults usually get IVs through macrodrip tubing sets. In fact, a 15 gtt/mL tubing set is frequently called a *standard set.*
- **Microdrip (smaller gtt/mL):** Microdrip tubing sets usually have drop factors of 60 gtt/mL. Pediatric patients typically get IVs through microdrip tubing sets.

Here's a quick and easy way to think about drop factors and drip rates:

- The drop factor (gtt/mL) lets you determine the drip rate (gtt/min).
- To calculate a drip rate, you need to know the total volume to be infused and the infusion time. Use this formula:

$$\text{drip rate (gtt/min)} = \frac{\text{total volume to be administered (mL)} \times \text{drop factor} \frac{\text{(gtt)}}{\text{(mL)}}}{\text{total infusion time (min)}}$$

- The total infusion time must be in minutes, not hours, for this formula to work. (This is different from the flow rate, which is in mL/hr.)

When you're using an infusion pump, you don't need to know the drop factor because the pump's computer does any needed calculations. All you need to know are the flow rate and the infusion time.

You're using a manual IV system and must give NS 1,000 mL over 12 hours. The drop factor is 20 gtt/mL. Calculate the drip rate.

To do so, follow these steps:

1. **Convert the total infusion time from hours to minutes.**

   $$x = 12 \text{ hr} \times \frac{60 \text{ min}}{1 \text{ hr}}$$

   $$x = \frac{720}{1} \text{ min}$$

   $$x = 720 \text{ min}$$

   The total time is 720 minutes.

2. **Use the drip rate formula to calculate the drip rate.**

   $$\text{drip rate (gtt/min)} = \frac{\text{total volume to be administered (mL)} \times \text{drop factor} \frac{\text{(gtt)}}{\text{(mL)}}}{\text{total infusion time (min)}}$$

   $$\text{drip rate (gtt/min)} = \frac{1{,}000 \times 20}{720}$$

   $$\text{drip rate (gtt/min)} = 27.78$$

   Round the number up. The drip rate is 28 gtt/min. (For drip rate, you're literally counting the number of drops entering the IV setup's drip chamber in one minute, so your answer needs to be a whole number.)

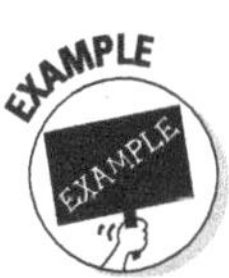

You've been ordered to administer 500 mg of a medication in 500 mL of D5W over 4 hours (see the section "Considering solution type" for details on D5W and other IV solutions). The drop factor is 10 gtt/mL. What's the drip rate in gtt/min?

To find out, follow these steps:

1. **Convert the total infusion time from hours to minutes.**

   $$x = 4\text{ hr} \times \frac{60\text{ min}}{1\text{ hr}}$$

   $$x = \frac{240}{1}\text{ min}$$

   $$x = 240\text{ min}$$

2. **Use the drip rate formula to calculate the drip rate.**

   $$\text{drip rate (gtt/min)} = \frac{500\text{ mL} \times 10\text{ gtt/mL}}{240\text{ min}}$$

   $$\text{drip rate (gtt/min)} = 20.83$$

   Round the number up. The drip rate is 21 gtt/min.

You do calculations for microdrip tubing sets the same way, except that they have a drop factor of 60 gtt/mL.

A doctor's order says to administer 1 L (1,000 mL) of normal saline over 10 hours. The drop factor is 60 drops per mL. What's the drip rate?

To find out, follow these steps:

1. **Convert the total infusion time from hours to minutes.**

   $$x = 10\text{ hr} \times \frac{60\text{ min}}{1\text{ hr}}$$

   $$x = \frac{600}{1}\text{ min}$$

   $$x = 600\text{ min}$$

2. **Use the drip rate formula to calculate the drip rate.**

   $$\text{drip rate (gtt/min)} = \frac{1{,}000\text{ mL} \times 60\text{ gtt/mL}}{600\text{ min}}$$

   $$\text{drip rate (gtt/min)} = 100$$

   The drip rate is 100 gtt/min.

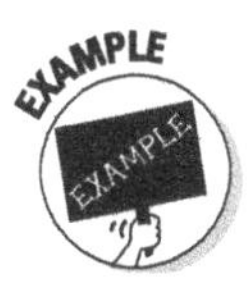

You're asked to administer 500 mL of lactated Ringer's solution to be given over 8 hours. If the drop factor is 10 gtt/mL, what's the drip rate?

In this problem you're given the volume to be administered, the infusion time, and the drop factor. One way to approach this problem is to use the drip rate formula to directly calculate the drip rate. Just follow these steps:

1. **Convert the total infusion time from hours to minutes.**

   $$x = 8\text{ hr} \times \frac{60\text{ min}}{1\text{ hr}}$$

   $$x = \frac{480}{1}\text{ min}$$

   $$x = 480\text{ min}$$

2. **Use the drip rate formula to calculate the drip rate.**

   $$\text{drip rate (gtt/min)} = \frac{500\text{ mL} \times 10\text{ gtt/mL}}{480\text{ min}}$$

   $$\text{drip rate (gtt/min)} = 10.42$$

   The drip rate is 10 gtt/min.

Another way to approach this problem is to first calculate the flow rate in mL/hr and then calculate the drip rate in gtt/min. To do so, use the ratio-proportion method and follow these steps (see Chapter 8 for more on calculation methods):

1. **Set up the following proportion to calculate the flow rate in mL/hr:**

   $$\frac{8\text{ hr}}{500\text{ mL}} = \frac{1\text{ hr}}{x\text{ mL}}$$

2. **Cross-multiply and solve.**

   $8x = 500$

   $x = 62.5$

   The flow rate is 62.5 mL/hr.

3. **Convert the flow rate from mL/hr to mL/min.**

$$\text{flow rate (mL/min)} = \frac{62.5\text{ mL}}{1\text{ hr}} \times \frac{1\text{ hr}}{60\text{min}}$$

$$\text{flow rate (mL/min)} = \frac{62.5}{60}$$

$$\text{flow rate (mL/min)} = 1.0416$$

The flow rate is 1.0416 mL/min.

4. **Use the drip rate formula to calculate the drip rate.**

$$\text{drip rate (gtt/min)} = \frac{1.0416\text{ mL} \times 10\text{ gtt/mL}}{1\text{ min}}$$

$$\text{drip rate (gtt/min)} = 10.416$$

Round down. The drip rate is 10 gtt/min.

You must administer 500 mL of NS over 4 hours. The drop factor is 60 gtt/min. What is the drip rate?

To find out, follow these steps:

1. **Use the flow rate formula to calculate the flow rate in mL/hr.**

   flow rate = 500 mL ÷ 4 hr

   flow rate = 125 mL/hr

   You infuse 125 mL/hr.

2. **Use the microdrip shortcut we describe in the sidebar "Drip rate shortcuts" to convert the flow rate to the drip rate.**

   Because the drop factor is 60 gtt/min, the drip rate is numerically equivalent to the flow rate. So the drip rate is 125 gtt/min.

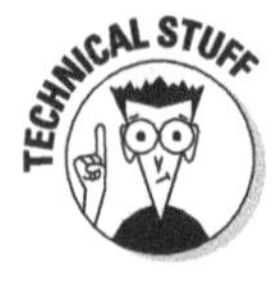

At this point you may be asking yourself, what's the difference between a flow rate and a drip rate? Both are ways of measuring the amount of fluid given to patients over a defined period of time. The difference is in the units: Flow rate is measured in mL/hr, and drip rate is measured in gtt/min.

Drip rate shortcuts

When the drop factor is 60 gtt/mL (as it is with microdrip tubing sets), you can use a shortcut to calculate the drip rate. The shortcut is this: With microdrip tubing sets, the drip rate and flow rate are numerically equivalent.

For example, if you're administering 1,000 mL over 10 hours, the flow rate is 100 mL/hr. Rewrite this rate as 100 mL/60 min. Because 1 mL equals 60 gtt, there are 6,000 gtt in 100 mL. Do the division, and you see that a flow rate of 100 mL/hr is equivalent to a drop rate of 100 gtt/min.

For macrodrip tubing sets, you can use the following three shortcuts:

- **Drop factor of 20 gtt/mL:** The hourly rate of 100 mL/hr equals 33.3 gtt/min.
- **Drop factor of 15 gtt/mL:** The hourly rate of 100 mL/hr equals 25 gtt/min.
- **Drop factor of 10 gtt/mL:** The hourly rate of 100 mL/hr equals 16.7 gtt/min.

Taking a Closer Look at IV Systems

You use one of two methods to administer IV fluids — the manual method (gravity flow) or the automated method (infusion pump). In a *manual IV system,* you control the flow rate of the infusion manually; in an *automatic IV system*, you program an electronic infusion pump to control the flow rate (see the section "Going with the flow: Calculating the flow rate" for more details). Both manual and automatic IV systems use IV bags, but the way they work is a little different.

Beginning with the IV bag

The IV route of administration, whether manual or automatic, starts with the IV bag. A fluid passes through some sophisticated equipment and ends up in the patient's vein, but it all starts with the bag.

An *IV bag* is a flexible plastic bag that contains fluids of various types, volumes, and concentrations (which we discuss in the following sections). Like the rest of the IV apparatus, the bag must be completely nonreactive with the fluid being dispensed. The bag hangs on a pole next to the patient's bed during administration (see the section "Going with gravity: Manual IV systems" for more details).

Some IV solutions are available in glass or plastic bottles.

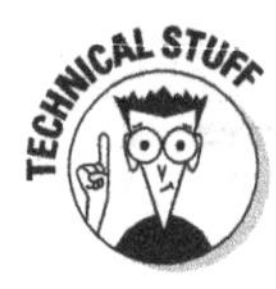

Per federal law, IV bags and their contents are considered prescription drugs.

Considering volume

Most bags of intravenous fluid come in volumes of 1,000 mL. But they can come in other volumes as well, including 500 mL, 250 mL, 150 mL, and 100 mL. Some medications are even diluted to volumes of 50–100 mL or come premixed at those volumes.

Considering solution type

IV solutions have different chemical makeups and various fluid concentrations. Common fluids include

- **NS:** Also called *normal saline,* this fluid contains 0.9% NaCl (sodium chloride) but no dextrose.
- **½ NS:** Also called *one-half normal saline,* this fluid contains 0.45% NaCl. It has half the amount of sodium as NS and no dextrose. Because it contains half the amount of saline, it's less concentrated than NS.
- **¼ NS:** Also called *one-quarter normal saline,* this fluid contains 0.35% NaCl. It also contains no dextrose and is more dilute than NS and ½NS.
- **D5W:** Any time you see a *D* as part of a fluid order, assume that the bag contains some concentration of dextrose. For example, D5W contains 5% dextrose in water. Other dextrose variants include D5NS (5% dextrose in normal saline), and D10NS (10% dextrose in normal saline).
- **Lactated Ringer's solution:** Also known as *LR,* this electrolyte solution is a little more dilute than 0.9% saline, but it's more concentrated than the other solutions we list here. It contains some potassium, calcium, and lactate. Dosing calculations for lactated Ringer's solution are similar to other IV fluid calculations (see the section "Infusion 101: Calculating Flow Rates, Infusion Times, and Drip Rates" for details).

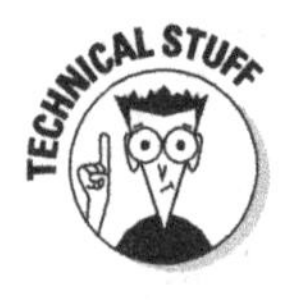

Crystalloid solutions are the most common type of IV fluids you'll administer. Examples of crystalloid solutions include normal saline, as well as the other solutions described in the preceding list. Crystalloids contain water-soluble molecules, usually mineral salts. However, you'll also have to administer *colloid fluids.* Colloids contain large insoluble molecules, and examples include albumin and hydroxyethyl starch (Hespan). Doctors order these fluids in the critical care unit (CCU) or on a medical-surgical floor.

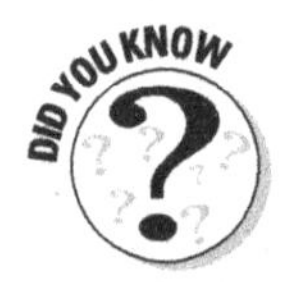

Banana bags are IV bags that contain a fluid made up of vitamins and minerals. Most commonly, they include thiamine, folic acid, a multivitamin, and magnesium. Physicians often order banana bags for those who are at risk of being severely malnourished, including those who abuse alcohol. The fluid in the banana bags can correct nutritional deficiencies, such as magnesium deficiencies. But (and we're not making it up) banana bags have made the news when super-skinny super models, movie stars, and rich people use nutrition IV drips to avoid eating. That practice is definitely not good for health because the fluid can't provide all the nutrition a person needs.

Going with gravity: Manual IV systems

Before the introduction of infusion pumps, nurses administered IV fluids manually (see the next section for details on automated IV systems). Most hospitals today use infusion pumps, but they aren't in universal use. You may find that smaller hospitals, extended care centers, hospices, and even some units in larger facilities don't have infusion pumps. So you need to know the basics of using a manual IV system. Following are the components of a manual IV system:

- **Pole:** In manual IV systems, gravity infuses the fluid in the IV bag. So the bag needs to hang from a *pole*.

  Keep in mind that a manual IV system is gravity dependent. The higher you hang the bag on the pole, the higher the pressure that's generated to force the fluid into the vein. Most IV bags are hung at least 3 feet above the patient's chest area.

- **IV bag:** The *IV bag* (or bottle) contains the medication or fluid. (See the section "Beginning with the IV bag" for more details.)
- **Lines:** The *lines* are plastic tubes that deliver the fluid to the needle.
- **Injection port:** The *injection port* is an opening in the line, where medical professionals can inject additional medications or fluids so they go into the patient via the IV.
- **Slide clamp:** The *slide clamp* is a small clamp that surrounds the line. You slide it to temporarily stop an IV infusion. It works the same way as when you kink a garden hose to temporarily stop the flow of water.
- **Drip chamber:** The *drip chamber* is a clear vessel located between the bag and the line. It allows air to rise from the fluid so it won't enter the patient's bloodstream. You use the drip chamber to count the number of drops that fall into it over a period of one minute.
- **Roller clamp:** The *roller clamp* (also called the *roller adapter* or *flow-control clamp*) is a mechanism you use to manually adjust the rate of the IV infusion. You use your thumb to move the roller, and the drip rate increases or decreases, depending on which way you move the roller.
- **Needle:** The *needle* introduces the IV fluid into the patient's vein. A 20-gauge (20 G) needle is the one most frequently used for manual infusions.

Figure 11-1 shows a schematic drawing of a manual IV setup.

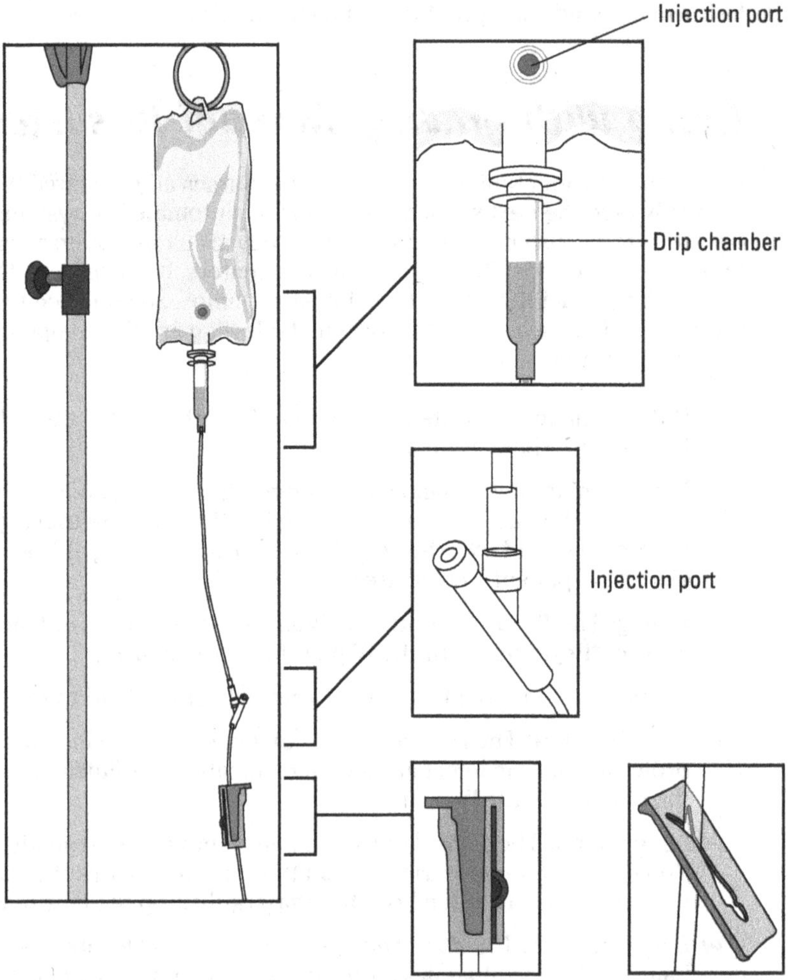

Injection port

Drip chamber

Injection port

Roller clamp

Slide clamp

Figure 11-1: Schematic drawing of an IV setup.

Getting pumped up: Automated IV systems

An *electronic infusion pump* (also called a *volumetric pump*) is a pump that calculates and delivers programmed flow rates and drip rates for IV fluids; it's controlled by a sophisticated multifeatured computer (see the section "Infusion 101: Calculating Flow Rates, Infusion Times, and Drip Rates" for details on flow rates and drip rates). The infusion pump doesn't depend on gravity to send fluid into the vein. Rather, the pump itself pushes the fluid into the vein. In general, infusion pumps are easier to program, easier to maintain, and a heck of a lot more accurate than their gravity-dependent counterparts. Figure 11-2 shows an electronic infusion pump.

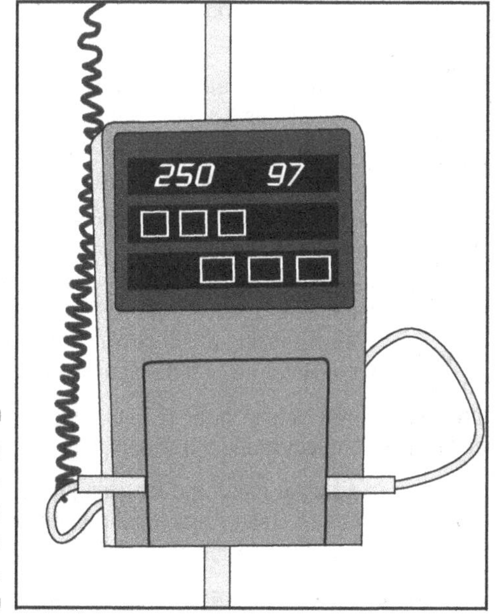

Figure 11-2: An electronic infusion pump.

Commonly, you see electronic infusion pumps in hospital settings and sometimes in extended care facilities and even in homes. Although infusion pumps may not be in every medical center, they are in the vast majority of hospital centers, so expect to work with them early on in your medical career.

Although infusion pumps can do a lot for you, you need to stay cautious and alert whenever you use them. Because they're automated systems, you need to monitor the IV site. Watch to make sure that the IV doesn't dislodge and cause a needle stick, leading to an infiltrated vein. If the vein becomes infiltrated, the site can become *extravasated* (a condition where fluid enters the tissue surrounding the vein).

Before you start using a modern electronic infusion pump, be sure to look at the user's manual. (It can contain between 50 and 200 pages!) You can choose many options when you program it, including units of delivery, timing, primary/secondary deliveries, and alerts. This wonder of modern medicine can be a real headache for you until you become familiar with it. But then it's easy to work with. Just remember: You can't afford to program the pump incorrectly.

What you need to know about IV history

To be a great success in the medical field, you only need to know, er, everything. Your focus must be on keeping patients safe, empathizing with patients, knowing your meds, knowing how to deliver them, knowing your calculations, and being a great administrator. Too much to ask? Yes, probably, but you're up to it, so let's add another element to the list — history, particularly IV history.

The history of IV infusions had a rocky start. At first, it was all about transfusing blood, and nobody knew anything about blood. The first recorded attempt was in 1492, when a doctor tried to give Pope Innocent VIII a blood transfusion. That didn't work out too well. The doctor administered the blood through the mouth. The Pope fell into a coma and died. The three boys the doctor took the blood from died, too.

Fast forward to 1656, when Sir Christopher Wren, the famous scientist and architect, used a quill attached to a pig's bladder to inject opium into a vein. It worked! He also successfully used a syringe to transfer blood from one dog to another.

In 1667, Dr. Jean-Baptiste Denis, physician to King Louis XIV of France, had another success. He transfused the blood of a sheep into a 15-year old boy, who recovered.

Leap ahead to the great cholera epidemics. In 1832, Dr. Thomas Latta gave a saline injection to a person with "blue" cholera and watched a miraculous recovery. By 1876, Dr. Sidney Ringer was proposing an electrolyte infusion of what would later be called *Ringer's solution.*

But it wasn't until 1933 that Baxter Travenol Company marketed IV solutions.

And what about the infusion pump? All credit goes to Dean Kamen, who invented the first wearable infusion pump in 1973.

Dosing Heparin, Insulin, and Other Infusions

In addition to intravenous fluids, you can administer diuretic infusions like furosemide (Lasix) or bumetanide (Bumex) via a continuous infusion. Other medications, such as heparin, insulin, and nutrition like total parenteral nutrition (TPN) can also be administered as continuous infusions. (Take a look at Chapters 13, 17, and 18 for a ton more details.

Heparin and insulin are measured in *units.* This can be a little confusing, especially since most calculations use mL/hr and gtt/min. For an IV continuous infusion, you're given the units and you need to calculate the flow rate in mL/hr.

You have to administer a premixed solution of heparin 25,000 units in 500 mL of NS at 1,200 units per hour. What's the infusion rate (flow rate)?

To solve this problem, use the ratio-proportion method and follow these steps:

1. **Set up the following proportion to calculate how many units are in 1 mL:**

   $$\frac{500 \text{ mL}}{25{,}000 \text{ units}} = \frac{1 \text{ mL}}{x \text{ units}}$$

2. **Cross-multiply and solve.**

   $500x = 25{,}000$

   $x = 50$

   There are 50 units in 1 mL.

3. **Set up the following proportion to calculate how many mL you give in an hour to administer 1,200 units in an hour:**

   $$\frac{50 \text{ units}}{1 \text{ mL}} = \frac{1{,}200 \text{ units}}{x \text{ mL}}$$

4. **Cross-multiply and solve.**

   $50x = 1{,}200$

   $x = 24$

   The flow rate is 24 mL/hr.

You're instructed to administer a continuous insulin infusion at 15 units/hr for a patient in diabetic ketoacidosis (DKA). The pharmacy prepares the insulin — 100 units of regular insulin in 100 mL of normal saline. What's the infusion rate (flow rate)?

To find out, use the ratio-proportion method and follow these steps:

1. **Set up the following proportion to calculate the infusion rate in mL/hr:**

   $$\frac{100 \text{ units}}{100 \text{ mL}} = \frac{15 \text{ units}}{x \text{ mL}}$$

   If you're wondering where these numbers come from, remember that the concentration of insulin is 100 units/100 mL and that the rate of unit/hr is given.

2. **Cross-multiply and solve.**

   $100x = 15 \times 100$

   $100x = 1{,}500$

   $x = 15$

   There are 15 units in 15 mL. The infusion rate is 15 mL/hr.

Note: Insulin is often dosed in a 1:1 ratio, as in the preceding example.

If you ever have any questions about any medication calculation, especially calculations for insulin and heparin, don't hesitate to ask a colleague or call the pharmacist. Solutions of insulin and heparin are prepared in concentrations that reduce calculation error, as the example of 100 units/100 mL shows. After all, a wrong dosage calculation of either medication could potentially be fatal. Heparin, being a blood thinner, can cause serious bleeding complications. Insulin can cause profound hypoglycemia if overdosed.

You're instructed to give a patient in congestive heart failure (CHF) furosemide (Lasix) as a continuous infusion at a dose of 20 mg/hr. The concentration of furosemide is 500 mg in 50 mL of NS. What's the infusion rate in mL/hr?

To find out, use the ratio-proportion method and follow these steps:

1. **Set up the following proportion to calculate the mg of furosemide in 1 mL:**

   $$\frac{500 \text{ mg}}{50 \text{ mL}} = \frac{x \text{ mg}}{1 \text{ mL}}$$

2. **Cross-multiply and solve.**

   $50x = 500$

   $x = 10$

   There are 10 mg of furosemide in 1 mL of solution.

3. **Set up the following proportion to calculate how many mL contain 20 mg:**

   $$\frac{10 \text{ mg}}{1 \text{ mL}} = \frac{20 \text{ mg}}{x \text{ mL}}$$

4. **Cross-multiply and solve.**

   $10x = 20$

   $x = 2$

   The infusion rate is 2 mL/hr.

Note: The pharmacy often prepares furosemide solution at a 10:1 concentration to reduce errors in dosage calculations.

Real-Life Practice: Finding the Drip Rate of a Dose of Albumin

You're instructed to administer albumin 25% in 50 mL over 2 hr. The drop factor is 20 gtt/mL. What's the drip rate?

To solve this problem, follow these steps:

1. **Convert the infusion time from hours to minutes.**

   $$x = 2 \text{ hr} \times \frac{60 \text{ min}}{1 \text{ hr}}$$

   $$x = \frac{120}{1} \text{ min}$$

   $$x = 120 \text{ min}$$

2. **Use the drip rate formula to calculate the drip rate.**

   $$\text{drip rate (gtt/min)} = \frac{50 \text{ mL} \times 20 \text{ gtt/mL}}{120 \text{ min}}$$

   $$\text{drip rate (gtt/min)} = 8.33$$

   The drip rate is 8 gtt/min.

Real-Life Practice: Calculating Infusion Time for D5W

You're asked to administer D5W 1,000 mL at 75 mL/hr. What's the infusion time?

To find out, just use the infusion time formula, like so:

infusion time (hr) = 1,000 mL ÷ 75 mL/hr

infusion time (hr) = 13.33

The infusion time is 13.33 hr, or 13 hours and 20 minutes.

Real-Life Practice: The Heparin Bolus and Maintenance Infusion

You're instructed to administer heparin via a weight-based regimen. First, you have to give an 80 unit/kg bolus, and then you have to start an infusion at 18 unit/kg/hr (units per kilogram of patient body weight per hour). The heparin is 25,000 units in 500 mL of 0.9% NS. The patient weighs 220 pounds. What's the flow rate in mL/hr?

To solve this problem, use a conversion factor and the ratio-proportion method. Follow these steps:

1. **Use the conversion factor 1 kg = 2.2 lb to convert the patient's weight from lb to kg.**

   $$x = 220 \text{ lb} \times \frac{1 \text{ kg}}{2.2 \text{ lb}}$$

   $$x = 100 \text{ kg}$$

   The patient weighs 100 kg.

2. **Set up the following equation to figure out how many units of heparin you need for the bolus, based on patient body weight:**

   100 kg × 80 units/kg = 8,000 units

3. **Set up the following proportion to figure out how many mL of solution you need for the bolus.**

   $$\frac{25{,}000 \text{ units}}{500 \text{ mL}} = \frac{8{,}000 \text{ units}}{x \text{ mL}}$$

4. **Cross-multiply and solve.**

   $$25{,}000x = 4{,}000{,}000$$

   $$x = 160$$

   You deliver the bolus of 8,000 units in 160 mL of solution.

5. **Set up the following equation to determine how many units of heparin you need for the infusion, based on patient body weight.**

   100 kg × 18 units/kg = 1,800 units

   You give 1,800 units per hour.

6. **Set up the following proportion to calculate how many mL of solution you need for the infusion of 18 units/kg/hr (1,800 units/hr):**

$$\frac{25{,}000 \text{ units}}{500 \text{ mL}} = \frac{1{,}800 \text{ units}}{x \text{ mL}}$$

7. **Cross-multiply and solve.**

$$25{,}000x = 900{,}000$$

$$x = 36$$

   The infusion rate is 36 mL/hr.

Chapter 12

Working with Reconstituted Solutions: It's like Magic

In This Chapter

- Considering the fundamentals of reconstituting a solution
- Reconstituting single-strength and multiple-strength medications
- Performing some medical dosing calculations using reconstituted solutions

Medications come in many forms: tablets, capsules, liquid suspensions, premixed intravenous (IV) solutions, topical gels, and irrigants. However, many medications that you dose in liquid form (especially antibiotics, such as amoxicillin) don't come as liquids; instead, they're manufactured and delivered to you as powders.

The powder form keeps these meds stable. When they become liquid solutions, they quickly lose stability. But to make a powder med usable, you have to *reconstitute* it (meaning, you have to turn it into a liquid solution).

In this chapter, we take a look at the parts of a reconstituted solution and show you how to prepare solutions. Specifically, we show you what mathematical calculations you need to do to reconstitute meds so you can properly administer them. Both the ratio-proportion and formula methods work well for these dosage calculations (see Chapter 8 for more on these methods).

When Solute Met Diluent: A Love Story

Reconstitution is the process of adding a liquid to a medication to turn it into a liquid suspension so that you can administer it to a patient. The route of administration for liquid suspensions is most often IV, but it may also be by injection or even by mouth.

Reconstitution has a few variants. For example, many moms reconstitute infant formula for oral administration, but this reconstitution is for feeding, not medicating, the baby. Changing the strength of a topical solution like hydrogen peroxide is like reconstitution, but it's more properly called *dilution*.

The three aspects of reconstitution are the components, the instructions, and the method. We look at each aspect in more detail in the following sections.

The components

Reconstitution has the following three components:

- **Solute:** The *solute* is the medication in powder form.
- **Diluent:** The *diluent* (sometimes called the *solvent*) is the liquid you mix with the solute.
- **Solution:** The *solution* is the liquid suspension that results from mixing the solute and the diluent.

What type of diluent do you use to create the solution you need to administer? It depends on the medication; find the answer on the med's label or package insert. Common diluents include sterile water, a 5% dextrose solution (D5W), or 0.9% isotonic saline (called *normal saline* or *NS*). Some medications allow you to use more than one diluent.

Normal saline is itself a reconstituted solution, but the manufacturer does the reconstitution work for you. NS contains 9 g of sodium chloride (NaCl) in 1 L of water.

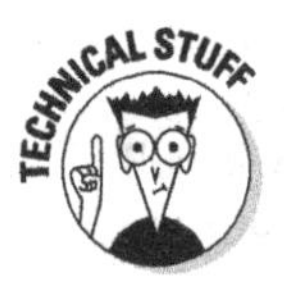

USP sterile water for injection is, well, water that's sterile. It has no buffer, antimicrobial agent, or *bacteriostat* (a substance that inhibits the growth of bacteria).

The instructions

To find out how much diluent to use to reconstitute a medication, read the med's label. If the info isn't on the label, read the package insert. Sometimes you can also consult a drug reference to find the instructions you need.

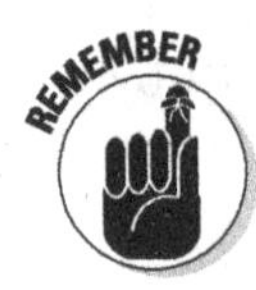

Before you reconstitute any solution, you must answer the following questions. The med's label or package insert has the answers.

- What type of diluent do you need?
- How much liquid do you need to dilute the solution?
- What's the total volume?
- What's the strength of the solution? Is it single strength or multiple strength? (See the sections "Reconstituting single-strength meds" and "Using the right concentration of a multiple-strength medication" for details.)
- After you reconstitute, how much time do you have to administer the solution before it becomes unstable? Can you refrigerate any extra solution?

The method

Here's a very general method for reconstituting a powder:

1. **Choose a syringe with the correct capacity.**
2. **Inject air into the diluent equal to the amount of diluent you will draw.**
3. **Draw out the diluent.**
4. **Squirt the diluent into the vial with the solute.**
5. **Shake well.**
6. **Draw out the amount of solution you need to administer.**

Be sure to check a med's label or package insert before you reconstitute it. Check this information every time you reconstitute a med; reconstitution instructions may change.

The story of magic powder

So you thought magic was a thing of fairy-tales and make-believe? Well, think again! Seventeenth-century medicine had its very own magic powder, called the *powder of sympathy*, or *weapon salve*. The powder of sympathy was a form of sympathetic magic. Surgeons applied the powder to the weapon that caused a wound, expecting that administering the med would heal the wound. No reconstitution required — all they had to do was sprinkle it on.

Rudolf Goclenius the Younger, a German physician and professor of medicine, first published the powder of sympathy idea in 1608. Robert Fludd brought the concept to England in the mid-1600s. His book about the salve was published in 29 editions.

We swear on the PDR (Physicians' Desk Reference) that we don't make these things up! Find out more about the powder of sympathy and other strange medical practices in Thomas Joseph Pettigrew's *On Superstitions Connected with the History and Practice of Medicine and Surgery*, published in 1844.

Working through the Process of Reconstitution

Reconstitution is generally a very straightforward process. To do successful reconstitutions, you must carefully read the medication labels and carefully measure the diluents. If you exercise care, your dosing will be successful. If you're careless, however, you run a real risk of making a serious dosing error.

Many times directions for reconstitution don't appear on the drug label itself, and you need to read the package insert for more information. If you have any questions after reading the package insert, call the pharmacist for more information.

The following sections show you how to reconstitute single-strength medications, explain the importance of concentration in multiple-strength meds, and discuss storage options for leftover reconstituted meds.

Reconstituting single-strength meds

A *single-strength medication* is reconstituted with a specific quantity of diluent to yield a precise concentration. The following sections walk you through four different reconstitution examples for single-strength meds.

Reconstituting amoxicillin

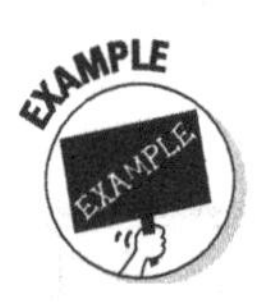

You're asked to administer amoxicillin 500 mg PO q12h (orally every 12 hours). The med comes in an oral suspension form that you must reconstitute to 250 mg/5 mL. How many teaspoons (tsp) will you administer with each dose?

To solve this problem, use the ratio-proportion method and follow these steps:

1. **Follow the instructions on the medication label to reconstitute the solution.**

   For a 100 mL bottle, you need 74 mL of water to reconstitute. For this particular medication, add ⅓ of the diluent at the beginning and shake the bottle vigorously. Then add the remaining ⅔ of the diluent and give the bottle another good shake.

   Note: As a practical matter, in most institutions, the pharmacist does the reconstitution.

2. **Use the ratio-proportion method to set up the following proportion:**

$$\frac{\text{known equivalent}}{\text{known equivalent}} = \frac{\text{known equivalent}}{\text{desired equivalent}}$$

$$\frac{250 \text{ mg}}{5 \text{ mL}} = \frac{500 \text{ mg}}{x \text{ mL}}$$

3. **Cross-multiply and solve.**

   $250x = 2{,}500$

   $x = 10$

   The answer is 10 mL. You must administer doses of 10 mL.

4. **Convert from mL to tsp by using the following equation and the conversion factor 1 tsp = 5 mL:**

   desired unit = given unit × conversion factor

   $$x \text{ tsp} = 10 \text{ mL} \times \frac{1 \text{ tsp}}{5 \text{ mL}}$$

   $$x \text{ tsp} = \frac{10 \text{ tsp}}{5}$$

   $$x \text{ tsp} = 2$$

   You give 2 tsp every 12 hours. This equation is easy to solve, and you can do it in your head. (Turn to Chapter 4 for more details on converting units.)

Reconstituting tobramycin

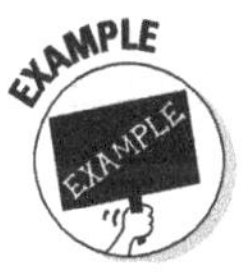

You're asked to administer tobramycin 100 mg IV q8h (intravenously every 8 hours) for a serious bacterial infection. Tobramycin comes in powder form, so you must reconstitute it. How many mL do you administer per dose?

Before you can start the dosing calculations for this problem, you must first evaluate the medication label, which appears in Figure 12-1, and then determine whether the prescribed dose is safe to administer to your particular patient.

Here's what the label tells you:

- You must add 30 mL of diluent.
- The diluent must be sterile water.
- The final concentration is 40 mg/mL.
- You must refrigerate the med after reconstitution and use it up within 24 hours.

Now it's time to determine whether the dose is safe to administer. Tobramycin is in a group of meds called the *aminoglycosides* (uh-*mee*-no-glike-o-sides). These meds are dosed based on patient weight. Your adult patient weighs 120 kg, and the package insert says that you can give no more than 3 mg/kg per day.

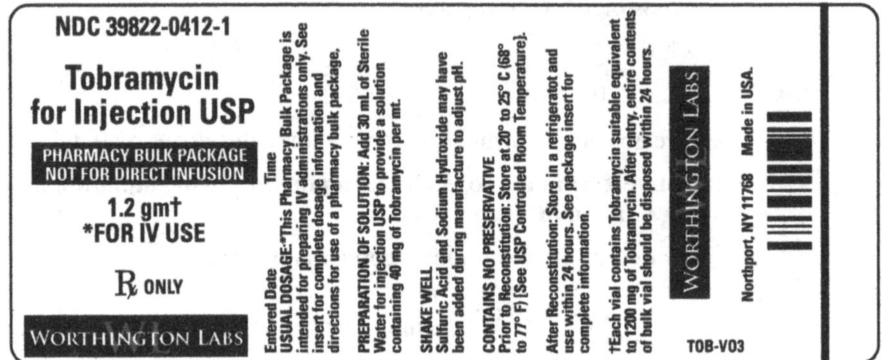

Figure 12-1: Tobramycin label.

Reprinted with permission from X-Gen Pharmaceuticals.

To find out if the prescribed dose (100 mg every 8 hours) is less than 3 mg/kg per day, calculate how many total mg are in the maximum daily dose compared to your prescribed dose.

- **Maximum dose:** $120 \text{ kg} \times \frac{3 \text{ mg}}{1 \text{ kg}} = 360 \text{ mg}$
- **Prescribed dose:** $\frac{100 \text{ mg}}{8 \text{ hr}} \times \frac{24 \text{ hr}}{1 \text{ day}} = \frac{2{,}400 \text{ mg}}{8 \text{ day}} = \frac{300 \text{ mg}}{1 \text{ day}}$

The prescribed dose of 100 mg every 8 hours totals 300 mg/day and is within the safe dosing range.

Finally, you're ready to start calculating the dose. You can use either the formula method or the ratio-proportion method to do so. Which one you use is truly a matter of preference, although we tend to use the ratio-proportion method in our calculations. (See Chapter 8 for more on these methods.)

To find out how many mL you need to administer for each dose of tobramycin, follow these steps:

1. **Use the formula method to calculate the dose in mL.**

   The label tells you that the final concentration is 40 mg/mL. You need to administer 100 mg, so set up the following equation:

$$D \text{ (dose)} = \frac{O \text{ (ordered)}}{H \text{ (have)}} \times Q \text{ (quantity)}$$

$$D \text{ mL} = \frac{100 \text{ mg (ordered)}}{40 \text{ mg (have)}} \times 1 \text{ mL (quantity)}$$

2. **Multiply and solve.**

   $$D \text{ mL} = \frac{100 \times 1}{40}$$

   $$D \text{ mL} = 2.5$$

   You must administer doses of 2.5 mL.

Alternately, you can use the ratio-proportion method to do the same thing by solving the following equation:

$$\frac{40 \text{ mg}}{1 \text{ mL}} = \frac{100 \text{ mg}}{x \text{ mL}}$$

$$40x = 100$$

$$x = 2.5$$

You must administer doses of 2.5 mL.

Reconstituting deferoxamine

You're asked to give deferoxamine 1 g (1,000 mg) IV to treat heavy metal poisoning. Deferoxamine comes in a 2 g (2,000 mg) vial. According to the drug label, you need to add 20 mL of sterile water for a final concentration of 95 mg/mL. How many mL do you need to administer?

To find out, use the ratio-proportion method and follow these steps:

1. **Set up the following proportion:**

   $$\frac{95 \text{ mg}}{1 \text{ mL}} = \frac{1{,}000 \text{ mg}}{x \text{ mL}}$$

2. **Cross-multiply and solve.**

   $$95x = 1{,}000$$

   $$x = 10.5$$

   You must administer a dose of 10.5 mL of deferoxamine.

Reconstituting hydrocortisone

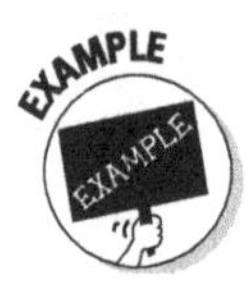

You're ordered to administer hydrocortisone (Solu-Cortef) 60 mg IV q8h. This hydrocortisone preparation is manufactured as a sterile powder. You read the package insert and see that the med needs to be reconstituted with 2 mL of either bacteriostatic water (Bacteriostatic Water for Injection, USP) or 0.9% sodium chloride (NS). The final concentration of this solution is 100 mg/mL. How many mL do you need to administer per dose?

To find out, use the ratio-proportion method and follow these steps:

1. **Set up the following proportion:**

   $$\frac{100 \text{ mg}}{1 \text{ mL}} = \frac{60 \text{ mg}}{x \text{ mL}}$$

2. **Cross-multiply and solve.**

   $100x = 60$

   $x = 0.6$

   You must administer 0.6 mL of hydrocortisone every 8 hours.

Using the right concentration of a multiple-strength medication

In contrast to the single-strength meds that we cover in the preceding section, *multiple-strength medications* can be reconstituted to different *concentrations* (or strengths). For example, some penicillins have as many as four possible concentrations on the label. The concentration you achieve through reconstitution depends on the amount of diluent you use.

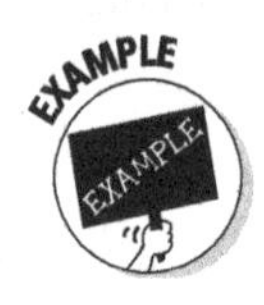

You're ordered to administer ceftriaxone (Rocephin) 250 mg IM times one dose. Ceftriaxone comes in 500 mg and 1,000 mg vials. According to the package insert, reconstituting the 500 mg vial with 1.8 mL of sterile water results in a final concentration of 250 mg/mL. The package insert also says that if you were to reconstitute the same 500 mg powder vial with 1.0 mL of sterile water, the final concentration would be 350 mg/mL. How many mL do you need to administer for a 250 mg IM dose?

To solve this problem, you don't even have to do any math because the package insert describes exactly what to do. Simply read the insert and follow the instructions for the 250 mg/mL concentration. Reconstitute the med with 1.8 mL of sterile water. Then withdraw 1.0 mL to administer.

Storing leftover meds

After you've given a medication to a patient, you often have some left over. The label or the package insert tells you what the "shelf life" of the reconstituted med is. Most med labels tell you how long they can be used if stored at room temperature and how long they can be used if refrigerated. Adhere to these instructions exactly.

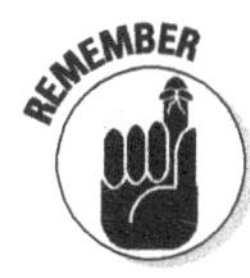

For any medication that's left over, label the vial with the following info and then store it according to its label's instructions:

- Name of the med administered
- Concentration of the med administered
- Date administered
- Expiration date of the med
- Route of administration (typically IM or IV)
- Your initials

Real-Life Practice: Reconstituting and Dosing Olanzapine

You're asked to administer 7.5 mg of olanzapine (Zyprexa), an antipsychotic, IM. It comes in powder form, and you must reconstitute it. According to the label, you must add 2.1 mL of sterile water to a 10 mg powder vial for a final concentration of 5 mg/mL. How many mL do you administer?

To solve this problem, use the ratio-proportion method and follow these steps:

1. **Set up the following proportion:**

   $$\frac{5 \text{ mg}}{1 \text{ mL}} = \frac{7.5 \text{ mg}}{x \text{ mL}}$$

2. **Cross-multiply and solve.**

   $5x = 7.5$

   $x = 1.5$

   You must administer 1.5 mL intramuscularly.

Real-Life Practice: Figuring the Dosage of Reconstituted Ampicillin

You need to administer ampicillin at a dose of 150 mg/kg of patient weight per day in divided doses to be given every 8 hours. Your patient weighs 80 pounds. The medication is available in 2 g (2,000 mg) powder. Use a diluent of 50 mL 0.9% NS (normal saline solution) for a final concentration of 40 mg/mL. What's the dose in mL?

To solve this problem, use some basic conversion factors and the ratio-proportion method. Follow these steps:

1. **Use the conversion factor 1 kg = 2.2 lb to convert the patient's weight from lb to kg.**

   $$\text{kg} = \text{lb} \times \frac{1\text{ kg}}{2.2\text{ lb}}$$

   $$\text{kg} = 80\text{ lb} \times \frac{1\text{ kg}}{2.2\text{ lb}}$$

   $$\text{kg} = 36.4$$

   The patient weighs 36.4 kg.

2. **Calculate the total dose for 24 hours.**

   $$36.4\text{ kg} \times \frac{150\text{ mg}}{1\text{ kg}} = 5{,}460\text{ mg}$$

   The maximum dose for 24 hours is approximately 5,400 mg. It's okay to round down from 5,460 mg to 5,400 mg because the difference of 60 mg is insignificant.

3. **Calculate the single dose to be given every 8 hours.**

   $5{,}400 \div 3 = 1{,}800$

   Each dose should contain 1,800 mg. (In case you're wondering, to find out how many single doses you have to give in one day, just divide 24 by 8 to get 3.)

4. **Convert mg to mL by setting up the following proportion:**

$$\frac{40 \text{ mg}}{1 \text{ mL}} = \frac{1{,}800 \text{ mg}}{x \text{ mL}}$$

5. **Cross-multiply and solve.**

$40x = 1{,}800$

$x = 45$

Each dose, given every 8 hours, is 45 mL.

Real-Life Practice: Reconstituting and Dosing a Multiple-Strength Medication

You're asked to administer pantoprazole (Protonix) 20 mg IV BID (twice daily). Protonix comes as a 40 mg powder; it's a multiple-strength med. How much you dilute the product depends on the type of infusion you're giving.

According to the package insert, you can reconstitute the med for both 2-minute and 15-minute infusions. For a 2-minute infusion, you must reconstitute 40 mg Protonix powder with 10 mL of 0.9% saline (NS) to achieve a final concentration of 4 mg/mL. For a 15-minute infusion, you dilute this solution further by combining it with 100 mg of 0.9% NS to get a concentration of 0.4 mg/mL.

How many mL do you administer for a 2-minute infusion? How many mL do you administer for a 15-minute infusion?

To calculate the mL you need for a 2-minute infusion, use the ratio-proportion method and follow these steps:

1. **Set up the following proportion:**

$$\frac{4 \text{ mg}}{1 \text{ mL}} = \frac{20 \text{ mg}}{x \text{ mL}}$$

2. **Cross-multiply and solve.**

$4x = 20$

$x = 5$

You administer 5 mL intravenously over 2 minutes.

To calculate the mL you need for a 15-minute infusion, use the ratio-proportion method and follow these steps:

1. **Set up the following proportion:**

   $$\frac{0.4 \text{ mg}}{1 \text{ mL}} = \frac{20 \text{ mg}}{x \text{ mL}}$$

2. **Cross-multiply and solve.**

   $$0.4x = 20$$

   $$x = 50$$

   You administer 50 mL intravenously over 15 minutes.

Part IV
Dosing in Special Situations

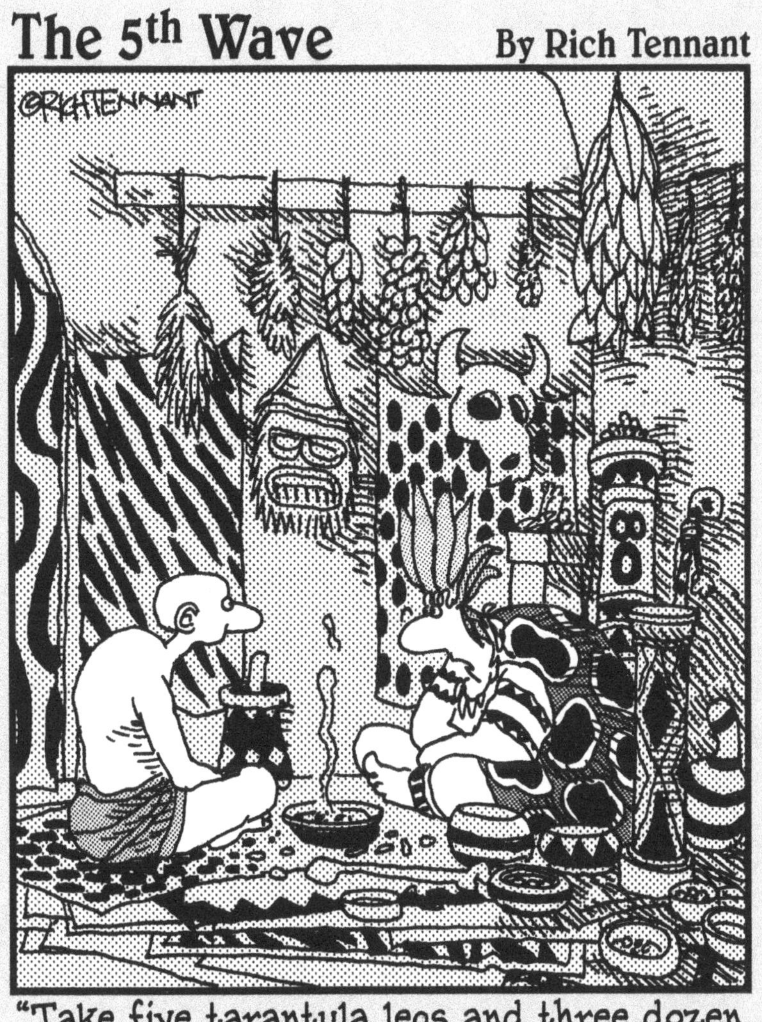

"Take five tarantula legs and three dozen fly eyes, and call me in the morning."

In this part . . .

Part IV looks at special medical situations. Chapter 13 is all about dosing insulin, and Chapter 14 shows you how to dose correctly for pregnant women. Chapter 15 is devoted to administering meds for children. In Chapter 16, you read about dosing changes and recalculating doses for changing patient conditions. Chapter 17 deals with the special requirements of critical care, and the part ends with Chapter 18, which looks at dosing for enteral and parenteral nutrition.

Chapter 13

Insulin: Call It a Miracle Drug

In This Chapter

- Dealing with diabetes
- Identifying different types of insulin
- Calculating insulin doses
- Simplifying insulin dosing with continuous infusions
- Practicing insulin dosage calculations with some real-life problems

Diabetes mellitus (the full name for diabetes) is a difficult disease, afflicting more and more people all the time. According to the American Diabetes Association (ADA), doctors diagnose more than 1.6 million new cases each year. It has reached epidemic proportions in the United States.

Diabetes is a metabolic disease in which the patient has high blood sugar (also known as a *high blood glucose level*) either because her body doesn't produce *insulin* (a hormone normally produced by the pancreas) or because her cells don't respond to it. As a result, the patient's body can't manage its blood sugar level.

Although diabetes has no cure, doctors can use medications and/or insulin to treat and manage it. If the body doesn't produce insulin, for example, medical science can help replace it. Insulin is a miracle drug because it can keep patients alive and productive.

In this chapter, you find out about the most important aspects of diabetes and the insulin you administer to treat it. We cover the different types of diabetes and insulin, explain how to measure and dose insulin, show how to administer it using an insulin syringe or IV, and, finally, provide some real-life practice problems to help you hone your dosage calculation skills.

Because insulin and diabetes are so prevalent today (and will surely be an important part of your medical career), make sure you don't skip this chapter!

Getting the Lowdown on Diabetes and Insulin

The insulin in a person's body is made by the *islets of Langerhans* (a region of specialized cells in the pancreas). What exactly does insulin do? Basically, its job is to facilitate glucose entry into the cells. After you eat a meal, the food is digested and glucose is a product of that digestion. Your cells need glucose as a fuel, just as a car needs gasoline. Without insulin, glucose can't get into your cells and do its job.

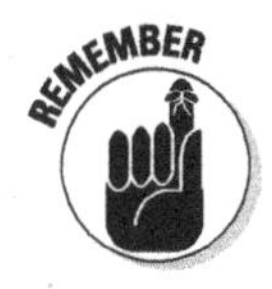

The three main types of diabetes mellitus are

- **Type 1 diabetes:** The body fails to produce insulin. With type 1 diabetes, the patient has to inject insulin.
- **Type 2 diabetes:** The body develops a resistance to the actions of insulin. Patients diagnosed with type 2 diabetes can often treat it by losing weight, changing their diet, and beginning an exercise program. Patients with type 2 diabetes also use medications, such as metformin (Glucophage), to help with blood sugar control. In very hard-to-control cases of type 2 diabetes, patients may need to use insulin.
- **Gestational diabetes:** A woman has a high blood glucose level during pregnancy. She needs to treat it with either a modified diet or insulin injections. This type of diabetes usually goes away after the woman gives birth.

Doctors can't precisely state the causes of diabetes, but a genetic predisposition in the patient appears to play some role. Type 1 diabetes may also be related to a bacterial or viral infection or to toxins. Type 2 diabetes seems to be connected more to age, obesity, and insufficient exercise (a difficult thing for coauthor Barry to write, given his age, weight, and lack of exercise). Other factors, including certain medications or illnesses involving the pancreas, may also be involved.

When the patient's body can't make insulin, or when the body develops a resistance to it, the patient — or you, if the patient is in a medical facility — must administer *exogenous* (outside the body) insulin. The most common route of administration for insulin is the subcutaneous injection (see the section "Getting the Most from the Dose with an Insulin Syringe" and Chapter 10 for details). But in critically ill patients, you may have to give insulin as a continuous infusion (see the section "Avoiding Confusion with the Continuous Infusion" and Chapter 11).

In the following sections, we introduce you to the basics of monitoring blood glucose and the types of insulin available for treating diabetes.

Diabetes can affect many organs in the body, but the principal organs include the eyes (*retinopathy*), the nerves (*neuropathy*), and the kidneys (*nephropathy*). In fact, diabetic nephropathy is a leading cause of kidney disease in the United States. People with diabetes also have an increased risk of coronary artery disease (CAD) as well as an increased incidence of peripheral arterial disease (PAD).

Monitoring blood glucose

Blood glucose level is the measurement of the amount of glucose in the blood. A normal level is about 4 mmol/L (millimoles/liter) or 72 mg/dL (milligrams/deciliter). A normal range for blood sugars is 70 to 100 mg/dL. Levels greater than 125 mg/dL on a fasting blood glucose test on two separate occasions is the definition of diabetes. While a patient's blood glucose level varies throughout the day, levels above or below the normal range indicate a medical problem.

Low blood glucose is called *hypoglycemia*. High blood glucose is called *hyperglycemia*. When a person's blood glucose level becomes very elevated (greater than 250 mg/dL), he can be at risk of a life-threatening medical condition called *diabetic ketoacidosis* (DKA). That's why you must pay close attention to blood glucose levels in your patients and monitor trends in blood sugar levels closely.

The *diabetic* (a person with diabetes) must monitor his blood glucose levels very closely to make sure they're in the normal range. To do so, he (or his healthcare professional, if the patient is in a clinic, hospital, or rehab center) uses an instrument called a *blood glucose meter* (sometimes called a Glucometer, which is a Bayer brand name).

Blood glucose meters come in all varieties, and some are really cool! For example, some meters store several months of readings, some create averages, some speak the reading to the patient, and some let the patient transfer readings to a computer.

The part that's not cool is that the patient must use a little spring-loaded *lancet* (a "finger pricker") to stab his finger to get a drop of blood for the test. Then he puts the drop on the meter's test strip, and the meter does the rest. Figure 13-1 shows a glucose meter.

The meter displays the test results in mg/dL or mmol/L. Whenever you're testing a patient's glucose levels, the only medical "dosing" task is to use the meter correctly and record the result. The amount of insulin you administer to the patient depends on the meter's reading.

If test results are below 50 mg/dL or above 250 mg/dL, the patient (if he's at home) or you (if he's in a hospital setting) must call the doctor right away!

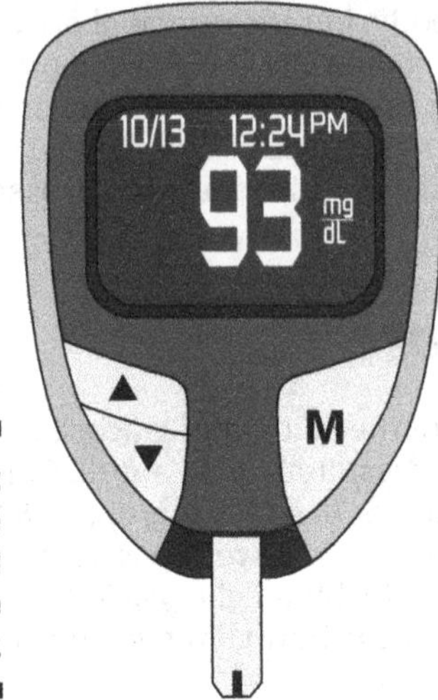

Figure 13-1: An example of a blood glucose meter.

Often the doctor orders the patient to check his blood glucose level before meals and at night. Sometimes the doctor may order the patient to check his *post-prandial* (meaning after meals) blood glucose level, too. Both fasting and post-prandial blood glucose levels can help determine insulin dosage.

The doctor often asks the patient to adjust his insulin dose, depending on his blood glucose levels. In the hospital setting, doctors often use a sliding scale for this purpose; see the section "Using the Sliding Scale for Insulin Doses" for details.

Typecasting insulin

Various types of insulin differ in their onset of action, peak, and duration of action. All medications are characterized by these three properties:

- **Onset of action:** When a drug first takes effect. For example, insulin lispro (Humalog) can begin to take effect in as little as 15 minutes. On the other hand, insulin glargine (Lantus) takes a couple of hours before it starts to kick in.
- **Peak:** When a medication exerts its maximum effect. For example, insulin lispro may take only about 15 minutes to first take effect, but its peak effect occurs approximately 1 to 2 hours after being injected subcutaneously.
- **Duration of action:** How long a medication stays in the body. Insulin lispro, for example, stays in the body for about 4 to 5 hours.

Some insulins go to work very rapidly and others are slower to act. Each type has a useful purpose.

Working fast with rapid-acting insulin

Rapid-acting (or *fast-acting*) *insulins* have an onset of action of about 15 minutes. They peak a couple of hours after administration. Examples include insulin lispro, insulin aspart (NovoLog), and insulin glulisine (Apidra). Because they have such short durations (only 4 to 5 hours), you (or the patient) usually administer them with meals.

Noticing the "R" in regular insulin

The most common type of insulin you administer is called *regular insulin.* Examples of this *short-acting insulin* include Novolin R and Humulin R. Regular insulins have an *R* in their names.

Regular insulin takes a little longer to kick in than rapid-acting insulin. The onset is about 30 minutes. It exerts its maximum effect about 2 to 4 hours after administration and stays in the body for about 6 hours before being eliminated.

Doctors often order regular insulin for sliding scale orders (see the later section "Using the Sliding Scale for Insulin Doses" for details).

Identifying interesting intermediates

NPH (Neutral Protamine Hagedorn) insulin (Humulin N, Novolin N, and Novolin NPH) is the quintessential example of an *intermediate-acting insulin.* Its onset is 1 to 2 hours, and it has its maximum effect anytime from 4 to 10 hours after administration. NPH can stay in the body for as long as 24 hours. An NPH insulin has an *N* or *NPH* on the drug label.

Looking at the long-acting insulins

The *long-acting insulin* glargine (Lantus) requires only one injection a day because it can last up to 24 hours. Lantus doesn't have a separate *L* on the drug label because it already starts with *L.*

But if you do see an *L* on the drug label (for example, Humulin L), it stands for *lente,* which means long acting. By the same token, a *U* on the label (for example, Humulin U) stands for *ultralente,* which means very long-acting.

The body eliminates insulin via the kidneys. If the patient who's getting insulin has kidney disease, the doc may need to reduce the insulin dosing. Why? Because the insulin will hang out longer in the body if the kidneys aren't working properly. The risk of hypoglycemia is a lot higher when you administer insulin to someone with kidney disease. Be aware of the patient's kidney function before dosing insulin. If you have any question about the insulin dosage, don't hesitate to contact the doctor or pharmacist.

Measuring Insulin in Units

Insulin isn't dosed in mg or mL. Instead, it's dosed in *units*. Only a few other medications are measured in units (heparin and vasopressin, for example, which you can read about in Chapter 17).

The majority of insulins come in a strength of 100 units/mL to make administering them easier. The label on the vial of 100 units/mL insulin often says "U-100" or "Use with U-100 insulin syringes only." The expectation is that you'll dispense it using a U-100 syringe (see the next section for details on this syringe). Figure 13-2 shows an insulin label.

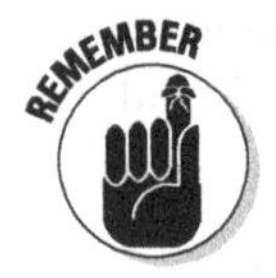

The *U* in U-100 on insulin's drug label isn't the same as the *U* that means the ultralente (or super-long-acting) type of insulin. U-100 refers to the insulin syringe you have to use to administer it.

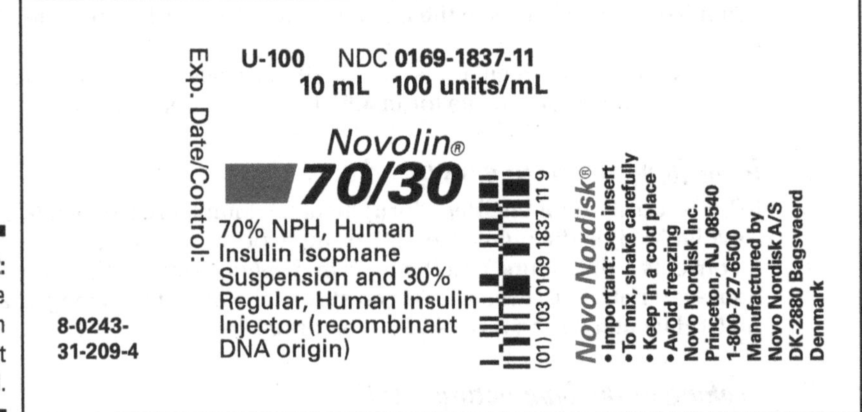

Figure 13-2: An example of an insulin product label.

Reprinted with permission from Novo Nordisk Pharmaceuticals.

Insulin is commonly dosed at 100 units/mL. Most vials contain 10 mL. How many units are in a vial?

To find out, use the ratio-proportion method and follow these steps (see Chapter 8 for details on this calculation method):

1. **Set up the following proportion:**

$$\frac{\text{known equivalent}}{\text{known equivalent}} = \frac{\text{desired equivalent}}{\text{known equivalent}}$$

$$\frac{100 \text{ units}}{1 \text{ mL}} = \frac{x \text{ units}}{10 \text{ mL}}$$

2. **Cross-multiply and solve.**

   $x = 100 \times 10$

   $x = 1{,}000$

   Each 10 mL vial contains 1,000 units.

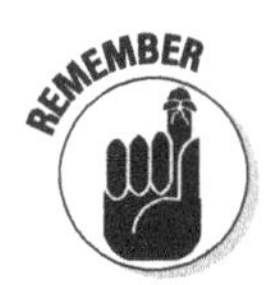

Everyone's insulin needs are different. So you need to know how many units are in a vial to make sure each at-home patient has an adequate supply of insulin.

You're discharging a patient, and the doctor writes an order for the patient to take NPH 30 units subcutaneously each day in the morning and 30 units subcutaneously before dinner. How many units is this for the month? How many vials will this person need every month?

To find out, follow these steps:

1. **Calculate the total units the patient needs each day.**

   30 units × 2 times/day = 60 units/day

2. **Calculate the total units the patient needs in a month; assume each month has 30 days.**

   60 units/day × 30 days = 1,800 units

   The patient will use 1,800 units every 30 days, or 1,800 units/month.

3. **Set up the following proportion to calculate how many vials the patient needs:**

   $$\frac{1{,}000 \text{ units}}{1 \text{ vial}} = \frac{1{,}800 \text{ units}}{x \text{ vial}}$$

4. **Cross-multiply and solve.**

   $1{,}000x = 1{,}800$

   $x = 1.8$

   The patient will use 1.8 vials/month, so the patient needs 2 vials of insulin per month. The patient will have 200 units left over at the end of the month, assuming the insulin dosing regimen doesn't change.

Some people require a lot of insulin. They may be prescribed vials with a concentration of 500 units/mL, which means that each 10 mL vial contains 5,000 units. Be careful when dosing insulin in a strength greater than 100 units/mL; there's no "standard" relationship of 100 units/mL. The concentration of 500 units/mL is five times stronger, and there's potential for overdosing the insulin.

Getting the Most from the Dose with an Insulin Syringe

To get the insulin from the vial into the patient's body, you (or the patient) usually have to administer it parenterally via subcutaneous injection into the fatty tissue beneath the skin. For this injection, you need a specially calibrated syringe called an *insulin syringe*. The *U-100 syringe*, as it's also called, is calibrated in units. (Sometimes you administer insulin intravenously. See the section "Avoiding Confusion with the Continuous Infusion" and Chapter 11 for details.)

On a standard 1 mL U-100 insulin syringe, the numbers start at 0 and go to 100 and correspond to units of insulin. Each line represents 2 units. This calibration makes it very easy to figure out how much insulin to administer.

Figure 13-3 shows an example of a U-100 insulin syringe.

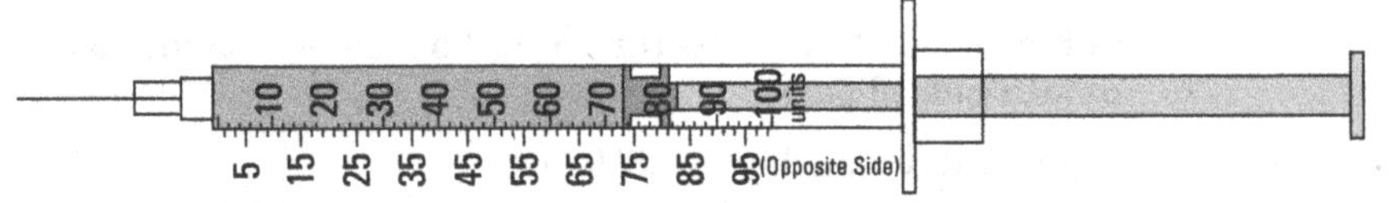

Figure 13-3: A U-100 insulin syringe.

The U-100 syringe comes in three sizes: 0.3 mL, 0.5 mL, and 1 mL. The calibration for each syringe is the same, but the syringe you use depends on the amount of insulin you're giving the patient:

- A 0.3 mL U-100 syringe holds up to 30 units of insulin. The marks go up to 30 on the syringe barrel.
- A 0.5 mL U-100 syringe holds up to 50 units of insulin. The marks go up to 50 on the syringe barrel.
- A 1 mL U-100 syringe holds up to 100 units of insulin. The marks go up to 100 on the syringe barrel.

You're ordered to administer 56 units of NPH insulin. How many mL is that?

This is so easy your eyes will fall out and you will develop hives if you don't get it. Just kidding, but really, this problem is super simple. Just use the ratio-proportion method and follow these steps:

1. **Set up the following proportion:**

$$\frac{100 \text{ units}}{1 \text{ mL}} = \frac{56 \text{ units}}{x \text{ mL}}$$

2. **Cross-multiply and solve.**

   $100x = 56$

   $x = 0.56$

   The 56 units of NPH insulin are equivalent to 0.56 mL.

Because you need to inject 56 units (or 0.56 mL) of NPH insulin, you use a 1 mL U-100 syringe. In between the large numbers that appear in multiples of 5 or 10 on the standard U-100 syringe, you see lines for every two units. These lines make it possible to accurately draw up 56 units from the vial.

Why would the doctor order such a unique insulin number for the patient? Well, everyone has different insulin requirements for both the short-acting and long-acting types. For this reason, insulin dosing is very individualized. No matter what dose a patient needs, you (and the patient) need to closely monitor the patient's blood glucose level and adjust (or *titrate*) the insulin dose until the blood glucose level is in an acceptable range.

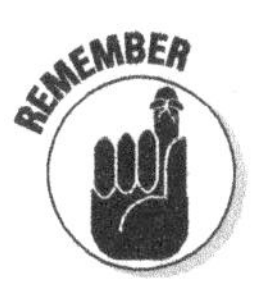

Although you may be interested in knowing how many mL you're injecting, as a practical matter, insulin orders call for units and the syringe is calibrated in units, so you don't need to do any calculating.

Combining Insulins

Insulins are separate entities, but you or the patient can combine them in a single injection. The doctor may order a combined dose if he believes the patient will benefit from getting a short-acting insulin and an intermediate-acting insulin in the same injection. After all, combining insulins means fewer injections for the patient to administer during the day.

This approach doesn't work for everyone; often it involves a discussion and teamwork between the doctor, patient, and dietitian to find out which insulin regimen works best for a particular individual. Often the doctor prescribes a combined insulin to be administered around mealtimes.

Some combinations of insulin are available as premixed solutions. For example, Humulin 70/30 is a premixed solution. Each unit of Humulin 70/30 contains 70% NPH insulin and 30% regular insulin. Here, the manufacturer has combined a short-acting insulin with an intermediate-acting insulin. The dosing is the same as regular insulin because Humulin 70/30 is supplied in vials with a concentration of 100 units/mL.

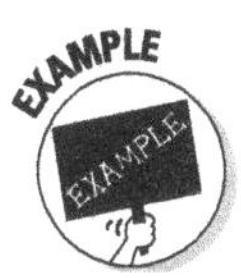

You're asked to administer 24 units of Humulin 70/30 in the morning and 24 units before dinner. The concentration of Humulin 70/30 is 100 units/mL. Using a 0.3 mL U-100 syringe, how many units would you draw up?

This question is a piece of cake! All you have to do is read the prescription. Draw up 24 units for the morning injection. Draw up 24 units for the evening injection.

Note: Humulin 70/30 comes as a suspension that settles between doses. You need to resuspend the insulin before each injection. Roll the vial between your hands until the insulin is uniformly cloudy.

When an insulin combination isn't premixed, you have to draw up two different types into one syringe to make whatever combination the doc prescribed.

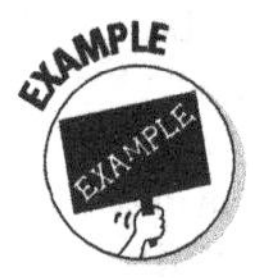

A doctor's order states to administer 30 units of NPH insulin and 26 units of Novolin R. How many units do you administer? What size syringe do you use?

1. **Determine the total to administer by adding the two insulin doses from the order.**

   30 units + 26 units = 56 units.

   You administer 56 units.

2. **Determine the syringe size, based on the total dose.**

   The dose of 56 units won't fit in a 0.3 mL syringe or a 0.5 mL syringe. So you must use a 1 mL U-100 syringe.

Giving it your best shot: Mixing insulins in a syringe

Here's a quick look at how to mix insulins in a syringe. Say you need to mix regular insulin (which is short acting and clear) with NPH (which is long acting and cloudy). Just follow these steps:

1. **Make sure your hands are clean, and use an alcohol pad to wipe off the vial tops.**
2. **Resuspend the NPH (the cloudy insulin) by rolling the vial between your hands.**
3. **Draw back the syringe to a position equal to the amount of NPH you'll inject, and inject the air into the NPH vial.**

   For example, if you're injecting 30 units of NPH, fill the syringe with air to the 30-unit mark and inject it into the vial.

4. **Draw back the syringe to a position equal to the amount of regular insulin you'll inject, and inject the air into the regular insulin vial.**

   For example, if you're injecting 16 units of regular insulin, fill the syringe with air to the 16-unit mark and inject it into the vial.

5. **Withdraw the regular insulin (the clear insulin) from its vial into the syringe.**

   In the example of 16 units, the syringe must fill to the 16-unit mark.

6. **Withdraw the NPH (the cloudy insulin) from its vial into the syringe.**

   In the example of 30 units, the syringe must fill to the 46-unit mark because 46 is the sum of the two insulin doses.

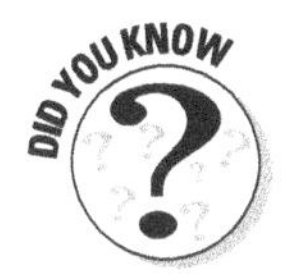

Did you know that insulin has another purpose besides lowering high blood glucose levels? Regular insulin, given intravenously, is a very effective method of treating *hyperkalemia* (very high potassium levels) in the body. Doctors usually order this insulin treatment as a single IV push, along with an ampule of glucose to make sure the blood glucose stays at a safe level while you're treating the high potassium level. An example of an order is 10 units of regular insulin with 50 mL 50% dextrose (D50).

Using the Sliding Scale for Insulin Doses

Many doctors write insulin orders with sliding scales to help medical professionals and patients know how much insulin to take, based on their blood glucose levels. A *sliding scale* is a table of dosages of regular insulin, based on the individual patient's blood glucose levels.

An example of a doctor's sliding scale order is

- If blood glucose is 150 or less, give no insulin.
- If blood glucose is 151–200, give 2 units regular insulin.
- If blood glucose is 201–250, give 4 units regular insulin.
- If blood glucose is 251–300, give 6 units regular insulin.
- If blood glucose is greater than 300, call the doctor.

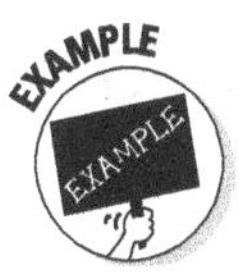

You check a diabetic patient's blood glucose level before her dinner and discover that it's 297. The doctor has provided the preceding sliding scale with his order. How much insulin do you administer?

This question is as easy as pie. Just read the sliding scale in the doctor's order to determine the insulin doses for each glucose level. The patient's blood glucose level is between 251 and 300 on the sliding scale, so you must give 6 units of regular insulin subcutaneously.

Avoiding Confusion with the Continuous Infusion

Sometimes doctors order continuous insulin therapy, particularly when the patient requires an alternative to multiple daily injections, has hyperglycemia, or is being treated for DKA. In these situations, the doctor orders the use of an insulin drip or an insulin pump. With either approach, you must pay close attention to the patient's blood glucose level. You likely need to monitor blood glucose levels every hour (q1h) initially and adjust the insulin drip as needed.

Close monitoring of the blood glucose level is especially important if the patient has DKA — a life-threatening condition that requires the patient to be on an insulin drip.

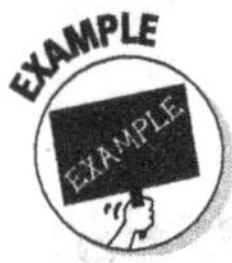

You're taking care of a patient on an insulin drip that consists of 50 units of regular insulin in 50 mL of normal saline at 12 units/hr. What's the infusion rate?

To solve this problem, use the ratio-proportion method and follow these steps:

1. **Set up the following proportion to convert units to mL:**

$$\frac{50\text{ units}}{50\text{ mL}} = \frac{12\text{ units}}{x\text{ mL}}$$

2. **Cross-multiply and solve.**

$$50x = 600$$

$$x = 12$$

The infusion rate is 12 mL/hr.

The concentration of the insulin infusion is 1:1 to minimize the risk of error and to simplify dosing calculations.

Real-Life Practice: Administering an Insulin Infusion to Treat DKA

You're taking care of a patient admitted to the ICU with DKA. He weighs 197 lb. The doctor's order says to give a regular insulin bolus of 0.15 units/kg followed by a regular insulin infusion of 100 units in 100 mL of normal saline at 0.1 units/kg/hr. How many units of insulin are in the bolus? How many mL make up the bolus? What's the flow rate of the drip?

To answer these three questions, use the basic conversion formula and the ratio-proportion method. Follow these steps:

1. **Use the conversion factor 1 kg = 2.2 lb to convert pounds to kg.**

desired unit = given unit × conversion factor

$$x \text{ kg} = 197 \text{ lb} \times \frac{1 \text{ kg}}{2.2 \text{ lb}}$$

$$x \text{ kg} = \frac{197}{2.2}$$

$$x \text{ kg} = 89.54$$

The patient weighs 89.54 kg.

2. **Set up and solve the following proportion to calculate the insulin bolus in units:**

$$\frac{1 \text{ kg}}{0.15 \text{ units}} = \frac{89.54 \text{ kg}}{x \text{ units}}$$

$$x = 0.15 \times 89.54$$

$$x = 13.431$$

Give the patient a bolus of 13 units of regular insulin.

3. **Set up and solve the following proportion to calculate the flow rate of the drip in units:**

$$\frac{1 \text{ kg}}{0.1 \text{ units}} = \frac{89.54 \text{ kg}}{x \text{ units}}$$

$$x = 0.1 \times 89.54$$

$$x = 8.954$$

The drip is 8.954 units for a patient weighing 89.54 kg. Administer 9 units/hr. (Notice that you can ignore the *hr* part of 0.1 units/kg/hr until you're finished calculating the units.)

4. **Set up and solve the following proportion to convert the flow rate of the drip from units/hr to mL/hr:**

$$\frac{100 \text{ units}}{100 \text{ mL}} = \frac{8.954 \text{ units}}{x \text{ mL}}$$

$$100x = 895.4$$

$$x = 8.954$$

The 8.954 units are equivalent to 8.954 mL. Infuse 9 mL/hr.

Real-Life Practice: Adjusting Insulin Levels Based on Glucose Levels

In a patient with DKA, the blood glucose levels gradually decrease toward normal. Your most recent measurement of blood glucose level is 234. The doctor's order states that if the blood glucose level is less than 250 mg/dL, you're to administer 1 L (1,000 mL) D5 ½ NS over 8 hours. You're also instructed to decrease the patient's insulin drip to 6 units/hr. The concentration of this drip is 100 units/100 mL. What are the flow rates for the two infusions?

To solve this problem, use the flow rate formula (see Chapter 11) and the ratio-proportion method. Follow these steps:

1. **Use the flow rate formula to calculate the flow rate for the dextrose (D5 ½ NS) infusion.**

   flow rate (mL/hr) = total volume ÷ designated time

   flow rate (mL/hr) = 1,000 mL ÷ 8 hr

   flow rate (mL/hr) = 125 mL/hr

   The flow rate of the D5 ½ NS infusion is 125 mL/hr.

2. **Set up the following proportion to calculate the flow rate for the insulin drip of 6 units/hr.**

   $$\frac{100 \text{ units}}{100 \text{ mL}} = \frac{6 \text{ units}}{x \text{ mL}}$$

3. **Cross-multiply and solve.**

   $100x = 600$

   $x = 6$

   The 6 units are equivalent to 6 mL. Adjust the flow rate to be 6 mL/hr.

Adjusting an insulin flow rate is fairly easy, given the 1:1 strength of insulin drips. Also, most protocols for patients in DKA order that you start a dextrose infusion after the blood glucose level falls to less than 250 because, while the blood sugar is at an acceptable level, the doctor won't stop the infusion until other blood chemistries normalize.

Chapter 14

Dosing for Two: The Pregnant Patient

In This Chapter

- Doing basic obstetrical dosing computations
- Observing both mother and fetus during and after medication administration
- Considering how nonpregnancy-related prescriptions can affect pregnant women
- Dosing for basic obstetrical complications with three pregnancy-related examples

Dosing medications for pregnant women is a two-sided puzzle because you need to know how any prescribed medication will affect both mother and fetus. You also have to consider the effects of the medications prescribed to the mother in conjunction with the pregnancy as well as those medications prescribed for other reasons, such as a chronic condition like hypertension, diabetes, or hypothyroidism. It's not uncommon for moms to be on multiple medications to manage these medical problems prior to becoming pregnant. You may be instructed to change a medication dose, discontinue it, or administer a safer and more appropriate substitute in order to avoid "double trouble!"

This chapter gives you the basics about dosing for the pregnant patient and her baby. Here, we give you a sense of which medications are commonly ordered during pregnancy and offer plenty of experience with dosing calculations for them. We provide some advice on monitoring Mom and baby during and after a medication has been administered. We also discuss the importance of being aware of any other medications Mom may be on and knowing the risks they may pose to her or the baby. Finally, we provide some example dosing scenarios for you to work through to get additional practice.

Calculations for Pregnancy-Related Situations

You can expect to see certain medications ordered during a pregnancy. Most of these pills and infusions relate to pregnancy-specific situations like the pregnancy itself, labor, and delivery. This section shows you how to calculate dosages related to the following four conditions common during pregnancy:

- Pregnancy-induced high blood pressure
- Eclampsia
- Cessation of uterine contractions
- Induction of uterine contractions

Reducing hypertension

Hypertension, also known as high blood pressure, is a problem that can develop before pregnancy, early in the pregnancy, or later in the second or third trimester. Hypertension that develops during pregnancy, usually after the 20th week of gestation (late in the second trimester), is called *gestational hypertension.*

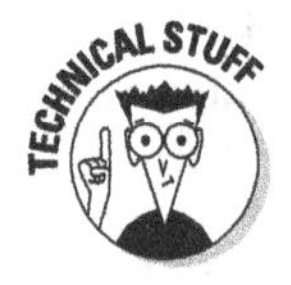

Gestational hypertension is defined as a BP (blood pressure) that's higher than 140/90. If you aren't fully up to speed on blood pressure measurements, head over to Chapter 3 for details on how to write true ratios and vital signs as ratios.

Many times you have to administer medications to help pregnant women lower their blood pressure. Pay attention to the signs of uncontrolled blood pressure, which can include headaches and double vision. If the mother-to-be had high blood pressure before her pregnancy, the doctor may have to change the medications when she becomes pregnant because certain high blood pressure medications (like ACE inhibitors, for example) are very bad for the fetus.

Some of the most common oral meds used to treat high blood pressure during pregnancy are labetalol (Normodyne), amlodipine, methyldopa (Aldomet), and hydralazine (Apresoline). They're considered safe for both the mom and the fetus.

In pregnancy, to get the dosage of these and other meds right, the physician sometimes has to do intricate dosing adjustments. To give you a little practice with making these adjustments, try the following example.

Ms. Jones has been recently diagnosed with pregnancy-induced high blood pressure. You must administer labetalol 150 mg BID (twice a day). The minimum dose of the drug is 100 mg tablets. How many tablets do you need to give Ms. Jones? The following two sections walk you through two formulas you can use to answer this question.

Using dimensional analysis

Although you can find elaborate definitions of dimensional analysis that apply to higher mathematics, in nursing, it comes down to this: Dimensional analysis is a simple way of calculating doses. The units are included and treated as numbers (see Chapter 8 for more details). To use dimensional analysis to find out how many tablets you need to give Ms. Jones, follow these steps:

1. **Set up the following equation:**

$$\text{Dose} = \frac{\text{factor}}{\text{factor}} \times \frac{\text{factor}}{\text{factor}}$$

$$x\,\frac{\text{tablet}}{\text{dose}} = \frac{1\ \text{tablet}}{100\ \cancel{\text{mg}}} \times \frac{150\ \cancel{\text{mg}}}{1\ \text{dose}}$$

2. **Multiply and solve.**

$$x = \frac{150}{100}$$

$$x = 1.5$$

The units cancel out. The patient dose is 1.5 tablets, meaning that you need to give Ms. Jones 1.5 tablets of labetalol twice a day.

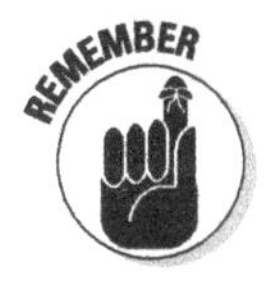

Before physically cutting any pill in half, make sure it's been scored so that you can cut the pill exactly in half (refer to Chapter 9 for more details). If you have any questions about administering a split tablet, call the doctor or pharmacist.

Using the formula method

As an alternative, you can do the same calculation using the formula method. At its simplest, the formula method of calculation means "take what you want and divide by what you have" (see Chapter 8 for more details). To use the formula method to find out how many tablets you need to give Ms. Jones, follow these steps:

1. **Set up the following equation:**

$$D\ (\text{dose}) = \frac{O\ (\text{ordered})}{H\ (\text{have})} \times Q\ (\text{quantity})$$

$$x = \frac{150\ \cancel{\text{mg}}}{100\ \cancel{\text{mg}}} \times 1\ \text{tablet}$$

2. **Divide and solve.**

$$x = \frac{150}{100}\ \text{tablet}$$

$$x = 1.5\ \text{tablet}$$

The units cancel out. The patient dose is 1.5 tablets, meaning that you need to give Ms. Jones 1.5 tablets of labetalol twice a day.

Preventing eclampsia

Preeclampsia and eclampsia are two serious medical conditions that can occur during pregnancy. *Preeclampsia* can first occur during or after the 20th week of gestation. Patients suffering from this condition can experience weight gain, swelling (called *edema*), really high blood pressure, and protein in the urine. Sometimes other body organs, like the liver and kidneys, are also affected. *Eclampsia* is the dreaded complication of preeclampsia. This life-threatening condition is characterized by seizures and coma and must be treated aggressively.

Magnesium sulfate is often used to prevent eclampsia from occurring, but the only known treatment for either preeclampsia or eclampsia is delivery of the baby, often by C-section.

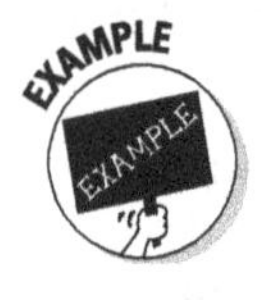

Ms. Smith is admitted to the hospital for preeclampsia. You're instructed to administer magnesium sulfate 40 g in 1 L (1,000 mL) of D5W at 2,000 mg an hour. The supplied volume of 1 L (1,000 mL) contains 40 g (40,000 mg) of magnesium sulfate. At what rate (how many mL/hour) should the magnesium sulfate be infused?

The ratio-proportion method is the best calculation method to use here because all the units are clearly displayed as an equation (refer to Chapter 8 for details on this calculation method). To calculate the rate of infusion, follow these steps:

1. **Set up the following proportion:**

$$\frac{\text{known equivalent}}{\text{known equivalent}} = \frac{\text{known equivalent}}{\text{desired equivalent}}$$

$$\frac{40{,}000\ \text{mg}}{1{,}000\ \text{mL}} = \frac{2{,}000\ \text{mg}}{x\ \text{mL}}$$

2. **Cross-multiply and solve.**

$$40{,}000x = 2{,}000{,}000$$
$$x = 50$$

The quantity 2,000 mg is contained in 50 mL of solution. Because the order is to infuse 2,000 mg/hr, the flow rate for the magnesium sulfate solution should be 50 mL/hr.

The total dose of magnesium sulfate should never exceed 40 grams over a 24-hour period. The doctor may need to reduce the dose if kidney disease is present. Magnesium sulfate is excreted almost entirely by the kidneys whether the patient has kidney disease or not. When a patient has severe kidney disease, excretion may be slowed, and the doctor may need to reduce the total dose by half.

Magnesium sulfate comes as a premixed solution, and it's available in many different dosages (40 g in 1,000 mL, like the example earlier in this section, or 20 g in 500 mL, just to name a couple). Doctors often order infusions to be given at 1 to 2 mg/hr. Notice we said *mg,* not *mL,* meaning there are two ways of ordering the same medication.

For any mom-to-be who's on a magnesium sulfate infusion, pay close attention to her vital signs as well as her neurological status, and make sure you've taken seizure precautions (like adding padded side rails and headboard to her bed and suction and oxygen to her bedside). One important way to assess the mom's neurological activity is by testing her *patellar reflex,* or knee jerk, safely and frequently. If you can't get a reflex, stop the magnesium sulfate infusion. If No Reaction Then No Mag Action! The doctor may also instruct you to check the magnesium level.

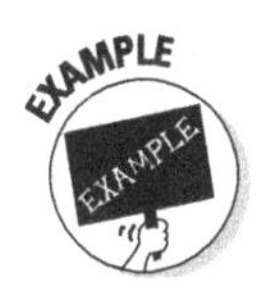

Say you're giving Ms. Smith 50 mL of magnesium sulfate an hour. You perform a neurological examination on Ms. Smith and find that her patellar reflex is absent. The doctor tells you to stop the infusion for one hour and then restart the infusion at 1 g/hr (1,000 mg/hr). What's your new flow rate in mL/hr?

From the previous magnesium sulfate example, you know that the premixed infusion is 40 g in 1,000 mL of D5W. With that in mind, follow these steps to determine the new flow rate by using the ratio-proportion method:

1. **Set up the following proportion:**

$$\frac{40{,}000 \text{ mg}}{1{,}000 \text{ mL}} = \frac{1{,}000 \text{ mg}}{x \text{ mL}}$$

2. **Cross-multiply and solve.**

$$40{,}000x = 1{,}000{,}000$$
$$x = 25$$

The new flow rate is 25 mL/hr.

Stopping early contractions

Terbutaline (Brethine) is a drug doctors often use to stop premature labor, and, thus, prevent the baby from escaping too early.

Technically speaking, terbutaline is a *bronchodilator* — it helps improve airflow — so it's no surprise that doctors often use it to treat patients with asthma and emphysema. Terbutaline is also prohibited for use by Olympic athletes; maybe it helps improve airflow too much!

The doc wants you to administer terbutaline sulfate 30 mg in 500 mL of ½ NS (5 percent dextrose in ½ normal saline) at a rate of 10 mcg/min. What's your infusion rate in mL/hr?

Follow these steps to use the ratio-proportion method to determine the infusion rate:

1. **Set up the following proportion to find the concentration of the terbutaline sulfate solution:**

   Concentration is expressed as mg/mL.

   $$\frac{30\text{ mg}}{500\text{ mL}} = \frac{x\text{ mg}}{1\text{ mL}}$$

2. **Cross-multiply and solve.**

   $$500x = 30$$
   $$x = 0.06$$

   The concentration of the solution is 0.06 mg/mL.

3. **Convert milligrams (mg) to micrograms (mcg).**

   $0.06\text{ mg} \times 1{,}000 = 60\text{ mcg}$

4. **Set up the following proportion to calculate the volume (in mL) that contains 10 mcg:**

   $$\frac{60\text{ mcg}}{1\text{ mL}} = \frac{10\text{ mcg}}{x\text{ mL}}$$

Remember that the doctor specified a rate of 10 mcg/min.

5. **Cross-multiply and solve.**

$$60x = 10$$
$$x = 0.167$$

The volume 0.167 mL contains 10 mcg, meaning that you dispense 0.167 mL (containing 10 mcg) per minute.

6. **Set up the following proportion to convert the per-minute rate to an hourly rate:**

$$\frac{1 \text{ min}}{0.167 \text{ mL}} = \frac{60 \text{ min}}{x \text{ mL}}$$

7. **Cross-multiply and solve.**

$x = 60 \times 0.167$

$x = 10.02$

The infusion rate is 10 mL/hr.

When a mother's on terbutaline, check on her frequently. Pay close attention to her vital signs, the contractions, and the fetal heart rate on the fetal monitor. If you notice any change in the mother's condition, such as a change in her breathing pattern or in the frequency or duration of her contractions, call the doctor immediately.

Inducing labor

When the doctor wants to induce labor, she stimulates the uterus to contract. You may have to administer the drug oxytocin to encourage this stimulation. Commonly, doctors use it to induce uterine contractions when the mom is past due and waiting for natural labor may be harmful to both Mom and Baby. Another reason to induce is when the mom has preeclampsia (see the earlier section "Preventing eclampsia" for details).

You're attending to Ms. Snyder. She's ten days beyond her due date, and your mission, should you choose to accept it, is to administer 30 units of oxytocin in 1 L of lactated Ringer's solution at an initial rate of 1 milliunit per minute for 30 minutes (1 unit is equivalent to 1,000 milliunits). What's your infusion rate for those first 30 minutes?

Follow these steps to use the ratio-proportion method to calculate your infusion rate:

1. **Set up the following proportion to determine the oxytocin solution strength in units/mL:**

   $$\frac{30 \text{ units}}{1{,}000 \text{ mL}} = \frac{x \text{ units}}{1 \text{ mL}}$$

2. **Cross-multiply and solve.**

   $$1{,}000x = 30$$
   $$x = 0.03$$

   The solution strength is 0.03 units/mL.

   Note that 0.03 units × 1,000 = 30 milliunits. The solution strength is better expressed as 30 milliunits/mL.

3. **Calculate the infusion rate.**

   The ordered dose of oxytocin is 1 milliunit/min for 30 minutes, so the total dose is 30 milliunits for 30 minutes. What's that in mL? You don't need an equation. You know from Step 2 that there are 30 milliunits/mL. So the infusion rate is 1 mL over 30 minutes.

   Because you're using an infusion pump, you need to convert the rate of 1 mL/30 minutes to an hourly rate.

4. **Set up the following proportion to calculate the hourly rate:**

   $$\frac{1 \text{ mL}}{30 \text{ min}} = \frac{x \text{ mL}}{60 \text{ min}}$$

5. **Cross-multiply and solve.**

   $$30x = 60$$
   $$x = 2$$

   The hourly infusion rate is 2 mL/hr.

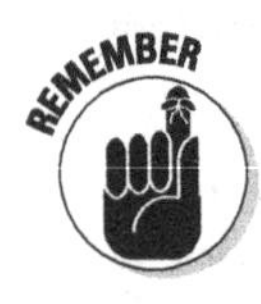

Be aware that, like magnesium sulfate and terbutaline infusions, a continuous infusion of oxytocin needs to be adjusted. The changes made to the doses of all these continuous infusions depend on how the patient responds. Be sure to monitor your patient closely and adjust the doses of the medications as needed. For example, you may need to adjust the dose of terbutaline to retard the uterine contractions.

Note: As with terbutaline, you need to monitor the mother's vital signs, the fetal heart rate, and the uterine contractions frequently whenever you're dealing with oxytocin infusions. If the contractions get too fast (more frequent than every 120 seconds) or if you notice changes in the fetus's heart rate, call the doctor immediately. You'll likely need to stop the oxytocin infusion.

Monitoring Mom and Junior When Administering Meds

Dosing the medications is just half the battle. You also need to pay close attention to the condition of both the mother and fetus whenever you're administering medications during pregnancy. The following sections show you just what to look for.

Checking Mom's vitals and examining her body

When administering medications to pregnant women, you need to routinely check their vital signs. Here's what you need to look for:

- **Temperature:** The mother should not have a fever.
- **Blood pressure:** Blood pressure readings must be consistent with expectations for the mother. They will either be in the normal range or be elevated if the mom has chronic or gestational hypertension.
- **Heart rate:** Be aware of the normal heart rate ranges for women at different stages of pregnancy and of the acceptable ranges for fetal heartbeat at difference stages of the pregnancy. 120 to 160 BPM is a good normal fetal heart rate.
- **Respiratory rate:** Expect a normal rate of 12 to 20 breaths per minute. You can use a pulse oximeter to assess Mom's oxygen level. A *pulse oximeter* is a medical device that measures the patient's oxygen saturation. This handy doohickey fits on the patient's index finger, and you follow her oxygen level on the monitor. Cool!

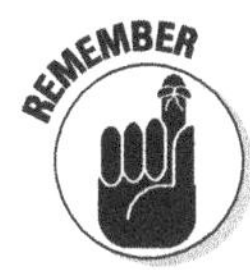

If any of the ranges go outside of normal, call the doctor immediately.

In addition to monitoring their vital signs, you need to do the following for all moms to whom you're administering medications:

- **Perform a brief physical exam that includes listening to the heart and lungs with your stethoscope.** The heart sounds should be regular, and the lungs should be clear. If the heart sounds are irregular or sound diminished, call the doctor. For the lung exam, listen for signs of fluid in the lungs, including diminished sounds at the lung bases and/or *rales* (an abnormal rattling), which are Velcro-like sounds that you can hear when a patient takes a deep breath. This can be a sign of pulmonary edema.

- **Listen to the bowels for bowel sounds.** Do bowels really make sounds? Absolutely! If you don't hear any, do a double-take and listen again! If you still don't hear any, call the doctor.

For moms who have preeclampsia or hypertension, add the following assessments to your to-do list:

- **Assess the patient's legs for any kind of swelling (or edema).** *Edema* is the buildup of fluid that occurs in the "third" or interstitial space of the body. Although edema is an accepted normal of pregnancy, you need to make sure the edema you find isn't early preeclampsia (see the earlier section "Preventing eclampsia" for details). If the swelling is confined to a particular area, call the doctor as it may suggest a problem with venous flow.
- **Do a neurological exam.** Make sure that your patient is alert and oriented to person, place, and time. Assess her reflexes and strength; look for any focal signs of weakness. If there's a problem, call the doctor. In particular, test for DTRs (deep tendon reflexes). You're looking for the degree of response when testing the patellar reflex, from absent to almost hyperreflexic. For a mother on magnesium sulfate, the response to DTR testing allows you to judge how to adjust your infusion. (See the section "Preventing eclampsia" for more details on this medication.)
- **Monitor pedal pulses in the feet to make sure the mom has adequate blood flow.** If you're unable to detect a pulse, call the doctor. If you're in a hospital setting, you may be asked to try to find the pulse with a machine called a Doppler. If you're unable to do so, notify the doctor, as this could be a medical emergency.

Here's a hint for how to find pedal pulses. Place your three middle fingers on top of your patient's foot; move your fingers back and forth across the foot in both directions until you find a pulse.

Using the fetal monitor to keep an eye on the baby

Monitoring Mom is important, but don't forget about Baby! You can use the *fetal monitor* (also known as a *Doppler fetal heart rate monitor*) to help you detect the fetus's heartbeat. This handheld ultrasound device gives you an audible simulation of what Baby's heartbeat sounds like.

Make sure the fetus's heart rate isn't too fast or too slow. Although the ideal heart rate varies depending on the stage of pregnancy, it should be in the range of 120 to 160 BPM by week 12.

Watch for changes in the fetal heart rate, especially when Mom is on the meds described in the section "Calculations for Pregnancy-Related Situations." You're basically monitoring for two important things: the heart rate itself and sudden changes in the heart rate. A heart rate that's too slow (usually less than 100 BPM) or a rate that's too fast (greater than 160 BPM) is a sign that something may be wrong with the baby. For example, the baby may not be getting the amount of oxygen it needs. If you notice any significant change in the baby's heart rate from baseline, call the doctor right away.

Dealing with Medications That Aren't Related to the Pregnancy

Pregnancy doesn't come into play just when you're administering drugs specifically related to pregnancy, labor, and delivery. Sometimes Mom is already on other meds for other conditions. Before administering any medication or performing a dosage calculation, you need to know whether the particular medication is *safe* for moms to take during pregnancy. To find out, ask yourself this question: What trimester is the mother in? The doctor knows and you should know, too.

The fetus is very susceptible to the effects of medications in the first and third trimesters. During the first trimester, in particular, the fetus is just beginning to develop, and many medications can radically affect its growth and development. For example, ACE (angiotensin-converting enzyme) inhibitors are drugs like quinapril (Accupril) and benazepril (Lotensin) that doctors often use to treat high blood pressure. Although they work fine for many patients, you never want to administer ACE inhibitors to a pregnant woman because they can really mess things up (as we say in precise medical terms) in the first trimester. They can even contribute to neonatal death or congenital malformations.

In the third trimester, the fetus may not be able to completely handle and effectively eliminate some meds. For example, Prozac is a commonly prescribed antidepressant, but if a pregnant woman takes Prozac in the third trimester, the fetus is at higher risk of complications such as premature labor.

Always be aware of any and all medications that a pregnant woman is taking. Double-check the safety and potential risk to the fetus of any medication before dosing it. After all, you're affecting a whole other life whenever you administer anything to Mom. (Check out the nearby sidebar "Categorizing meds according to their effects on the fetus" for details on how to tell which medications are safe for the fetus and which ones aren't.)

Categorizing meds according to their effects on the fetus

The U.S. Food and Drug Administration (FDA) puts all drugs into one of five categories based on how big a risk they pose to the fetus. Drugs in Category A are the safest, while drugs in Category X are known to be unsafe. This five-category system isn't foolproof, but it does help determine whether or not a medication may be harmful to the fetus. For your convenience and your patients' safety, every prescription your patients take should have a label that states which category that particular medication is in.

The following list summarizes the FDA use-in-pregnancy categories:

- **Category A:** No risk. Based on studies done in humans, these drugs pose little or no risk of harm to the fetus in any trimester. Medications in this category are considered safe for pregnant women to take.
- **Category B:** No evidence of risk in humans. This category has a double definition. There is either no risk to animals or no risk to humans even if animal studies showed an adverse effect.
- **Category C:** Some risk. There may be some risk in laboratory animals with this category drug, with limited human data available, but it's generally considered safe. If the doctor prescribes a medication in this category to a pregnant woman, she likely has a medical condition that justifies use of that drug despite the possible risk to the fetus.
- **Category D:** Evidence of risk. Some human studies show evidence of fetal risk, but if the possible benefits of taking the medication outweigh the possible fetal risk, a doctor may still prescribe a drug in this category to a pregnant woman.
- **Category X:** Contraindicated in pregnancy (see the section "Checking for contraindications" for what this term means). Both animal and human studies show evidence of fetal risk. The bottom line for medications in this category is: Don't let a pregnant patient take them.

Checking for contraindications

An *indication* is a symptom. It comes from the Latin word *indicare,* meaning "to show" or "to point out." A *contraindication* is a factor that argues against dosing a drug or performing a procedure. Doctors have used the word since the 1620s.

So how do you know a drug's contraindications? They're listed on the *package insert* — the literature that comes with the medication. Unfortunately, this literature is often printed in a type that's way too tiny to read. But, lucky for you, you can use the Internet or a drug reference to find the data you need in a more readable format.

The *Physicians' Desk Reference (PDR)* is an excellent resource for learning about medications, side effects, and interactions. Go to `www.pdrhealth.com` for details.

Figure 14-1 is an extract from an online file for the drug pitavastatin (Livalo). The manufacturer's literature says exactly the same thing as its FDA filing. We've boldfaced the contraindications for pregnant and lactating women.

Livalo (Pitavastatin)

CONTRAINDICATIONS

* Known hypersensitivity to product components (4)
* Active liver disease, which may include unexplained persistent elevations in hepatic transaminase levels (4)
* **Women who are pregnant or may become pregnant (4, 8.1)**
* **Nursing mothers (4, 8.3)**
* Co-administration with cyclosporine (4, 7.1, 12.3)

Figure 14-1: An example of the contraindications for pitavastatin (Livalo).

Don't let the reference to women who "may become pregnant" make you crazy! In theory, all noncelibate women between puberty and menopause may become pregnant; however, in daily practice, this phrase refers only to women who tell their doctors that they're trying to have a baby in the next year or so. If a woman says she hopes to become pregnant any time in the next few months, her doctor needs to review all her medications and discontinue any that are potentially *teratogenic* (tur-*rat*-o-gen-ic). Teratogenic is doctor talk, meaning "harmful to the fetus."

Minimizing the number and amount of meds pregnant women take

Your common sense pays off when you look carefully at the meds your pregnant patients are taking. Generally speaking, the less medication (dosage size) and the fewer meds (number of medications) a pregnant woman takes, the better both Mom and fetus will be. By minimizing medications, you reduce the risk to the fetus and the risk of possible drug-drug interactions. Doing so helps reduce the number of variables you have to consider when medicating pregnant women.

A conscientious OB/GYN in an outpatient practice will likely keep the meds to a minimum. If you notice the dosages are somewhat high (for example, a pregnant woman is taking the maximum daily dose of medication for hypertension), you may sense the reason for it. For instance, you may know the doctor is trying to balance the health of the mom against the risk to the fetus. But if you don't sense the reason for the high dosages, consult the doctor.

Similarly, in a clinic where the mom's doctor is a family practice physician or an internist (in other words, not an OB/GYN), as soon as the doctor learns that a patient is pregnant, you expect the doctor to review the pregnant woman's meds and make some adjustments, if possible.

The goal of any conscientious physician is to minimize the number and amount of medication a mother takes during pregnancy. All nonessential medications should be discontinued.

The situation is a lot different in a hospital. If a pregnant woman is admitted because of either illness or trauma, doctors have a different (and more dramatic) exercise in managing medications. In life-critical situations, balancing the mother's health against risk to the fetus is more important than minimizing meds. In life-critical situations, the list of variables really increases!

Real-Life Practice: Treating Hyperemesis Gravidarum

In pregnancy, many moms-to-be have a love-hate relationship with food. Sometimes they crave funky food combinations like peanut butter and pickles or pickles and ice cream. Many times, though, moms (especially early in pregnancy) experience nausea and vomiting, often called *morning sickness.* At those times, they don't even want to think about pickles! Sometimes pregnant women get so dehydrated from intractable vomiting that they have to go to the hospital for hydration. This severe form of morning sickness is called *hyperemesis gravidarum.*

Here's an example of what you may see in the hospital setting. A patient is admitted dehydrated, and you must rehydrate her. The doctor wants you to administer 1 L (1,000 mL) of D5NS at 125 mL/hr. What is the total time for the infusion?

To find out, use the ratio-proportion method and follow these steps:

1. **Set up the following proportion:**

$$\frac{125 \text{ mL}}{1 \text{ hr}} = \frac{1{,}000 \text{ mL}}{x \text{ hr}}$$

2. **Cross-multiply and solve.**

$$125x = 1{,}000$$
$$x = 8$$

The total time is 8 hours.

When doctors write IV orders, they often make the math easy to calculate for themselves. IV fluids can be written as 40 mL/hr, 80 mL/hr, or 125 mL/hr. The total amount infused for each dose for a 24-hour period is 1 liter, 2 liters, and 3 liters, respectively. For example, the quantity 1,000 mL (or 1 L) delivered at 125 mL/hr would take 8 hours. Infusing 3,000 mL (or 3 L) would take 24 hours.

Real-Life Practice: Fighting Infection by Wiping Out the Germs

Sometimes moms-to-be get infections. The best way to treat those infections is to administer an antibiotic, typically penicillin, which is where this real-world example comes in.

You must administer penicillin V to a mom-to-be who has a fever. Because she doesn't like pills, the doctor says to give her 250 mg every 8 hours in an oral solution for 7 days. Penicillin V potassium for oral solution is pinkish colored, and when you reconstitute it, you get a cherry-flavored red solution. Each 5 mL of the solution contains the equivalent of 125 mg. How much solution will you give in total?

To find out, use the ratio-proportion method and follow these steps:

1. **Set up the following proportion:**

$$\frac{125 \text{ mg}}{5 \text{ mL}} = \frac{250 \text{ mg}}{x \text{ mL}}$$

2. **Cross-multiply and solve.**

$$125x = 1{,}250$$
$$x = 10$$

The answer is 10 mL. Give the patient 10 mL of solution three times a day (every 8 hours).

Real-Life Practice: Wiping Out Even More Germs

In a scenario that's similar to the one you see in the preceding section, you're instructed to give Mom penicillin G 500,000 units every 6 hours. The penicillin G preparation you use comes as a premixed solution of 2,000,000 units per 50 mL vial. How many mL do you give?

To find out, use the ratio-proportion method and follow these steps:

1. **Set up the following proportion:**

$$\frac{2{,}000{,}000 \text{ units}}{50 \text{ mL}} = \frac{500{,}000 \text{ units}}{x \text{ mL}}$$

2. **Cross-multiply and solve.**

$$2{,}000{,}000x = 25{,}000{,}000$$
$$x = 12.5$$

You must administer 12.5 mL every 6 hours.

If units of penicillin were dollars, you would be a millionaire. After all, while oxytocin is administered in milliunits, intravenous penicillin is dosed in millions of units per vial. That's a lot of units!

Chapter 15

Kid Stuff: Pediatric Calculations

In This Chapter

- Understanding how dosing meds for kids is different from dosing for adults
- Dosing based on weight, age, and BSA
- Using caution when dosing and administering IV meds for children and infants
- Practicing some real-life medical dosage calculations for infants and children

When it comes to medical care, infants and children are special. Like most patients, they need you to help take care of them, but they aren't adults. Their bodies are different, and they have different medication requirements. So be sure to think of kids as more than "little adults" whenever you work with them.

Preemies are different from infants, who are different from children, who are different from preteens and teens, who are different from adults. Whole lotta difference, right? Right!

Much of this book is about doing dosage calculations for and administering to the adult, but this chapter is here to give you a different perspective. Here, you see the importance of a child's weight, age, and body surface area (BSA) in dosing. You also get a plethora of information you need to know when doing medical dosing calculations for infants and children. Finally, you get some dosing practice with a few real-life, kid-focused problems.

Realizing the Dosing Differences from Child to Child and Adult to Child

The first thing you must ask when you're administering a medication to a nonadult patient is, "How old is the patient?" Is she an infant — perhaps a preemie? Maybe she's a preteen. Children's ages are important to know because they affect how kids can absorb or metabolize medications. Starting from the teenager and working backward, here are the main age groups:

- **Teenager:** A *teenager* is younger than 18 but older than 12. Not only are teenagers' hormones starting to "kick in," but they're close to adults in terms of drug absorption, metabolism, and elimination.
- **Child:** A *child* is a young person from 1 year of age to about 12 years of age; this group includes the preteen. If you were to tell a 12-year-old to "stop acting like a child," technically you'd be wrong, because she still is a child.
- **Infant:** An *infant* is less than 1 year old but has been around for at least a month.
- **Newborn:** A *newborn* (also called a *neonate*) has been "walking the earth" for less than a month.
- **Preemie:** A *preemie* is a premature newborn, defined as being born before the 38th week of pregnancy.

Children are different from adults in many ways, and the doctor's prescriptions need to reflect this difference. Here's what you need to be aware of when dosing medications for children:

- For the most part, the *drug metabolism* (the biochemical modification of substances by an organism) of medications occurs in the liver while elimination occurs in the kidneys. But the actual drug metabolisms of infants and children are different from those of adults. And infants may not have the same enzymatic activity to process a medication as children.
- In adults, 60 percent of the total body volume is water, although this amount can differ a little according to age and gender. In infants, the water components of total body volume can be as much as 75 percent of their weight. The amount of water making up total body weight decreases over the first few months of their lives as body fat increases. (This increased water percentage can also explain why children and infants are more susceptible to dehydration than adults. They carry a lot more water, and bam! — When that water disappears, they're dehydrated.)

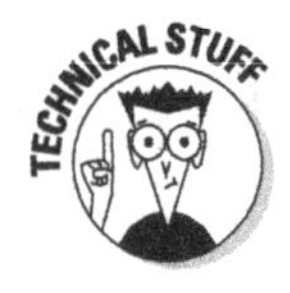

Medications can be either *hydrophilic* (water loving) or *lipophilic* (fat loving). Given the differences in body fat and water weight in children and infants compared to adults, differences in how a drug is distributed in a child's body are only natural. For instance, younger children may require higher doses of water-soluble medicines because they have more water weight.

Simply put, children and infants absorb medications differently than adults do:

- Infants and children absorb medication through the skin faster than adults.
- The child's gastrointestinal (GI) tract is likely to absorb more of a medication than an adult's. The immature GI system of a child may not produce as much gastric acid as an adult, which can alter the absorption of some oral medications.
- A child has a slower *peristalsis* (the contraction of muscles to move contents through the GI tract), which can change the absorption of a medication in a child compared with the absorption in an adult.

To address the differences in medication absorption between children of different ages and between children and adults, when you do medical dosage calculations for infants and children, you almost always begin by calculating either weight in kg or body surface area (BSA) in m^2. The next two sections show you how to do so.

Weighing and Going Metric: Dosing Meds for Kids

You need to know how to convert pounds to kg (refer to Chapter 4 for more on converting units).

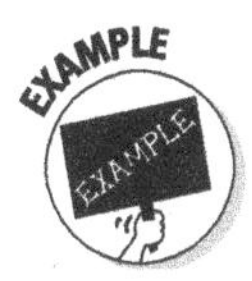

You weigh an 8-year-old child and find that he weighs 54 pounds. What's his weight in kg?

Use the ratio-proportion method (see Chapter 8) and follow these steps to find out:

1. **Set up the following proportion using the conversion factor 1 kg = 2.2 lb:**

$$\frac{\text{known equivalent}}{\text{known equivalent}} = \frac{\text{known equivalent}}{\text{desired equivalent}}$$

$$\frac{2.2 \text{ lb}}{1 \text{ kg}} = \frac{54 \text{ lb}}{x \text{ kg}}$$

2. **Cross-multiply and solve.**

$2.2x = 54$

$x = 24.5$

The answer is 24.5 kg.

A simpler way to do this calculation is to divide lb by 2.2 to get kg; see Chapter 4 for more on conversion factors.

After you know the patient's weight, you use it to calculate how much medication to administer. The rest of this section shows you how.

Using weight when you calculate

Most of the time when you dose for kids, you administer medication in doses of mg/kg. (For an alternate method, see the section "Trying Another Way: Calculating BSA.") Depending on the medication, you either have to figure out how many mg to give in a single dose or calculate the safe dosage for 24 hours.

Determining total dosage

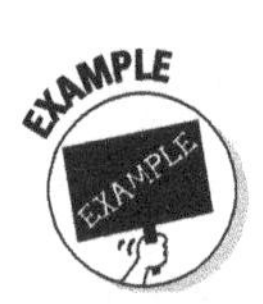

A child weighs 24.5 kg. You're asked to administer erythromycin suspension at a total dose of 40 mg/kg per day. What's the total amount of erythromycin you can give in a 24-hour period?

To solve this problem, use the ratio-proportion method and follow these steps:

1. **Set up the following proportion:**

   $$\frac{1\text{ kg}}{40\text{ mg}} = \frac{24.5\text{ kg}}{x\text{ mg}}$$

2. **Cross-multiply and solve.**

   $x = 40 \times 24.5$

   $x = 980$

   The answer is 980 mg. Round that up to 1,000 mg. You administer 1,000 mg over a 24-hour period.

A faster way to solve this problem is to just multiply 40 × 25, giving you 1,000.

Figuring out specific doses

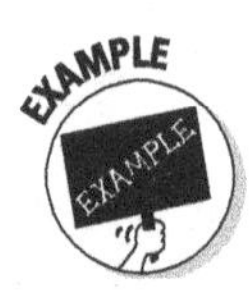

For the child in the preceding example, you need to dose the erythromycin every 8 hours. You know that the total amount of medication to administer is 1,000 mg over 24 hours. It's available in suspension form 200 mg/5 mL. How much medication, in mL, do you give at each dose?

To find out, use simple division and the ratio-proportion method. Follow these steps:

1. **To determine the number of dosing periods in a day, divide the total hours in a day by the dosing interval.**

   $24 \div 8 = 3$

   You administer 3 doses over a 24-hour period.

2. **To determine how much medication you administer at each dose, divide the total amount of medication per day by the number of doses you have to give per day.**

   $1{,}000 \div 3 = 333.3$

   You administer 333 mg for each dose.

3. **To convert the dose from mg to mL, set up the following proportion:**

   $$\frac{200 \text{ mg}}{5 \text{ mL}} = \frac{333 \text{ mg}}{x \text{ mL}}$$

4. **Cross-multiply and solve.**

   $200x = 1{,}665$

   $x = 8.325$

   The answer is 8.325 mL. You'd give 8.33 mL for each dose to provide the needed 333 mg.

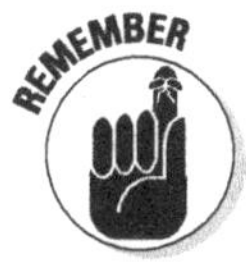

This example is typical of most dosing calculations. You determine how much of a med to administer in mg over a 24-hour period and then determine how much to give in mg or mL per dose.

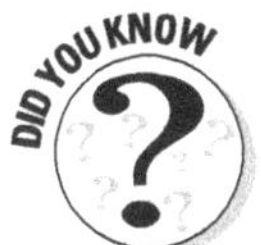

Obesity isn't just a problem with adults; it can affect children as well. An obese child may metabolize drugs at a different rate than his skinnier counterpart. In one study, scientists from the University of Minnesota found that obese children handled caffeine and dextromethorphan (dex-tro-me-*thor*-phan), a common ingredient in cough medicine, differently than other children.

Dosing safely for kids' safety

In the preceding example, you calculate the amount of erythromycin to give, based on the doctor's order. But is it a proper dose to administer to the patient?

Check a drug reference to find out. For a child, the dose of erythromycin can range from 30 to 50 mg/kg per day, with a maximum dose of 3.2 g (3,200 mg) per day for the suspension form. Is a dose of 1,000 mg/day safe to give to a child who weighs 24.5 kg?

To answer this question, all you have to do is multiply the maximum safe drug amount by the child's weight, like so:

$$\text{Max dose/day} = 50 \text{ mg} \times 24.5 \text{ kg}$$

$$\text{Max dose/day} = 1{,}225 \text{ mg/day}$$

The maximum safe dose is 1,225 mg/day. A dose of 1,000 mg/day is less than the maximum, so it's safe to give.

Note: Most pediatric-based medications have safe-dosing ranges. Some are age based, and some are weight based. Ranges vary depending on whether you're treating newborns, infants, children, or adults. Phenobarbital and azithromycin (Zithromax) have very specific dosing ranges, whereas erythromycin has a wider dosage range of 30 to 50 mg/kg/day. Whenever you're dealing with a patient in the pediatric age group, calculate and then double-check your calculations. If you have any questions, never hesitate to contact the pharmacist or prescribing physician. (See Chapter 6 to review the patient safety "mantra": Check, check, and check yet again.)

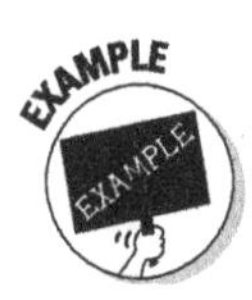

You're asked to administer azithromycin 500 mg daily for 3 days to a child who weighs 90 pounds to treat *otitis media* (middle-ear infection). Is this a safe dose to administer?

To find out, use the basic conversion formula (see Chapter 4) and follow these steps:

1. **Convert the child's weight from lb to kg using the conversion factor 1 kg = 2.2 lb.**

   $$90 \div 2.2 = 40.9$$

   The patient weighs 40.9 kg. Round up to 41 kg.

2. **Calculate the maximum single dose you can administer.**

   A reference book tells you that for a child older than 6 months you shouldn't administer more than 10 mg/kg/day as a single dose. Multiply that maximum single dose by the child's weight to find out the maximum dose for the child.

   $$\frac{10 \text{ mg}}{1 \text{ kg}} \times 41 \text{ kg} = 410 \text{ mg}$$

   The maximum allowable dose for a child of this weight is 410 mg/day. The order of 500 mg is too much, so you can't carry out the doctor's order. Consult the doctor immediately.

You can use many reference handbooks to calculate safe doses. Also, don't forget to use resources you have close at hand — your local pharmacist or your hospital pharmacist if you work in or are affiliated with a medical center. Sometimes they can be your best resources.

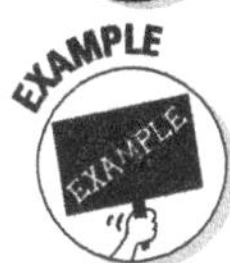

A doctor's order says to administer phenobarbital to a 58-pound child 100 mg 3 times a day. Is this a safe dose?

To find out, follow these steps:

1. **Convert the child's weight from lb to kg using the conversion factor 1 kg = 2.2 lb.**

   $58 \div 2.2 = 26.4$

   The child weighs 26.4 kg.

2. **Calculate the maximum single dose you can administer.**

   You look in a drug reference and it tells you that the safe dosage for oral phenobarbital for a child is no more than 2 mg/kg 3 times a day. Multiply that maximum dose by the child's weight to find out the maximum dose for this child.

   $$\frac{2\text{ mg}}{1\text{ kg}} \times 26.4\text{ kg} = 52.8\text{ mg}$$

   The maximum allowable dose for a child of this weight is no more than 52.8 mg 3 times per day. A dose of 100 mg 3 times a day is too much, so it isn't safe to administer. Consult the doctor right away.

Trying Another Way: Calculating BSA

Body surface area (BSA) offers an alternate way to calculate medication doses. Instead of dosing in mg/kg of body weight, you dose per square meter (m^2) of body surface area. Although you do most dosing based on body weight, you still need to be familiar with dosing based on BSA.

In adults, you calculate the BSA based on height and weight. Fortunately, you can find formulas, online calculators, and even smartphone apps that help you do so. However, in pediatrics, you frequently have to use a nomogram to do BSA calculations.

A *nomogram* is a graph or table that shows the relationship between two different measurements. It's sort of a diagram on a piece of paper or plastic that you can use for calculations. Figure 15-1 shows an example of a West nomogram.

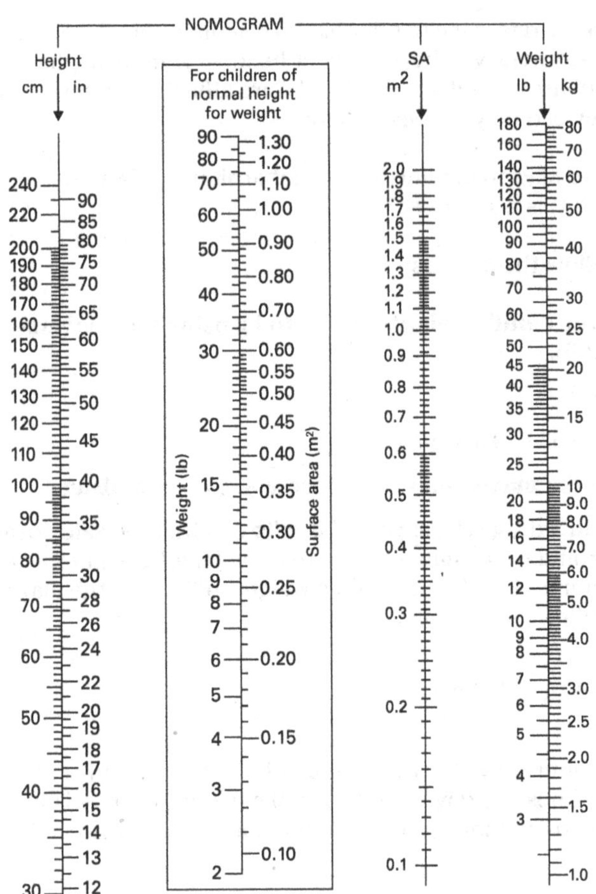

Figure 15-1: A West nomogram.

To use the West nomogram, you need to know the weight and height of a patient. After you know these numbers, lay a ruler on the child's height, and angle it so that it also lies on the child's weight. Then look at where the ruler intersects a BSA value. For example, if a child has a height of 40 inches and weighs 36 lb, the BSA is 0.67 m^2.

After you know the child's BSA, you can use it in your dosing calculations by comparing the child's BSA to the average adult BSA.

In addition to finding BSA for dosing "regular" meds, you commonly use a nomogram to administer chemotherapy. You can also use it in calculating a child's hydration needs.

A child is 50 inches tall and weighs 80 pounds. If a normal adult dose of a medication is 600 mg, what's a safe dose to administer to this child?

To find out, first use a nomogram to find the child's BSA. In case you don't have a nomogram handy, the child's BSA is 1.1 m^2. Then calculate the dose based on the child's BSA compared to the "standard" adult BSA, which is defined as 1.73 m^2:

$$\frac{\text{child BSA}\left(\text{m}^2\right)}{\text{adult BSA}\left(\text{m}^2\right)} \times \text{adult dose (mg)} = \text{child dose (mg)}$$

$$\frac{1.1\ \text{m}^2}{1.73\ \text{m}^2} \times 600\ \text{mg} = 381.5\ \text{mg}$$

The safe dose for the child is 318.5 mg.

Considering Some Other Rules of Dosing

Medical dosing calculations for pediatric patients based on mg/kg and BSA are the most accurate dosing methods because they give you the exact amounts to administer.

Sometimes, however, you can use one of these other, less exact dosing rules:

- **Clark's rule:** Approximate dosing based on weight
- **Fried's rule:** Approximate dosing based on age
- **Young's rule:** Approximate dosing based on age

Keep in mind that these three rules are for approximate dosing and aren't as accurate as mg/kg- and BSA-based dosing. Practitioners can use them to determine the correct dosing in particular dosing situations. Be aware of all three of these dosing calculations; the more pediatric dosage "rules" you know, the better you can check your own calculations as well as those of your colleagues. Remember: Checks and balances are the key to patient safety!

The following sections show you how to use these rules in your dosing calculations.

Clark's rule

To approximate a child's dose of a medication based on weight, all you need is the child's weight in pounds. Simply divide the child's weight by 150, and multiply the adult dosage in mg by the result to estimate the dose you should give:

$$\frac{\text{child's weight (lb)}}{150\text{ (lb)}} \times \text{adult dose (mg)} = \text{child dose (mg)}$$

You're asked to administer amoxicillin/clavulanate (Augmentin), which is a combination antibiotic used to treat respiratory infections, to a child patient every 8 hours. The adult dose is 875 mg every 12 hours (1,750 mg/day). The child weighs 70 lb. Based on Clark's rule, how much would you administer to the child per dose? Is that dose safe?

To find out, follow these steps:

1. **Use Clark's rule to calculate the approximate dose.**

   $$\frac{\text{child's weight (lb)}}{150\text{ (lb)}} \times \text{adult dose (mg)} = \text{child dose (mg)}$$

   $$\frac{70\text{ lb}}{150\text{ lb}} \times 1{,}750\text{ mg} = 817\text{ mg}$$

   The approximate dose for the child is 817 mg given over 24 hours, or 272 mg given every 8 hours (817 ÷ 3 = 272.3).

2. **Convert the child's weight from lb to kg.**

   70 ÷ 2.2 = 31.8 kg

   The child weighs about 32 kg.

3. **Calculate the maximum safe dose you can administer using mg/kg dosing.**

   You look in a drug reference and find that for children 3 months of age or older, amoxicillin/clavulanate should be dosed in an amount no greater than 45 mg/kg/day, divided in 3 doses and given every 8 hours. Simply multiply this maximum safe dose by the child's weight to calculate the maximum safe dose for the child. (See the earlier section "Dosing safely for kids' safety" for more details.)

   $$\frac{45\text{ mg}}{1\text{ kg}} \times 32\text{ kg} = 1{,}440$$

   Give no more than 1,440 mg per day, divided in 3 doses:

   1,440 ÷ 3 = 480 mg/dose

   The maximum safe single dose is 480 mg.

4. **Compare 480 mg maximum safe dose with the 272 mg approximation you got from Clark's rule in Step 1.**

   The 272 mg/dose is safe to administer.

Fried's rule

Fried's rule is similar to Clark's rule, except that you use age rather than weight. You use it mainly to approximate dosing for infants and children up to 2 years of age. The rule assumes that an adult dose would be appropriate for a child who is 12.5 years (150 months) old. Younger children, therefore, get a smaller dose.

To calculate a child's dose of a medication based on age, divide the child's age in months by 150 and multiply the adult dose by the result:

$$\frac{\text{child's age (months)}}{\text{150 (months)}} \times \text{adult dose (mg)} = \text{child dose (mg)}$$

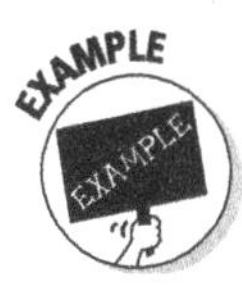

You need to dose amoxicillin/clavulanate to a 23-month-old child for an upper respiratory tract infection. The adult dose is 875 mg every 12 hours (1,750 mg/day). According to your drug reference, for children 3 months of age or older, amoxicillin/clavulanate should be dosed in an amount no greater than 45 mg/kg/day, divided into 3 doses and given every 8 hours. Use Fried's rule to calculate the required dosage. Then double-check to make sure the dosage is safe.

To solve this problem, follow these steps:

1. **Use Fried's rule to calculate the approximate dose.**

   $$\frac{\text{child's age (months)}}{\text{150 (months)}} \times \text{adult dose (mg)} = \text{child dose (mg)}$$

   $$\frac{23\text{ mo}}{150\text{ mo}} \times 1{,}750\text{ mg} = 268\text{ mg}$$

   The approximate dose for the child is 268 mg given over 24 hours, or 89 mg given every 8 hours (268 ÷ 3 = 89.3).

2. **Calculate the maximum safe dose you can administer using mg/kg dosing.**

   Because you don't have the child's weight, assume that an average weight for a male child who is 23 months old is about 26.5 lb, or 12 kg (26.5 ÷ 2.2 = 12). Multiply that weight by the maximum safe daily dose of amoxicillin/clavulanate.

   $$\frac{45\text{ mg}}{1\text{ kg}} \times 12\text{ kg} = 540\text{ mg}$$

The safe maximum dose is 540 mg/day, divided into 3 doses:

540 ÷ 3 = 180 mg

The maximum safe single dose is 180 mg, given every 3 hours.

3. **Compare 180 mg maximum safe single dose with the 89 mg approximation you got from Fried's rule in Step 1.**

   The 89 mg/dose is safe to administer.

Young's rule

You can use Young's rule to calculate pediatric dosage for children from 1 year of age up to 12 years of age. For Young's rule, you divide the child's age in years by the same value plus 12; then you multiply the adult dosage by the result to estimate the dose you should give:

$$\frac{\text{child's age (years)}}{\text{child's age (years)} + 12\text{ (years)}} \times \text{adult dose (mg)} = \text{child dose (mg)}$$

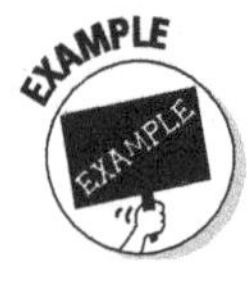

You must give amoxicillin/clavulanate to a 6-year-old child for an upper respiratory tract infection. The adult dose is 875 mg every 12 hours (1,750 mg/day). According to your reference book, for children 3 months of age or older, amoxicillin/clavulanate should be dosed in an amount no greater than 45 mg/kg/day, divided into 3 doses and given every 8 hours. Use Young's Rule to calculate the required dosage. Then double-check to make sure the dosage is safe.

To solve this problem, follow these steps:

1. **Use Young's rule to calculate the approximate dose.**

$$\frac{\text{child's age (years)}}{\text{child's age (years)} + 12\text{ (years)}} \times \text{adult dose (mg)} = \text{child dose (mg)}$$

$$\frac{6\text{ yr}}{6\text{ yr} + 12\text{ yr}} \times 1{,}750\text{ mg} = 583.33\text{ mg}$$

   The approximate dose is 583 mg given over 24 hours, or 194 mg every 8 hours (583 ÷ 3 = 194.3).

2. **Calculate the maximum safe dose you can administer using mg/kg dosing.**

Assume that the average weight for a 6-year-old is 46 lb, or 21 kg ($46 \div 2.2 = 20.9$). According to the drug reference, you're to give no more than 45 mg/kg/day. Multiply the average weight by the maximum safe daily dose of amoxicillin/clavulanate.

$$\frac{45\text{ mg}}{1\text{ kg}} \times 21\text{ kg} = 945\text{ mg}$$

The maximum safe dose to give is 945 mg/day, divided into 3 doses:

$945 \div 3 = 315$ mg

The maximum safe single dose is 315 mg, given every 8 hours.

3. **Compare 315 mg maximum safe dose with the 194 mg approximation you got from Young's rule in Step 1.**

   The dose of 194 mg every 8 hours is safe.

Looking at Special Considerations for Four Routes of Administration

You can use the same four routes of medication administration for children and infants that you use for adults: PO (oral), IM (intramuscular), subq (subcutaneous), and IV (intravenous). But you need to be aware of a few key differences between adults and children for each one:

- **Oral:** With children, you may need to use an oral syringe for oral administration. Do so when the child isn't yet able to use a cup to take a liquid. You can also use a dropper.
- **Intramuscular:** Infants and newborns don't have much muscle or fatty tissue. For the most part, if you need to administer an IM injection in young children, you really don't give any more than 1 mL. Measure the amount carefully — you need to be exact in your dose. Even in older children — up to the preteen years — you often administer 1 mL IM injections. That being said, you sometimes need to account for body type when administering an injection.
- **Subcutaneous:** As with the intramuscular injection, administering a subq injection of more than 1 mL isn't recommended for young children up to the preteen years. But again, you sometimes need to account for body type when administering an injection.
- **Intravenous:** Giving IV fluids to kids is such a specialized process that we dedicate the next two sections to this topic.

When you give a med to a child, be sure she doesn't choke. If you're administering a liquid form of a medication, put it in the center of the child's tongue. You can also get permission from the doc to use applesauce or custard to help get the medication "down the hatch." Doing so can be doubly helpful since some meds taste downright awful.

Managing IV Fluids for Infants and Children

Because infants and children carry more water than their adult counterparts, they're more susceptible to dehydration. In a hospital setting (where you're most likely to administer IV fluids), calculating a child's maintenance fluid needs is paramount.

Because you need to be very exact when calculating pediatric fluid needs, your dosing relies mainly on the child's weight in kg. The following sections show you how to determine children's maintenance fluid needs based on their weight, caloric needs, and BSA.

The kilogram bands

Think about children's maintenance fluid needs in terms of each 10 kg of child body weight. Use kilogram bands (1–10 kg, 11–20 kg, and above 21 kg) to make calculations about maintenance fluid needs. These bands provide the best approximation for fluid maintenance; it would be cumbersome and unnecessary for medical professionals to devise narrower bands.

1–10 kg

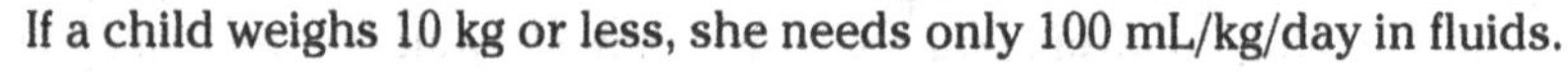

If a child weighs 10 kg or less, she needs only 100 mL/kg/day in fluids.

You have a child who weighs 20 pounds. What are his maintenance fluid needs per day?

To find out, follow these steps:

1. **Use the conversion factor 1 kg = 2.2 lb to convert the child's weight from lb to kg.**

   20 ÷ 2.2 = 9.1 kg

   The child weighs 9.1 kg.

2. **Calculate the child's maintenance fluid needs by multiplying his weight by the daily fluid needs for a child who weighs less than 10 kg.**

   $$\frac{100 \text{ mL}}{1 \text{ kg}} \times 9.1 \text{ kg} = 910 \text{ mL}$$

   You administer 910 mL over 24 hours to meet this child's maintenance fluid needs.

11–20 kg

When you're attending to a child who weighs between 11 and 20 kg, the fluid equation changes a bit. A child who weighs between 11 and 20 kg needs 1 L (1,000 mL) of fluid, plus an additional 50 mL for any kg over 10 kg, each day. The formula for this is

> $F = 1{,}000 + (50(w - 10))$, where F is the fluid requirement in mL and w is the child's weight in kg

You have a child who weighs 15 kg. What are his maintenance fluid needs?

All you have to do is plug the child's weight into the given formula, like so:

$$F = 1{,}000 + (50(15 - 10))$$

$$F = 1{,}000 + (50 \times 5)$$

$$F = 1{,}000 + 250$$

$$F = 1{,}250$$

Here's a step-by-step approach:

1. **Subtract the first 10 kg from the total weight to find the remaining weight to be calculated.**

   15 kg – 10 kg = 5 kg

   Remember that the first 10 kg demand 1,000 mL in fluids.

2. **Calculate the fluid requirement for the remaining 5 kg by multiplying the weight by the amount of fluids needed per kg.**

   $$\frac{50 \text{ mL}}{1 \text{ kg}} \times 5 \text{ kg} = 250 \text{ mL}$$

   You need to administer an additional 250 mL for this child's fluid maintenance.

3. Add the two fluid amounts together.

1,000 mL + 250 mL = 1,250 mL

You need to administer 1,250 mL over 24 hours.

21 kg and beyond

Children who weigh 21 kg or more need 1.5 L (1,500 mL) of fluid daily. They also need an additional 20 mL for any kg over 20 kg. The formula for this is

$F = 1{,}500 + (20(w - 20))$, where F is the fluid requirement in mL and w is the child's weight in kg.

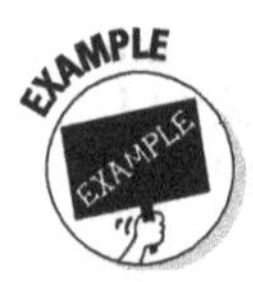

You have a child who weighs 35 kg. What are her maintenance fluid needs?

To find out, just plug the child's weight into the given formula, like so:

$F = 1{,}500 + (20(35 - 20))$

$F = 1{,}500 + (20 \times 15)$

$F = 1{,}500 + 300$

$F = 1{,}800$

You must administer 1,800 mL over 24 hours.

Counting calories

Nope, this section isn't about how adults count calories when they're dieting. Here, we're talking about another way to determine a child's maintenance fluid requirements, based on his caloric needs: For every 100 kilocalories (kcal) a child metabolizes in a day, the child should receive 120 mL of fluid.

How do you determine a child's caloric needs or caloric expenditure? You simply look at a caloric chart. For example, the American Heart Association (AHA) recommends that the average caloric requirement for a 2- to 3-year-old child be 1,000 kcal/day, regardless of gender. Compare that amount to a child between the ages of 4 and 8, who requires a higher caloric intake. Find out more about children's caloric requirements at `http://www.heart.org/HEARTORG/GettingHealthy/Dietary-Recommendations-for-Healthy-Children_UCM_303886_Article.jsp`.

If you have questions about pediatric caloric needs, ask your facility's dietitian or nutritionist. Most medical centers have one on staff.

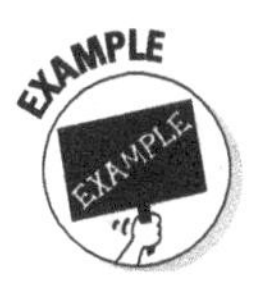

The hospital dietitian determines that a 4-year-old child uses 1,300 calories a day. What are the fluid needs of the child?

To find out, use the ratio-proportion method (see Chapter 8) and follow these steps:

1. **Set up the following proportion:**

   $$\frac{100 \text{ kcal}}{120 \text{ mL}} = \frac{1{,}300 \text{ kcal}}{x \text{ mL}}$$

2. **Cross-multiply and solve.**

   $100x = 156{,}000$

   $x = 1{,}560$

   The child requires 1,560 mL of fluid a day.

Using the BSA

You can also use the child's BSA to figure out a child's fluid needs. The formula for doing so is

> $F = 1{,}500 \times BSA$, where F is the fluid requirement in mL and BSA is the child's body surface area in m^2

To find BSA, use a nomogram, an online calculator, or a smartphone app (see the earlier section "Trying Another Way: Calculating BSA" for more details).

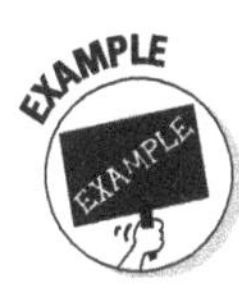

You determine that a child's BSA is 0.63 m^2. What's the child's fluid requirement?

To find out, simply plug the BSA into the given formula, like so:

$F = 1{,}500 \times BSA$

$F = 1{,}500 \times 0.63$

$F = 945$

The child requires 945 mL of fluid a day.

Being Extra Careful When Administering Meds or Fluids Intravenously

Be very careful when you administer meds or other fluids intravenously to pediatric patients. You must carefully regulate how much fluid is being administered — both the amount and the flow. Usually, you need some special equipment to do so.

Expect to use a volume-control device, such as a Soluset or a Buretrol. Both of these volume-control devices have chambers that can hold up to 150 mL. Figure 15-2 shows a Buretrol.

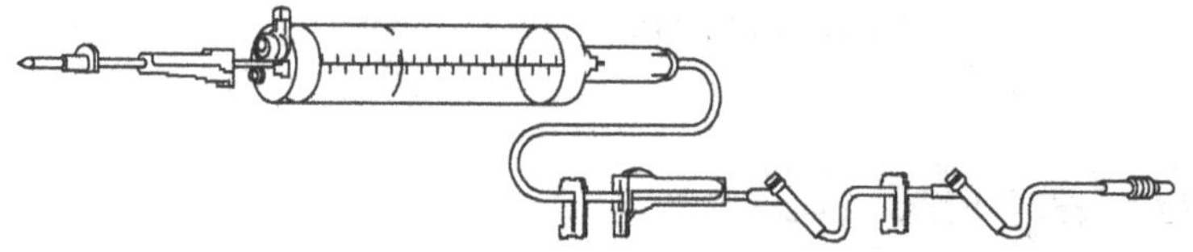

Figure 15-2: A volume-control device.

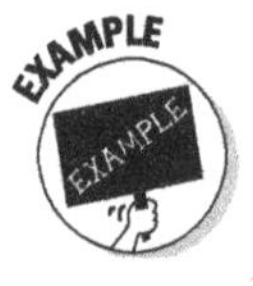

You're asked to administer ampicillin 500 mg IV every 8 hours in D5 ½ NS (dextrose and saline) 50 mL to infuse over 30 minutes. Then you're to follow the infusion with a 15 mL flush. For the infusion, you're to use a volume-control device. Like most volume-control devices, this one has a drop factor of 60 gtt/mL. The child weighs 16 kg. Is this dose safe to administer? What's the drip rate of the infusion?

Note: Ampicillin comes as a powder that you must reconstitute. A standard dose of 500 mg is available and requires that you add 1.8 mL of *diluent* (fluid that you add to turn the powder into a liquid). In this case, the diluent is D5 ½ NS. To prepare the 500 mg dose, just "draw up" (or remove) 1.8 mL of liquid from the ampicillin vial after you reconstitute it. (For more about reconstituting meds, see Chapter 12.)

To solve this problem, follow these steps:

1. **Calculate the maximum safe dose you can administer using mg/kg dosing (see the section "Dosing safely for kids' safety" for more details).**

   The total ordered dose is 500 mg, given every 8 hours, or 1,500 mg/day (500 mg × 3 times/day = 1,500 mg/day). Your drug reference tells you that for children weighing less than 40 kg, a safe dose of ampicillin is 100–200 mg/kg a day, divided every 6 to 8 hours.

To determine the maximum total safe dose for 24 hours, multiply the child's weight in kg by the mg/kg dose recommendation.

$$\frac{100 \text{ mg}}{1 \text{ kg}} \times 16 \text{ kg} = 1{,}600 \text{ mg}$$

The total safe dose is 1,600 mg a day, so it's okay to dispense the ordered 1,500 mg/day, provided that you divide it into 3 doses/day, as ordered.

2. **To determine the drip rate of the infusion, use the drip rate formula from Chapter 11 to set up the following equation.**

   Remember that the majority of volume-control devices for pediatric administration have a drop factor of 60 gtt/mL.

$$\text{drip rate (gtt/min)} = \frac{\text{total volume to be administered (mL)} \times \text{drop factor } \frac{\text{(gtt)}}{\text{(mL)}}}{\text{total infusion time (min)}}$$

$$\text{drip rate (gtt/min)} = \frac{50 \text{ mL} \times \frac{60 \text{ gtt}}{1 \text{ mL}}}{30 \text{ min}}$$

   In case you're wondering where we get 50 mL, the total volume to be infused is the sum of 1.8 mL (ampicillin) + 48.2 mL (D5 ½ NS), which equals 50 mL.

3. **Multiply and solve.**

$$x = \frac{3{,}000 \text{ gtt}}{30 \text{ min}}$$

$$x = 100 \text{ gtt/min}$$

   The drip rate is 100 gtt/min.

It's easy to create a 500 mg dose when you reconstitute a 500 mg vial of ampicillin powder. But what if only 1 g vials of ampicillin were available? This little change makes a big difference in the amount you need to withdraw. What is the new volume of ampicillin you need to administer? What is the new drip rate?

A drug reference tells you that for a 1 g (1,000 mg) vial, you may add 7.5 mL of sterile water for reconstitution. The volume you need to remove from the vial is different than it was in the preceding example.

Follow these steps to solve this problem:

1. **To find the volume of ampicillin that you need to administer, set up the following ratio-proportion equation:**

$$\frac{1{,}000\text{ mg}}{7.5\text{ mL}} = \frac{500\text{ mg}}{x\text{ mL}}$$

2. **Cross-multiply and solve.**

$$1{,}000x = 7.5 \times 500$$

$$1{,}000x = 3{,}750$$

$$x = 3.75$$

You remove 3.75 mL of the medication from the vial.

3. **To find the drip rate, use the drip rate formula from Chapter 12 to set up the following equation:**

$$\text{drip rate (gtt/min)} = \frac{50\text{ mL} \times \frac{60\text{ gtt}}{1\text{ mL}}}{30\text{ min}}$$

Where did we get 50 mL? The total volume to be infused is the sum of 3.75 mL (ampicillin) + 46.25 mL (D5 ½ NS), which equals 50 mL.

4. **Multiply and solve.**

$$x = \frac{3{,}000\text{ gtt}}{30\text{ min}}$$

$$x = 100\text{ gtt/min}$$

The drip rate is 100 gtt/min.

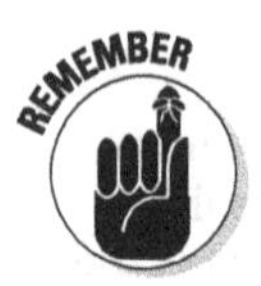

With pediatric dosing, you need to carefully monitor all the fluid being administered to the child, especially if the child has any kidney or heart problems. Incorporate all the fluid into your dosing calculations, including the volume to be flushed, the mL of medication itself, and the diluent.

Real-Life Practice: Determining Whether an Ordered IV Dosage Is Safe

You're asked to administer oxacillin 750 mg IV every 6 hours (3,000 mg/day) to a child who weighs 75 pounds. Is it a safe dose to give to this child?

To find out, just follow these steps:

1. **Convert the child's weight from lb to kg using the conversion factor 1 kg = 2.2 lb.**

   75 ÷ 2.2 = 34.09

   75 lb = 34.1 kg

2. **Calculate the maximum safe dose you can administer using mg/kg dosing.**

   According to the drug reference guide, a safe dose for a child weighing less than 40 kg is 100–200 mg/kg/day, given every 4 to 6 hours in divided doses. Simply multiply this mg/kg dose recommendation by the child's weight to calculate the maximum safe dose for the child. (See the earlier section "Dosing safely for kids' safety" for more details.)

   $$x = \frac{200 \text{ mg}}{1 \text{ kg}} \times 34.1 \text{ kg}$$

   $$x = 6{,}820 \text{ mg}$$

   The maximum safe dose is 6,820 mg/day. So it's okay to dispense this med at the ordered 3,000 mg/day, provided that you divide it into 4 doses/day (every 6 hours), as ordered.

Real-Life Practice: Figuring a Ped Patient's Fluid Needs

You have a child who weighs 43 kg, and you need to administer IV fluids. What are his maintenance fluid needs?

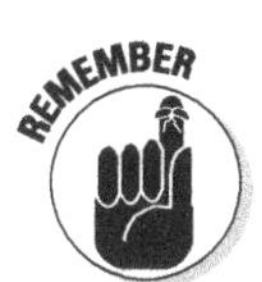

The rule for administering IV fluids is that children weighing more than 20 kg need 1.5 L (1,500 mL) of fluid plus an additional 20 mL for any kg over 20 kg. (See the section "The kilogram bands" for more details.)

To solve this problem, all you have to do is plug the child's weight into the formula for a child weighing more than 20 kg, like so:

$$F = 1{,}500 + (20(43 - 20))$$

$$F = 1{,}500 + (20 \times 23)$$

$$F = 1{,}500 + 460$$

$$F = 1{,}960$$

You must administer 1,960 mL over 24 hours.

Real-Life Practice: Safely Administering an IV Infusion

You need to administer 500 mg/2 mL of a medication in D5 ½ NS 75 mL over 30 minutes. Then you must follow it with a 15 mL flush. You're to use a volume-control device with a drop factor of 60 gtt/mL for the infusion. What's the total volume that you put into the volume-control chamber? What's the drip rate?

The first question is easy to answer. The dose is 75 mL over 30 minutes. So all you have to do is add 2 mL of the medication to 73 mL D5 ½ NS for a total of 75 mL.

To determine the drip rate of the infusion, follow these steps:

1. **Use the drip rate formula from Chapter 11 to set up the following equation:**

   $$\text{drip rate (gtt/min)} = \frac{75\text{ mL} \times \frac{60\text{ gtt}}{1\text{ mL}}}{30\text{ min}}$$

2. **Multiply and solve.**

   $$x = \frac{4{,}500}{30}$$

   $$x = 150$$

   The drip rate is 150 gtt/min.

Chapter 16

Adjusting Dosages for People in Special Situations

In This Chapter

- Understanding how medical conditions like kidney and liver diseases affect drug dosing
- Dosing for people with bowel diseases or malabsorption
- Considering older patients when dosing meds
- Practicing dosing in special situations with a couple of real-life problems

Medications differ in how the body metabolizes and excretes them. Some depend more on the liver for metabolism and elimination, while others depend more on the kidney. The patient's age and weight also affect the dosage and frequency of medication administration.

When you're dosing and administering medications, you need to be aware of any medical conditions your patients have, because a certain medication may or may not be okay to give, based on those medical conditions. Abnormalities in absorption, liver problems, and kidney disease dramatically affect how, when, and if you can (or should) administer a medication. If a patient is on dialysis, you must review the dosage of all meds before you administer them. For example, gabapentin (Neurontin), a commonly prescribed antiseizure medication, depends primarily on the kidney for elimination, so the doctor needs to decrease the dose if kidney disease is present.

In this chapter, we review various medical conditions that can affect how and when you give a medication. All health professionals must be aware of these factors (and usually are) before prescribing or dosing any medication.

Even though doctors often are aware of changes in liver function or kidney function and the other factors that can affect how the body handles a medication (and, thus, make the necessary dosing changes), it's important that you're also aware of such conditions and factors as well as the possible risk of side effects associated with different medications. The mantra is "Check, double-check, and check again!"

Keeping Up with the Kidneys

For any medication, how well the patient's kidneys are working is an important dosing consideration. The best way to determine a patient's kidney function is by looking at her *glomerular* (glow-*mair*-u-ler) *filtration rate,* or GFR. The GFR is a measure of how well your kidneys are acting like a filter (in other words, how well your kidneys are working). Measured in mL/min, you can find a patient's GFR on a certain blood chemistry panel, commonly referred to either as a *basic metabolic panel* or as a *chem-7,* depending on the hospital system in which you work.

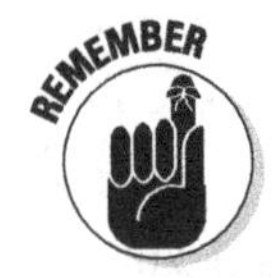

Before dosing any medication, you must know your patient's GFR.

In drug references, you often see the term *creatinine clearance rate* (CrCl), which is just a way of measuring kidney function. There are subtle differences between the terms CrCl and GFR, but when you see *creatinine clearance,* assume it to be the level of kidney function for dosing medications.

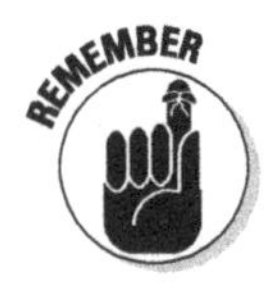

Don't hesitate to call the doctor or pharmacist if you have a question about dosing a medication for a patient with kidney problems. Remember the mantra "patient safety first."

Dosing considerations and changes for folks with kidney disease

The keys to making dosages right for those with kidney disease are knowing the patient's age, the extent of the patient's renal impairment, and the metabolism of commonly-dosed medications, and observing patient reactions. With that knowledge, you can dose and administer meds with ease.

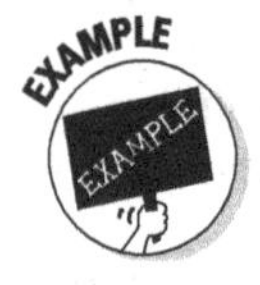

You're taking care of an 80-year-old woman with a history of kidney disease and are asked to administer gabapentin (Neurontin) 300 mg PO tid (orally, three times daily). What do you need to be aware of before administering this drug?

You don't have to do any math to find this answer. You just need to do the following:

1. **Know the patient's level of kidney function.**

   The doc needs to adjust the dose depending on the level of kidney function. Chronic kidney disease (CKD) is identified by five stages (Stage 1 through Stage 5), each with a different GFR value. Knowing the patient's stage of CKD by knowing the GFR helps you determine the proper dose.

2. **Know the patient's age.**

   Both younger and older patients with CKD may need a dosage adjustment. Differences in muscle mass, absorptive and elimination capacity, as well as other factors, can affect how well the body handles a medication. (See the section "Dosing for the Elderly" for more details.)

3. **Observe and take action.**

   You read in a drug reference that potential side effects of gabapentin include somnolence (drowsiness), confusion, and dizziness. These effects can be amplified, depending on the other medications the patient is taking.

   The next morning you notice that your patient is confused, compared to the previous day. You call the doctor, and she tells you to hold the medication until the confusion disappears.

In many cases of patients with kidney disease, the doctor will start a very low dose of gabapentin and slowly titrate up.

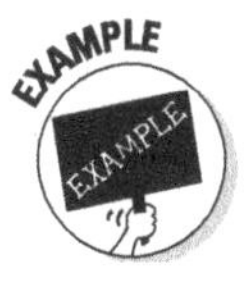

The doctor's order says to administer cephalexin (Keflex) 500 mg oral suspension PO q6h (every 6 hours). Cephalexin is available in a concentration of 250 mg/5 mL. You notice that on the patient's blood work the GFR is 30 mL/min (not very good). You reference a drug handbook, which states that a cephalexin dose should be reduced to 500 mg every 8 to 12 hours for a GFR in this range. You call the doctor and he asks you to decrease the dose to 500 mg every 12 hours. How many mL do you administer with each dose?

To find out, use the ratio-proportion method (see Chapter 8) and follow these steps:

1. **Set up the following proportion to determine how many mL contain 500 mg:**

   $$\frac{\text{known equivalent}}{\text{known equivalent}} = \frac{\text{known equivalent}}{\text{desired equivalent}}$$

   $$\frac{250 \text{ mg}}{5 \text{ mL}} = \frac{500 \text{ mg}}{x \text{ mL}}$$

2. **Cross-multiply and solve.**

   $250x = 5 \times 500$

   $250x = 2{,}500$

   $x = 10$

   You give 10 mL orally twice a day.

Because you double-checked, the patient received a safe but effective dose of the antibiotic.

A doctor's order says to give levofloxacin (Levaquin) 500 mg IV q24h (every 24 hours). Levofloxacin is available as a premixed infusion 500 mg in 100 mL D5W. You note that the patient's GFR is 25 mL/min. Is this an appropriate dose? If not, how much should you administer, in mL?

To solve this problem, use the ratio-proportion method and follow these steps:

1. **Know the level of kidney function.**

   You check a drug handbook (and the package insert) and see that the dose should be reduced for renal impairment (a GFR between 20 and 50 mL/min). You call the doctor, and he decreases the dose to 250 mg IV q24h.

2. **Set up the following proportion to determine how many mL contain 250 mL:**

   $$\frac{500 \text{ mg}}{100 \text{ mL}} = \frac{250 \text{ mg}}{x \text{ mL}}$$

3. **Cross-multiply and solve.**

   $500x = 100 \times 250$

   $500x = 25{,}000$

   $x = 50$

   You infuse 50 mL once a day.

Many other medications besides the three we mention in the preceding examples often require dosage adjustments based on kidney function. One of the most common ones that you'll deal with is insulin (see Chapter 13 for more details).

You're instructed to administer Humulin 70/30 (a mixed insulin) 26 units in the morning and 24 units in the afternoon. This regimen is similar to what the patient follows at home. The patient has acute kidney failure. You monitor the patient's blood glucose level before meals and at night, and you have to call the doctor a few times because the blood glucose levels are 50 to 60 mg/dL (that's very low). The doctor orders you to reduce the doses of Humulin 70/30 by fifty percent. What happened? What's the new, reduced dose?

To answer these questions, follow these steps:

1. **Know the level of kidney function.**

   The patient has had an acute worsening of his kidney function compared to his prior baseline. Because the kidneys clear and eliminate insulin from the body, the patient's reduced kidney function allows the insulin to hang around in the body longer than it should, thus driving the blood glucose level too low.

2. **To calculate the reduced dose, set up and solve the following simple equations:**

   26 units (morning) × 0.5 = 13 units (morning)

   24 units (afternoon) × 0.5 = 12 units (afternoon)

   Inject 13 units of Humulin in the morning and 12 units in the afternoon.

Dealing with dialysis

Dialysis is a type of artificial kidney filter that does what diseased kidneys can no longer do — cleans the blood by filtering and eliminating toxins from the body. Doctors often have to alter medication dosage and frequency of administration when a patient is on dialysis.

If you plan to work in a hospital or rehabilitation setting, prepare to work with the following two types of dialysis:

- **Hemodialysis (HD):** This type uses a dialysis machine to "clean the blood" three times a week. Most people on hemodialysis come to the hospital three times a week, either Monday-Wednesday-Friday or Tuesday-Thursday-Saturday. Often, doctors try to maintain a similar schedule when a person is in the hospital.
- **Peritoneal dialysis (PD):** This type is a more continuous type of dialysis, during which a solution is run through the patient's peritoneal cavity. This type is done by the patient's bedside over a 24-hour period in the hospital.

If you're taking care of a patient who's on dialysis, be aware of the following:

- Dialysis either partially or fully removes many medications. They may need to be re-dosed after dialysis. Examples of such meds include commonly prescribed antibiotics.
- Medications that are more "kidney dependent" for processing and elimination need to be dosed for a GFR (or creatinine clearance) of less than 10 mL/min for patients on dialysis.

The doctor's order says to administer cefepime (an antibiotic) 1 g IV q12h (every 12 hours) to a patient who's on hemodialysis. Cefepime is available as a 1 g (1,000 mg) vial that must be reconstituted within 100 mL isotonic saline. Is this an appropriate dose? If not, how much do you administer, in mL?

To answer these questions, use the ratio-proportion method and follow these steps:

1. **Know the impact of dialysis.**

   You research a drug reference and notice two things:

   First, dialysis removes the medication, so you need to administer it *after* dialysis on hemodialysis days.

   Second, the medication should be dosed for a creatinine clearance of less than 10 mL/min.

   You call the ordering doctor, and he changes the order to "Administer cefepime 500 mg IV q24h (every 24 hours) after dialysis on dialysis days. On other days, administer 500 mg IV q24h."

2. **Set up the following proportion to calculate the revised dose:**

   $$\frac{1{,}000\text{ mg}}{100\text{ mL}} = \frac{500\text{ mg}}{x\text{ mL}}$$

3. **Cross-multiply and solve.**

   $1{,}000x = 50{,}000$

   $x = 50$

   You infuse 50 mL every 24 hours.

HD versus PD

Medication dosage and frequency of administration can differ for a person on hemodialysis (HD) versus a person on peritoneal dialysis (PD). For instance, the cefepime example in the section "Dealing with dialysis" concerned a patient on HD. If you were taking care of someone who was on PD, the dose of cefepime would have to be adjusted further to 500 mg IV q48h.

If a facility has an electronic medical record (EMR) system or even just a computer-based ordering capability, built-in medical safety features will likely alert the ordering healthcare professional about potential medical interactions and will automatically adjust dosing regimens based on GFR level. Even so, be careful to double-check your dosing calculations for any patient who's on HD or PD.

Dosing for Liver Disease

In terms of medicine, the liver's primary responsibility is to metabolize and detoxify many medications. Liver disease affects its ability to do these jobs and, as a result, affects the dosage of those meds.

Cirrhosis is a chronic liver disease in which the liver becomes scarred. A cirrhotic or diseased liver doesn't work as well at metabolizing medications, so the doctor may need to make dosing adjustments for patients with cirrhosis.

Hepatitis, an acute inflammation of the liver, can also affect liver function. If you're taking care of someone with hepatitis, as with cirrhosis, you may be instructed to adjust medication dosages.

Hepatitis refers to an *acute* liver problem (predominantly one that develops severely and suddenly), while cirrhosis refers to a *chronic* problem (one that develops over time). Cirrhosis has many causes, and various forms of hepatitis can be among them.

Many classes of meds need dosing adjustments for patients who have liver and/or kidney impairment. Be on the lookout for antibiotics, heart medications, and antiseizure medications, among others.

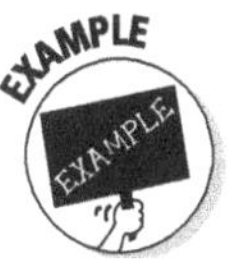

You're taking care of a patient admitted to the hospital with pneumonia. You read the medical record and learn that he has underlying cirrhosis. The medications ordered include erythromycin and lorazepam (Ativan). The lorazepam is ordered as an oral solution 2 mg PO q6h (every 6 hours). It's available in a concentration of 2 mg/mL. The erythromycin is ordered as an oral suspension 800 mg PO q6h. It comes as erythromycin ethylsuccinate (EES) 200 mg/5 mL. Are these appropriate and safe dosages, given the underlying cirrhosis? If not, how much lorazepam and erythromycin, in mL, should you administer?

To solve this problem, use the ratio-proportion method (see Chapter 8) and follow these steps:

1. **Research the lorazepam.**

   Consult a drug reference. The doc may need to reduce the med if the patient has problems with liver or kidney function. Because it's a sedative, you must use caution when dosing older patients (see the later section "Dosing for the Elderly" for more details). The hospital pharmacist confirms what you've read.

   You call the doctor, and he instructs you to decrease the dose to 1 mg q6h.

2. **Set up the following proportion to determine how many mL contain a 1 mg dose of lorazepam:**

   $$\frac{2\text{ mg}}{1\text{ mL}} = \frac{1\text{ mg}}{x\text{ mL}}$$

3. **Cross-multiply and solve.**

   $2x = 1$

   $x = 0.5$

   Administer 0.5 mL lorazepam every 6 hours.

4. **Research the erythromycin.**

   A drug reference tells you that erythromycin should be used cautiously in those with *hepatic impairment* (liver disease). You speak with the doctor, and he decreases the dosage from 800 mg to 400 mg PO q6h.

5. **Set up the following proportion to determine how many mL are in each 400 mg dose of erythromycin:**

   $$\frac{200\text{ mg}}{5\text{ mL}} = \frac{400\text{ mg}}{x\text{ mL}}$$

6. **Cross-multiply and solve.**

   $200x = 5 \times 400$

   $200x = 2{,}000$

   $x = 10$

   Administer the reduced dose of EES 10 mL every 6 hours.

You're instructed to administer phenytoin sodium (Dilantin) 150 mg PO tid (three times daily) to a hospitalized patient. You note in a drug reference that phenytoin sodium needs to be dosed cautiously for people with hepatic impairment.

You speak with the doctor, who decreases the dose to 100 mg PO tid. The patient has had difficulty with swallowing tablets, so you're ordered to administer the med in liquid form. It's available as an oral suspension 125 mg/5 mL. How many mL do you give?

To find out, use the ratio-proportion method and follow these steps:

1. **Set up the following proportion to determine how many mL contain 100 mg of phenytoin sodium:**

   $$\frac{125\text{ mg}}{5\text{ mL}} = \frac{100\text{ mg}}{x\text{ mL}}$$

2. **Cross-multiply and solve.**

   $125x = 5 \times 100$

   $125x = 500$

   $x = 4$

   Administer 4 mL phenytoin sodium PO tid.

Note: The examples in this chapter are meant to serve as a guide. However, some medications need to be dosed for patients with both liver and kidney impairment. Doctors use History and Physical forms (called H&Ps) to obtain all past medical and surgical problems as well as a list of meds taken at home so they can make sure that all medication dosing is safe and effective. The goal of doctors and other prescribing medical professionals is to ensure proper dosing of all medications. If you have any questions about the dosing of any med, don't hesitate to call the doctor.

Leveling the Playing Field

Doctors measure the effectiveness of some medications using *therapeutic drug monitoring* (a type of drug test that measures medication levels in the patient's blood). For certain medications that are metabolized and eliminated by the liver (such as phenytoin and theophylline) as well as those that are metabolized and eliminated by the kidneys (such as digoxin and lithium), you must adjust their doses if any liver or kidney disease is present.

Many drugs have a narrow *therapeutic range* (the range in which the med treats a disease effectively while remaining safe to use). If the medication level is beyond the therapeutic range, potentially dangerous effects to the body can occur.

You're taking care of a patient with congestive heart failure (CHF) who is admitted to the hospital for a CHF *exacerbation* (the CHF has grown more severe). The patient has a creatinine clearance of 30 mL/min. At home, the patient has been taking digoxin 0.125 mg PO daily. The doctor orders a digoxin level test, and it comes back at 3.2. What do you do?

You don't have to do any math to find the answer. Just follow these steps:

1. **Notice the digoxin level.**

   The level of 3.2 is higher than normal (which is between 0.8 and 2.0).

2. **Inform the physician.**

   You notify the doctor, and she says to hold the dose. She orders repeat drug level tests and follows up. Then the doctor reorders the dose as "digoxin 0.125 mg PO on Monday, Wednesday, and Friday."

Dosing for Patients Who Malabsorb Meds and Nutrients

Drug absorption refers to how well the body takes in and assimilates prescribed medications. If the patient can't absorb medication properly (or if she simply doesn't tolerate it), the doctor may need to adjust the dosage or administer the med another way for it to be effective.

Dosing with bowel diseases in mind

Many conditions, including any type of bowel disease (think Crohn's disease or inflammatory bowel disease, IBD), malabsorption syndromes (think celiac disease or gluten-mediated disease), or prior bowel surgery, can lead to the body's not absorbing meds (or nutrients) very well.

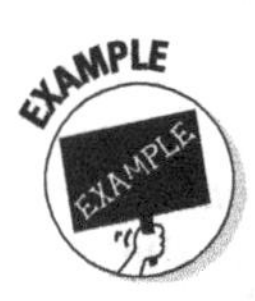

You're attending to a patient with Crohn's disease. The doctor's orders state to administer magnesium oxide (MgO) 400 mg PO tid. After two doses, the patient refuses to take the medication because the MgO made his diarrhea worse. The doc instructs you to give 4 g magnesium sulfate intravenously over 6 hours. It's available as a premixed solution of 2 g in 100 mL. How many mL do you administer? What's the flow (or infusion) rate?

To solve this problem, use the ratio-proportion method (see Chapter 8) and the basic flow rate formula (see Chapter 11). Follow these steps:

1. **Set up the following proportion to calculate the mL of magnesium sulfate to give:**

   $$\frac{2\text{ g}}{100\text{ mL}} = \frac{4\text{ g}}{x\text{ mL}}$$

2. **Cross-multiply and solve.**

   $2x = 400$

   $x = 200$

   Administer 200 mL magnesium sulfate. In other words, administer two 100 mL containers of the 2 g premixed solution.

3. **Calculate the flow rate.**

   flow rate (mL/hr) = total volume ÷ designated time

   flow rate (mL/hr) = 200 mL ÷ 6 hr

   flow rate (mL/hr) = 33.33 mL/hr

   The flow rate is 33 mL/hr.

You may often administer substances other than medications. For example, you may need to dose electrolytes and other nutrients *parenterally* (outside the digestive system) if a patient can't take them another way because of an absorption problem.

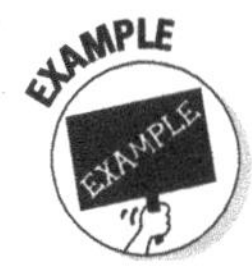

You're taking care of a patient with a malabsorption syndrome and severe iron deficiency. You need to replace the iron parenterally. The doctor's order tells you to administer iron sucrose (Venofer) 300 mg in 250 mL normal saline IV over 3 hours times 1 dose. What's the flow rate?

To find out, all you have to do is use the basic flow rate formula from Chapter 11, like so:

flow rate (mL/hr) = 250 mL ÷ 3 hr

flow rate (mL/hr) = 83.33 mL/hr

The flow rate is 83 mL/hr.

Factoring in other causes of decreased absorption

Not all causes of decreased absorption are the result of a bowel disease. For example, older patients experience a slowdown in *bowel motility* (movement of food through the intestines), as well as a decrease in the synthesis of stomach acid, which can decrease the absorption. Diabetes can also lead to decreased gastrointestinal (GI) motility, which can affect the absorption of medications.

Another cause may be related to congestive heart failure (CHF). CHF is a common reason why patients are admitted to the hospital, and it can certainly affect the heart and lungs. But it can also affect other organs, one of which is the intestine. Fluid can build up in the intestine (creating an *edematous,* or edema-related, state), thus affecting the absorption efficacy of many medications.

One class of medications that can be affected by edematous states is diuretics. Doctors prescribe medications like furosemide (Lasix) and metalozone (Zaroxolyn) to get rid of excess fluid from the body, but a lot of intestinal edema in a patient may affect absorption.

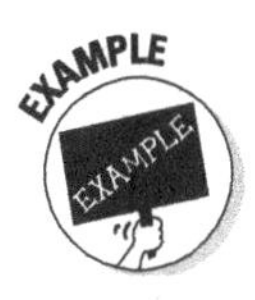

You're instructed to administer furosemide (Lasix) 80 mg PO bid to an 85-year-old patient with kidney dysfunction and diabetes, who was admitted to the hospital for a CHF exacerbation. What are some factors that will determine how well the furosemide will be absorbed?

To answer this question, apply critical thinking, not math.

- **Consider the kidney dysfunction.**

  The doctor prescribing the med will need to evaluate the GFR. With a lower GFR, the patient may need larger doses of furosemide for it to be effective. (See the earlier section "Keeping Up with the Kidneys" for more details.)

- **Consider the diabetes.**

  Decreased stomach acid secretion or decreased bowel motility accompany diabetes, although the doctor will not rule out a decrease for other reasons. Such a decrease can cause decreased absorption, so the furosemide may not be as effective as it should be.

- **Consider the CHF.**

  The intestinal edema (which is related to CHF), may affect the absorption of the furosemide.

Dosing for the Elderly

Today's population includes an increasing number of elderly patients. As people age, their body compositions and overall physiologies change, and these changes can affect the absorption, metabolism, and excretion of many medications. It's important to be aware of these changes when you calculate medication dosages for your elderly patients.

Considering the changing body physiology

The body of an older person contains less muscle mass and an increase in fat, and the digestion process and stomach movement slow down. In turn, older people also experience changes in the ability to absorb medications.

Even in the absence of other medical conditions, older people experience an age-related lessening of kidney function. This decrease in function can impact eliminating certain medications. Liver metabolism can also slow down.

Be sure to keep all these variables in mind when you dose medications for older patients.

Knowing the albumin level

Another important factor is how much a medication is bound to plasma proteins, principally albumin. (*Albumin* is a protein in the blood.)

Some medications, like digoxin, phenytoin, and lorazepam, are partially bound to albumin. If the albumin level in the patient's body is low, the amount of the medication that is protein-bound decreases, while the unbound portion of the medication increases. The unbound portion of the medication is what exerts the med's effects, including side effects and potential adverse reactions.

Dosing smaller, not bigger

For any doctor or other healthcare professional who prescribes or doses medications, the challenge is to use the smallest (but still effective) dose to achieve the desired outcome. The higher the dose, more often than not, the greater the possibility that the patient will experience more side effects.

Being on the lookout for harmful drug interactions

The elderly patient has, on average, four chronic medical problems and nine different medications to treat them. *Polypharmacy* (taking many medications) increases the chances of side effects and drug interactions. So you need to be hyperaware of possibly harmful drug interactions when you're dosing for elderly patients.

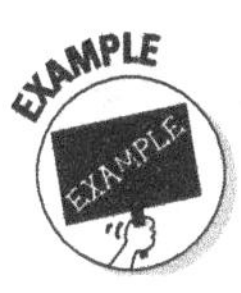

You're taking care of a 90-year-old woman and the doctor's order says to administer lorazepam (Ativan) 0.5 mg IV q8h (every 8 hours). What are some factors you need to consider when dosing this med in an elderly patient?

To work through this problem, put on your thinking cap instead of using your calculator.

- **Consider lorazepam.**

  Lorazepam is a *lipophilic* (fat-loving) medication. Changes in the body composition of elderly patients favor an increase in body fat and a decrease in muscle tissue. As a result, lorazepam may stay in the body longer and be harder for the body to eliminate.

- **Consider albumin.**

  If serum (blood) albumin is low, it can increase the protein-unbound portion of the medication in the body. The potential for side effects is, therefore, higher.

- **Consider any mix of meds.**

  Given the number of medications an elderly patient may be on, the potential for drug interactions definitely increases.

Real-Life Practice: Checking for Drug Interactions

You're taking care of a person admitted with pneumonia. He has a history of diabetes mellitus, chronic liver disease, and kidney disease with an estimated creatinine clearance of 25 mL/min (a low number). See if you can figure out what's wrong with these dosing orders.

The medications listed on his admission orders include the following:

- Ceftazidime (Fortaz) 1 g IV q8h
- Azithromycin 500 mg PO q24h
- Vancomycin 1 g IV times 1 dose
- Hydrocodone (Vicodin) 10/660 mg PO prn (as needed) for pain
- Insulin glargine (Lantus) 35 units subcut 1 time daily

Are the medications properly ordered, given this patient's medical problems? You get the answers by checking a drug reference. Here's what you find:

- **Ceftazidime:** For a creatinine clearance of 25 mL/min, the doctor needs to decrease the 1 g IV q8h dose. You call the doctor, and he changes the dose to 1 g IV q24h.
- **Azithromycin:** The doctor must reduce the azithromycin dose if any liver disease is present. The drug reference recommends that the doc decrease the dose to 250 mg daily and not exceed the maximum of 1.5 g over the course of treatment. You speak with the doctor, and, given the patient's history of liver disease, he changes the dose to 250 mg PO daily.
- **Vancomycin:** This one-time dose is appropriate for an admission order. Further dosing depends on the patient's kidney function.
- **Hydrocodone:** Hydrocodone preparations (such as Vicodin) are a combination of acetaminophen and hydrocodone. Because the patient has liver disease, you need to watch the acetaminophen (the 660 in the med's strength) closely. You speak with the doctor, and he discontinues the medication.
- **Insulin glargine:** You note that the patient has kidney disease. Watch his blood glucose levels over the next 24 hours and then reassess the insulin dose.

Real-Life Practice: Dosing Meds to a Patient on HD

You're taking care of a person who is on hemodialysis (HD). You look through the patient's chart and see the following new doctor's orders:

- Trimethoprim-sulfamethoxazole (Bactrim) 1 tablet DS (double-strength tablet containing 800 mg sulfamethoxazole and 160 mg trimethoprim) PO bid
- Spironolactone (Aldactone) 25 mg (1 oral tablet) PO bid
- Ceftriaxone (Rocephin) 1 g IV q24h

Are these medications okay to administer at these doses?

The key to dosing correctly is to recognize that your patient is on HD, to use a drug reference, and to communicate with the doctor. Here's what you find when you look in a drug reference:

- **Trimethoprim-sulfamethoxazole:** This med is contraindicated for patients with a GFR of less than 15 mL/min. You call the doctor, and she discontinues it.
- **Spironolactone:** This medication should generally be avoided if the patient has a GFR of less than 30 mL/min or is on dialysis. You call the kidney doctor, and he discontinues it.
- **Ceftriaxone:** The doctor needs to adjust this med for those on dialysis. The medication is prescribed correctly; however, it needs to be dosed *after* hemodialysis on dialysis days.

Chapter 17

Critical Care Dosing and Calculations

In This Chapter

- Knowing what to expect in the ICU
- Doing dosing calculations for patients with extremely low or high blood pressure
- Dosing for patients with heart failure or dysrhythmia
- Calculating heparin doses to treat serious medical conditions
- Getting some dosing practice with some real-life problems

You find most critically ill patients in a *critical care unit* (CCU), often also referred to as an *intensive care unit* (ICU). Often, critically ill patients have more than one body system affected, and these critical conditions require great care in drug dosing and constant monitoring.

Intensive care is usually indicated for patients who are *hemodynamically unstable*. In the critical care unit, you encounter patients who have problems with very low blood pressure (*shock*) or uncontrolled high blood pressure *(hypertensive crisis)*. You also take care of patients with respiratory failure, renal (kidney) failure, and/or cardiac problems, such as congestive heart failure (CHF), heart attack *(myocardial infarction)*, and *cardiogenic shock* (low blood pressure from the heart's failure to pump). Patients may be in a specialized unit, such as a coronary care unit (also abbreviated CCU), respiratory intensive care unit (RICU), neonatal intensive care unit (NICU), or trauma intensive care unit (TICU).

Critical care nursing can be very demanding. You need to be very careful but efficient with your dosage calculations because patients are critical and time is of the essence. In most critical care units, you use an infusion pump for IV therapy, and the pump does a lot of your work automatically. However, you still need to pay close attention to the meds you're administering and check and double-check your dosing calculations.

Whether you're working in the critical care unit or on a medical-surgical floor, as a medical professional, you must be familiar with your *scope of practice.* This means that you should never undertake any nursing action or perform any medical practice that you do not have sufficient knowledge of or are not qualified to do. For nurses, the scope of practice is determined by the state nursing board and can differ state by state.

In this chapter, you see and practice medical dosage calculations for critically ill patients. Critical care can be daunting, but don't stress out too much. Just gather up your knowledge and your skills, and you'll do fine.

Being Prepared for Intensive Work in Intensive Care

Patients in the critical care unit often have complicated cases. A whole lot is going on at once. The staff doesn't stand still for a single moment, so prepare yourself to be pulled in many directions at the same time. In the ICU, you face some tough conditions (which we cover in the next section), but we're here to help you overcome them.

What to expect in the ICU

In the ICU, be prepared to encounter these conditions:

- **Patient dosing requirements can change frequently.** As a result, your dosing calculations also change frequently.
- **A patient may *code* at any moment.** A *code* is an emergency announcement made on the hospital speaker system, such as "Code Black" (which often means bomb threat). *Coding* is slang for a patient emergency, such as "Code Blue" (which often means cardiac arrest). You must respond to all codes with both appropriate procedures and appropriate meds, correctly dosed.

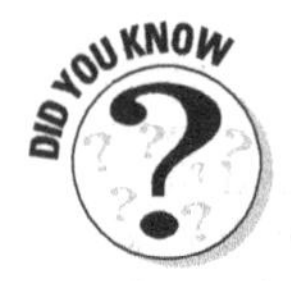

Codes vary widely from hospital to hospital for both patient emergencies and disasters. "Code Black" can mean "bomb threat" at one hospital and "child abduction" at another. This inconsistency can be a problem for a doctor who has privileges at multiple hospitals. The codes are supposed to prevent stress among visitors, but that may not work anymore. "Code Blue" is commonly associated with cardiac arrest, and the public knows it. Also, the public isn't deceived by pages for "Dr. Stillheart" or "Dr. Allcome."

- **Nursing coverage, even in the ICU, can be stretched during bad economic times.** Licensed Practical Nurses (LPNs) — also known as Licensed Vocational Nurses (LVNs) — are not permitted to work in some ICUs. The situation can increase the burden on the RNs.
- **Patients need to be monitored frequently.** Your monitoring of patients is critical because their conditions can change rapidly. You'll need to check the monitors or take vital signs frequently.

What to do to stay ahead of the game

How can you handle these difficult, demanding conditions? Experience, knowledge, and approach are your best tools. Here's what you need to do:

- **Get experience.** Experience in the ICU is the best teacher. The longer you do the work, the more you'll know.
- **Know your dosage calculations.** The more comfortable you are with medical dosage calculations, the less time you'll lose doing them.
- **Know your meds.** Be aware of the common medications ordered for ICU patients. In the ICU, you usually treat *hypertension* (high blood pressure), *hypotension* (low blood pressure), shock, heart failure, heart attack, kidney failure, and pain.
- **Know your procedures.** Become skilled at doing the common procedures ordered for ICU patients, including starting an IV, giving parenteral injections, and tube feeding.
- **Develop a calm approach.** Don't rush a calculation or a procedure. Be calm as you do your work. Consider the Japanese phrase *isogaba maware* which means, "When one rushes, instead of going in a straight line, one goes in a circle."

Raising a Shockingly Low Blood Pressure

In the ICU, you calculate flow rates and infusion times. In many cases, the flow rates are higher for critical patients, and the infusion times may vary, depending on how unstable the patient is.

Often, you have to deal with patients in shock, and doctor's orders reflect the need for aggressive volume resuscitation, often using normal saline (abbreviated NS). *Shock* (also known as circulatory shock) is a life-threatening condition, usually related to loss of blood volume. A patient's blood pressure may be so low that she requires liters of fluid before the BP stabilizes. Sometimes in cases like this, a doctor writes "1 L of fluids Wide Open." You set the infusion pump at 999 mL/hr to carry out this order.

To infuse fluids, you work with flow rate, infusion time, and total volume. Here are the formulas you need to know:

- Flow rate (mL/hr) = total volume (mL) ÷ infusion time (hr)
- Infusion time (hr) = total volume (mL) ÷ flow rate (mL/hr)
- Total volume (mL) = flow rate (mL/hr) × infusion time (hr)

You're asked to administer an NS bolus 500 mL over 30 minutes to a patient who's in shock. The patient's blood pressure is 80/40 mmHg. After the initial fluid bolus, the order states to administer another 1 L (1,000 mL) over 3 hours. What's the flow rate for both the initial fluid bolus and the subsequent maintenance infusion?

To solve this problem, follow these steps:

1. **Use the flow rate formula to calculate the flow rate of the bolus infusion.**

   flow rate (mL/hr) = total volume (mL) ÷ infusion time (hr)

   flow rate (mL/hr) = 500 mL ÷ 0.5 hr

   flow rate (mL/hr) = 1,000 mL/hr

   The flow rate of the bolus is 1,000 mL/hr, given over 0.5 hours.

2. **Use the flow rate formula to calculate the maintenance flow rate.**

   flow rate (mL/hr) = 1,000 mL ÷ 3 hr

   flow rate (mL/hr) = 333.3 mL/hr

   The flow rate of the maintenance fluid is 333 mL/hr, given over 3 hours.

   After the initial fluid bolus, you adjust the infusion pump to reflect the change for the maintenance flow rate.

The following sections show you what to do in critical situations that often accompany patient shock.

Dealing with acid buildup

Many patients in the critical care unit, especially those in shock, can develop problems with acid buildup in the body. Patients in shock often experience lactic acid buildup from the shocklike state or loss of bicarbonate (think baking soda) in the stool if significant diarrhea is present.

To treat these patients, doctors may order you to administer intravenous fluids with bicarbonate. You calculate the flow rates and infusion times the same way you do for fluids without bicarbonate.

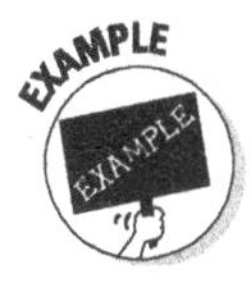

You're asked to administer 0.45% NaCl (also called ½ NS) with 75 mEq of sodium bicarbonate at 150 mL/hr for a 1 L (1,000 mL) bag only. What's the infusion time?

To answer this question, all you have to do is plug the given numbers into the infusion time formula, like so:

infusion time (hr) = total volume (mL) ÷ flow rate (mL/hr)

infusion time (hr) = 1,000 mL ÷ 150 mL/hr

infusion time (hr) = 6.67 hr

The infusion time is 6.7 hr, or 6 hr 42 min. (To see more about mEq, or milliequivalents, take a look at Chapter 18.)

Infusing pressors when other fluids aren't enough

Sometimes aggressive volume resuscitation with intravenous saline isn't enough to stabilize the blood pressure. In that case, the doctor may order you to administer other meds, called pressors, as continuous infusions to raise the BP.

A *pressor* is a substance that will raise blood pressure. Examples of pressors include dopamine, norepinephrine (Levophed), phenylephrine (Neo-Synephrine), and vasopressin. The following sections show you how to do dosage calculations for pressors.

Finding the flow rate when you know the dosage

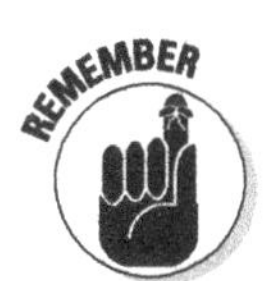

You frequently calculate the flow rate in mL/hr after you know the initial drug dosage. Most pressors are dosed in mcg either per unit of patient metric weight (kg), per unit of time (min), or both. For example,

- Dopamine is commonly dosed in mcg/kg/min.
- Norepinephrine is commonly dosed in mcg/min.
- Phenylephrine is commonly dosed in mcg/min.
- Vasopressin is commonly dosed in units/min.

You need to administer dopamine 800 mg in 500 mL 0.9% saline (NS) at 15 mcg/kg/min. The patient weighs 200 pounds. What's the flow rate in mL/hr?

Before you can find the flow rate, you have to do some converting. After you have the right units, use the ratio-proportion method and dimensional analysis (see Chapter 8) to find the flow rate. Follow these steps:

1. **Use the conversion factor 1 kg = 2.2 lb to convert the patient's weight from lb to kg.**

   desired unit = given unit × conversion factor

   $$x\text{ kg} = 200\text{ lb} \times \frac{1\text{ kg}}{2.2\text{ lb}}$$

   $$x\text{ kg} = \frac{200}{2.2}$$

   $$x\text{ kg} = 90.9$$

   The patient weighs 91 kg. (***Note:*** When converting from lb to kg, you can also just divide lbs by 2.2. See Chapter 4 for more on converting units.)

2. **Use the conversion factor 1 mg = 1,000 mcg to convert the dose (800 mg) from mg to mcg.**

   $$x\text{ mcg} = 800\text{ mg} \times \frac{1{,}000\text{ mcg}}{1\text{ mg}}$$

   $$x\text{ mcg} = \frac{800 \times 1{,}000}{1}$$

   $$x\text{ mcg} = 800{,}000$$

   The dose is 800,000 mcg in 500 mL NS.

3. **Multiply the patient's weight by the dose in mcg/kg to figure out the total dose for a patient weighing 91 kg.**

   15 mcg/kg × 91 kg = 1,365 mcg

   You infuse 1,365 mcg/min.

4. **Set up the following proportion to determine how many mL of solution contain 1,365 mcg:**

   $$\frac{\text{known equivalent}}{\text{known equivalent}} = \frac{\text{known equivalent}}{\text{desired equivalent}}$$

   $$\frac{800{,}000\text{ mcg}}{500\text{ mL}} = \frac{1{,}365\text{ mcg}}{x\text{ mL}}$$

5. **Cross-multiply and solve.**

   $800{,}000x = 682{,}500$

   $x = 0.853$

You infuse 0.85 mL/min to deliver 1,365 mcg/min.

6. **Set up the following dimensional analysis equation to convert the flow rate from mL/min to mL/hr:**

$$\text{Dose} = \frac{\text{factor}}{\text{factor}} \times \frac{\text{factor}}{\text{factor}}$$

$$x = \frac{0.85\text{ mL}}{1\cancel{\text{min}}} \times \frac{60\cancel{\text{min}}}{1\text{ hr}}$$

The min cancel out.

7. **Multiply and solve.**

$x = 0.85 \times 60$

$x = 51$

The flow rate is 51 mL/hr.

Calculating the dosage when you know the flow rate

Another typical pressor dosage calculation is the inverse of the calculation we use in the preceding example: You know the infusion rate in mL/hr and need to determine the dosage.

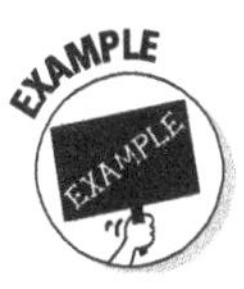

You're instructed to administer phenylephrine (Neo-Synephrine) 10 mg in 500 mL NS for a patient in septic shock. If the infusion rate is 15 mL/hr, what's the corresponding dosage in mcg/min?

To find out, use dimensional analysis, simple conversions, and the ratio-proportion method. Follow these steps:

1. **Set up the following dimensional analysis equation to convert the flow rate from mL/hr to mL/min:**

$$x = \frac{15\text{ mL}}{1\cancel{\text{hr}}} \times \frac{1\cancel{\text{hr}}}{60\text{ min}}$$

The hours cancel out.

2. **Divide and solve.**

$$x = \frac{15}{60}$$

$x = 0.25$

The flow rate is 0.25 mL/min.

3. **Use the conversion factor 1 mg = 1,000 mcg to convert the dose (10 mg) from mg to mcg.**

$$x \text{ mcg} = 10 \text{ mg} \times \frac{1{,}000 \text{ mcg}}{1 \text{ mg}}$$

$$x \text{ mcg} = \frac{10 \times 1{,}000}{1}$$

$$x \text{ mcg} = 10{,}000$$

The dose is 10,000 mcg in 500 mL NS.

4. **Set up the following proportion to determine how many mcg are in 0.25 mL:**

$$\frac{10{,}000 \text{ mcg}}{500 \text{ mL}} = \frac{x \text{ mcg}}{0.25 \text{ mL}}$$

5. **Cross-multiply and solve.**

$500x = 2{,}500$

$x = 5$

When you infuse 0.25 mL/min, you infuse 5 mcg/min of phenylephrine.

With each medical dosage calculation you do, you begin to develop your own thought process for approaching complex problems. This is especially true in critical care medicine. The key is breaking down a complex problem into its essential components.

Here's the preceding example with a simple twist. You're instructed to administer phenylephrine (Neo-Synephrine) 10 mg in 500 mg NS for a patient in septic shock. If the infusion rate is 15 mL/hr, what's the corresponding dosage in mcg/min?

To solve this problem, use dimensional analysis, simple conversions, and the ratio-proportion method. Follow these steps:

1. **Set up the following dimensional analysis equation to convert the flow rate from mL/hr to mL/min:**

$$x = \frac{15 \text{ mL}}{1 \cancel{\text{hr}}} \times \frac{1 \cancel{\text{hr}}}{60 \text{ min}}$$

The hours cancel out.

2. **Multiply and solve.**

$$x = \frac{15}{60}$$

$$x = 0.25$$

The flow rate is 0.25 mL/min.

3. **Set up the following proportion to calculate the concentration (the strength) of the solution in mg/mL:**

$$\frac{500 \text{ mL}}{10 \text{ mg}} = \frac{1 \text{ mL}}{x \text{ mg}}$$

4. **Cross-multiply and solve.**

$$500x = 10$$

$$x = 0.02 \text{ mg}$$

The concentration is 0.02 mg/mL.

5. **Use the conversion factor 1 mg = 1,000 mcg to convert the concentration from mg (0.02 mg) to mcg.**

$$x \text{ mcg} = 0.02 \text{ mg} \times \frac{1{,}000 \text{ mcg}}{1 \text{ mg}}$$

$$x \text{ mcg} = \frac{0.02 \times 1{,}000}{1}$$

$$x \text{ mcg} = \frac{20}{1}$$

$$x \text{ mcg} = 20$$

The concentration of 0.02 mg/mL is equal to 20 mcg/mL.

6. **Set up the following dimensional analysis equation to convert the dose (20 mcg/mL) to mcg/min; use the flow rate you calculated in Steps 1 and 2 (0.25 mL/min):**

$$x = \frac{0.25 \cancel{\text{mL}}}{1 \text{ min}} \times \frac{20 \text{ mcg}}{1 \cancel{\text{mL}}}$$

The mL cancel out.

7. **Multiply and solve.**

   $x = 0.25 \times 20$

   $x = 5$

   The dosage is 5 mcg/min.

What's different about this calculation? You determine the concentration of the solution before converting from mg to mcg. The concentration is the dosage of a medication (usually mg or mcg) divided by the volume of the solution (usually mL).

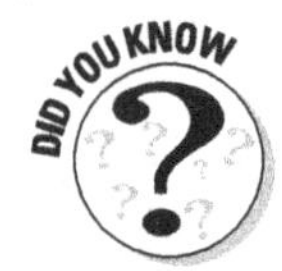

Did you know that dopamine can have different effects on the body, depending on the dose? Low-dose dopamine, usually dosed 1 to 5 mcg/kg/min, is sometimes referred to as *renal dose dopamine* because it increases blood flow to the kidneys. A higher dose, in the realm of 6 to 10 mcg/kg/min, is often called a *cardiac dose* because it can have effects on the heart. Higher doses, greater than 10 mcg/kg/min, have what are called *vasoconstrictor effects,* which help raise blood pressure.

Titrating the dose

In critical care, the dosing of many infusions isn't a static process but rather a dynamic one. Many medication orders are *titration orders,* which means the medication dosage can be altered to achieve a desired effect, depending on the infusion and the doctor's order. Pressors, infusions to treat high blood pressure, furosemide, and insulin infusions can be titrated. With the pressor medications that we describe in this chapter, the object is usually to achieve a goal blood pressure.

You're treating a patient admitted to the CCU with hypotension (low blood pressure). The doctor's order says to titrate dopamine 800 mg in 500 mL NS to achieve a mean arterial pressure (MAP) of greater than 65 mmHg. The patient's weight is 200 pounds (91 kg). The initial flow rate is 30 mL/hr, which corresponds to a dose of 9 mcg/kg/min. You titrate the flow rate to 50 mL/hr and are able to achieve the goal MAP with this flow rate. What is the corresponding dose in mcg/kg/min?

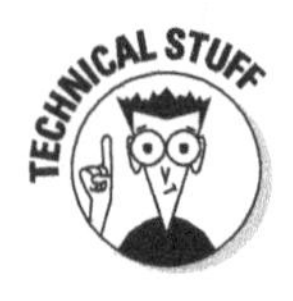

It's believed that a MAP greater than 60 mmHg is enough to sustain the organs of the average person. If the MAP falls significantly below this number for an appreciable time, the organs won't get enough blood flow and will become *ischemic* (restricted in blood supply) and, therefore, liable to damage or dysfunction.

To find out the corresponding dose in mcg/kg/min, use simple conversions and dimensional analysis and follow these steps:

1. **Use the conversion factor 1 kg = 2.2 lb to convert the patient's weight from lb to kg.**

   x kg = 200 lb ÷ 2.2

   x kg = 90.9

   The patient weights 91 kg.

2. **Use the conversion factor 1 mg = 1,000 mcg to convert from mg to mcg.**

   $$x \text{ mcg} = 800 \text{ mg} \times \frac{1{,}000 \text{ mcg}}{1 \text{ mg}}$$

   $$x \text{ mcg} = \frac{800 \times 1{,}000}{1}$$

   $$x \text{ mcg} = \frac{800{,}000}{1}$$

   $$x \text{ mcg} = 800{,}000$$

   There are 800,000 mcg in 800 mg.

3. **Set up the following dimensional analysis equation to convert the flow rate from mL/hr to mL/min.**

   $$x = \frac{50 \text{ mL}}{1 \cancel{\text{hr}}} \times \frac{1 \cancel{\text{hr}}}{60 \text{ min}}$$

4. **Divide and solve.**

   $$x = \frac{50}{60}$$

   $$x = 0.83$$

   The patient is receiving 0.83 mL/min.

5. **Set up the following dimensional analysis equation to convert the flow rate from mL/min to mcg/min:**

   $$x = \frac{0.83 \cancel{\text{mL}}}{1 \text{ min}} \times \frac{800{,}000 \text{ mcg}}{500 \cancel{\text{mL}}}$$

   The mL cancel out.

6. **Divide and solve.**

$$x = \frac{0.83 \times 800{,}000}{500}$$

$$x = 1{,}328$$

The flow rate is 1,328 mcg/min.

7. **Divide the flow rate by the patient's body weight to calculate how many mcg/min the patient is getting per kg.**

x = 1,328 mcg/min ÷ 91 kg

x = 14.59 mcg/kg/min

The adjusted dosage is 14.6 mcg/kg/min.

Lowering Skyrocketing High Blood Pressure

In the CCU, you see all variations of blood pressure, from the extremely low blood pressure (shock) to the *hypertensive crisis,* where the blood pressure has skyrocketed. You use the same calculations for meds that lower blood pressure that you use for meds that boost blood pressure (see the preceding section for details on raising blood pressure).

You can administer BP-lowering medications as single doses or as continuous infusions, depending on the doctor's orders. These medications can be titrated to achieve a goal pressure, as per a doctor's order. If the patient is critical enough to be kept in intensive care, in all probability she's likely to be on a continuous infusion, titrated to keep her blood pressure at a desired level.

The following sections show you how to do dosage calculations for some common BP-lowering meds.

Leading with labetalol

Labetalol is a very effective medication used to treat high blood pressure. In a CCU environment, it's a common medication that many doctors will initially prescribe. As a continuous infusion, labetalol is easily titratable and usually well tolerated by the patient.

Giving a single dose of labetalol

You need to administer labetalol 10 mg IV push to a patient who has an elevated blood pressure. Labetalol is available in a concentration of 5 mg/mL. How many mL do you administer?

To find out, use the ratio-proportion method and follow these steps:

1. **Set up the following proportion:**

   $$\frac{5\text{ mg}}{1\text{ mL}} = \frac{10\text{ mg}}{x\text{ mL}}$$

2. **Cross-multiply and solve.**

   $5x = 10$

   $x = 2$

   You give 2 mL IV push.

Figuring the infusion rate of labetalol

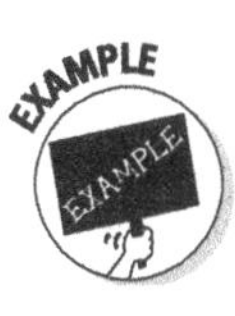

You notice that the patient's blood pressure decreases only for a short time. You notify the doctor immediately, and he instructs you to start a labetalol infusion at 2 mg/min and titrate to keep the systolic blood pressure (SBP) less than 190 mmHg. According to your drug reference, labetalol 200 mg is diluted in 160 mL D5W. What's the infusion rate?

To answer this question, use the ratio-proportion method and the flow rate formula. Follow these steps:

1. **Set up the following proportion to calculate the strength of the solution (in other words, to find out how many mg are in 1 mL):**

   $$\frac{160\text{ mL}}{200\text{ mg}} = \frac{1\text{ mL}}{x\text{ mg}}$$

2. **Cross-multiply and solve.**

   $160x = 200$

   $x = 1.25$

   There are 1.25 mg in 1 mL of solution.

3. **Set up the following proportion to determine how many mL/min you need to administer, given that you must give 2 mg/min and 1 mL contains 1.25 mg:**

   $$\frac{1\text{ mL}}{1.25\text{ mg}} = \frac{x\text{ mL}}{2\text{ mg}}$$

4. **Cross-multiply and solve.**

   $1.25x = 2$

   $x = 1.6$

   You need to infuse 1.6 mL/min to dose 2 mg/min of labetalol.

5. **Use the conversion factor 1 hr = 60 min to convert the flow rate from mL/min to mL/hr.**

   flow rate (mL/hr) = flow rate (mL/min) × 60 min/1 hr

   flow rate (mL/hr) = 1.6 × 60

   flow rate (mL/hr) = 96

   The patient should receive labetalol at 96 mL/hr.

Exploding with nitro

You can use two kinds of nitro to treat hypertensive crisis. (No, we aren't talking about dynamite, but it's a relative.) The meds are nitroprusside and nitroglycerin. Both are dosed in mcg/min.

Nitroglycerin can give the patient a headache, which may require you to lower the infusion rate, substitute another medication, or discontinue altogether if the headache doesn't go away.

Dynamic trio: A brief history of nitroglycerin

Here's the world's shortest history of dynamite and dosing.

Ascanio Sobrero synthesized glyceryl trinitrate (also known as *nitroglycerin*) in 1847. In the 1860s, Alfred Nobel was making nitroglycerin, and an explosion killed his younger brother. By 1867, his company had developed dynamite by mixing nitro with diatomaceous earth. Much safer!

Early on, people knew handling nitro could cause sudden intense headaches. Dr. William Murrell reasoned that the reason for these headaches was because the substance was working as a *vasodilator*, enlarging the blood vessels. Murrell experimented with using nitro to treat angina pectoris and began treating patients with small doses. He found no headaches (unless the dose was too high). He published his results in *The Lancet* in 1879.

Doctors called the med glyceryl trinitrate so the term *nitro* wouldn't alarm patients. It was a big success and is still in use today. And, of course, you've heard of the Nobel Prize in physiology or medicine.

You're asked to give nitroprusside to a patient in hypertensive crisis, starting at 0.3 mcg/kg/min. Then you must titrate the dose to maintain a SBP of less than 190 mmHg. The nitroprusside is 50 mg diluted in 1,000 mL of D5W. The patient weighs 190 pounds. If the flow rate is 20 mL/hr, what's the titrated dose in mcg/kg/min?

To solve this problem, do some basic converting, use the ratio-proportion method, and follow these steps:

1. **Use the conversion factor 1 kg = 2.2 lb to convert the patient's weight from lb to kg.**

   x kg = 190 lb ÷ 2.2

   x kg = 86.36

   The patient weighs 86 kg.

2. **Use the conversion factor 1 mg = 1,000 mcg to convert the solution's concentration from mg/mL to mcg/mL.**

   $$x \text{ mcg} = 50 \text{ mg} \times \frac{1{,}000 \text{ mcg}}{1 \text{ mg}}$$

   $$x \text{ mcg} = \frac{50 \times 1{,}000}{1}$$

   $$x \text{ mcg} = \frac{50{,}000}{1}$$

   $$x \text{ mcg} = 50{,}000$$

   There are 50,000 mcg in 1,000 mL D5W.

3. **Set up the following proportion to convert the flow rate from 20 mL/hr to mL/min:**

   $$\frac{20 \text{ mL}}{60 \text{ min}} = \frac{x \text{ mL}}{1 \text{ min}}$$

4. **Cross-multiply and solve.**

   $60x = 20$

   $x = 0.33$

   The flow rate is 0.33 mL/min.

5. **Set up the following proportion to determine how many mcg the patient is getting per min, given that 1,000 mL contain 50,000 mcg and the flow rate is 0.33 mL/min:**

$$\frac{50{,}000\text{ mcg}}{1{,}000\text{ mL}} = \frac{x\text{ mcg}}{0.33\text{ mL}}$$

6. **Cross-multiply and solve.**

   $1{,}000x = 0.33 \times 50{,}000$

   $1{,}000x = 16{,}500$

   $x = 16.5$

   The patient is receiving 16.5 mcg/min.

7. **Divide the dose by the patient's weight to determine how many mcg the patient is getting per kg per min.**

   $x = 16.5\text{ mcg/min} \div 86\text{ kg}$

   $x = 0.19\text{ mcg/kg/min}$

   The titrated dose is 0.19 mcg/kg/min.

You're asked to administer nitroglycerin IV to a patient with uncontrolled hypertension and new onset pulmonary edema. The nitroglycerin is 100 mg in 250 mg D5W. You must initially dose the nitro at 15 mcg/min. What's the infusion rate in mL/hr?

To find out, use the ratio-proportion method and follow these steps:

1. **Set up the following proportion to determine the concentration of the solution (in other words, how many mcg are in 1 mL):**

   $$\frac{250\text{ mL}}{100{,}000\text{ mcg}} = \frac{1\text{ mL}}{x\text{ mcg}}$$

2. **Cross-multiply and solve.**

   $250x = 100{,}000$

   $x = 400$

   There are 400 mcg in 1 mL of solution.

3. **Set up the following proportion to calculate the flow rate in mL/min, given that you must give 15 mcg/min and 1 mL contains 400 mcg:**

   $$\frac{1\text{ mL}}{400\text{ mcg}} = \frac{x\text{ mL}}{15\text{ mcg}}$$

4. **Cross-multiply and solve.**

   $400x = 15$

   $x = 0.0375$

You infuse 0.0375 mL/min when you infuse 15 mcg. Round that up to 0.04 mL/min.

5. **Convert the flow rate from mL/min to mL/hr.**

   flow rate (mL/hr) = flow rate (mL/min) × 60 min/1 hr

   flow rate (mL/hr) = 0.04 × 60

   flow rate (mL/hr) = 2.4

   The patient should receive 2.4 mL/hr.

Nitroprusside is a very potent blood pressure medicine. Because it can really lower blood pressures in a short period of time, a doctor may use a device called an arterial line to follow the blood pressure closely. An *arterial line* is a catheter that the doctor places in an artery, usually the radial artery in the forearm. It allows the medical team to closely follow the patient's blood pressure minute by minute.

Dosing Meds That Fight Heart Failure

Medications that help to get a failing heart started are called *inotropes* (*eye-no-tropes*). Positive inotropic agents increase myocardial contractility; in other words, they increase the strength of the heart muscle contractions. Examples of positive inotropic agents include dopamine, dobutamine, milrinone, and epinephrine (Adrenalin). The following sections show you how to do dosage calculations for some of these meds.

Calculating the dosage of epinephrine

Epinephrine is used in the CCU, often for patients after heart surgery. Like dopamine, different dosages can have different effects on the body. Also, patients on epinephrine are often on other meds, like milrinone, dopamine, or dobutamine. These medications are frequently titrated, based on readings from a Swan-Ganz catheter. Epinephrine is dosed in mcg/min.

A *Swan-Ganz catheter* is a device that measures, among other things, the filling pressure ("wedge" pressure) of the heart. Doctors use different measurements to titrate post-heart surgery meds, including the *pulmonary capillary wedge pressure* (PCWP) or *cardiac index* (CI). A typical order may read, "Titrate to keep the PCWP > 20 mmHg."

You're treating a patient with decompensated heart failure (functional deterioration). You're ordered to start epinephrine 3 mg in 250 mL D5W at 2 mcg/min. What is the flow rate in mL/hr?

To solve this problem, first do some simple converting and then use the ratio-proportion method. Follow these steps:

1. **Use the conversion factor 1 mg = 1,000 mcg to convert from mg to mcg to determine how many mcg are in the 250 mL solution.**

   $$x \text{ mcg} = 3 \text{ mg} \times \frac{1{,}000 \text{ mcg}}{1 \text{ mg}}$$

   $$x \text{ mcg} = \frac{3 \times 1{,}000}{1}$$

   $$x \text{ mcg} = \frac{3{,}000}{1}$$

   $$x \text{ mcg} = 3{,}000$$

   There are 3,000 mcg in 250 mL D5W.

2. **Set up the following proportion to convert 2 mcg/min to mL/min:**

   $$\frac{3{,}000 \text{ mcg}}{250 \text{ mL}} = \frac{2 \text{ mcg}}{x \text{ mL}}$$

3. **Cross-multiply and solve.**

   $3{,}000x = 500$

   $x = 0.167$

   The volume 0.167 mL, or 0.17 mL, contains 2 mcg.

4. **Set up the following dimensional analysis equation to convert the flow rate from mL/min to mL/hr:**

   $$x = \frac{0.17 \text{ mL}}{1 \cancel{\text{min}}} \times \frac{60 \cancel{\text{min}}}{1 \text{ hr}}$$

   The min cancel out.

5. **Multiply and solve.**

   $x = 0.17 \times 60$

   $x = 10.2$

   The patient should receive 10 mL/hr.

Figuring the dosages for milrinone

Milrinone (Primacor) is a heart medication that does many things. Not only does it increase the contraction strength of the heart muscle (like epinephrine, a positive inotrope), but it can also help increase the blood supply to the heart with minimal effects on the heart rate. It can be used in conjunction with other positive inotropic medications or can be used solely on its own. It is often used in patients with very advanced systolic heart failure (meaning the heart is not working well as a pump) and also in patients after heart bypass and/or valvular surgery. Milrinone is dosed as mcg/kg/min after an initial (loading) dose in mcg/kg.

Note: Dopamine and dobutamine are also dosed in mcg/kg/min but without the need to administer a loading dose.

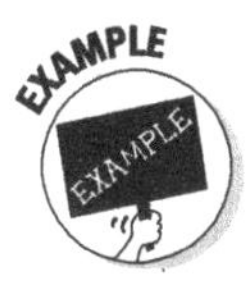

You're taking care of a patient who is S/P heart surgery (status post heart surgery) and has a Swan-Ganz catheter. You're asked to titrate milrinone 20 mg in 100 mL D5W, starting at 0.4 mcg/kg/min to maintain a cardiac index (CI) > 2.0. The patient weighs 180 pounds. What's the initial flow rate?

To solve this problem, you need to do some simple converting and then use the ratio-proportion method. Follow these steps:

1. **Use the conversion factor 1 kg = 2.2 lb to convert the patient's weight from lb to kg.**

   x kg = 180 lb ÷ 2.2

   x kg = 81.8

   The patient weighs 82 kg.

2. **Use the conversion factor 1 mg = 1,000 mcg to convert from mg to mcg.**

   $$x \text{ mcg} = 20 \text{ mg} \times \frac{1{,}000 \text{ mcg}}{1 \text{ mg}}$$

   $$x \text{ mcg} = \frac{20 \times 1{,}000}{1}$$

   $$x \text{ mcg} = \frac{20{,}000}{1}$$

   $$x \text{ mcg} = 20{,}000$$

3. **Multiply the dose in mcg/kg by the patient's weight to calculate the initial dose in mcg/kg/min.**

   x mcg/kg = 0.4×82

   $x = 32.8$

   The dosage of milrinone is 33 mcg/min for a patient who weights 82 kg.

4. **Set up the following proportion to determine the flow rate in mL/min, given that you're to dose at 33 mcg/min and the 100 mL solution contains 20,000 mcg:**

   $$\frac{20{,}000 \text{ mcg}}{100 \text{ mL}} = \frac{33 \text{ mcg}}{x \text{ mL}}$$

5. **Cross-multiply and solve.**

   $20{,}000x = 100 \times 33$

   $20{,}000x = 3{,}300$

   $x = 0.165$

   There are 33 mcg in about 0.16 mL of solution. Infuse at a rate of 0.16 mL/min.

6. **Convert the flow rate from mL/min to mL/hr.**

   flow rate (mL/hr) = flow rate (mL/min) × 60 min/1 hr

   flow rate (mL/hr) = 0.16×60

   flow rate (mL/hr) = 9.6

   The patient should receive milrinone at 10 mL/hr.

Treating a Dysrhythmia

When you take a patient's vital signs, you note whether he has a very fast pulse or a very slow one. A fast pulse — greater than 100 beats per minute (bpm) — is called *tachycardia.* A slow heart rate — less than 60 bpm —is called *bradycardia*. These terms are from Greek words that literally mean "rapid heart" and "slow heart."

Restrictive parameters apply for medications that can slow down the heart rate (or have a *chronotropic* effect). You will read doctor's orders that say "Do not give this medication if the heart rate is less than 50 bpm." Although the true definition of bradycardia is <60 BPM, for the purpose of administering many heart medications, a cutoff of 50 or 55 bpm is often used.

For patients in critical care units, or on any *telemetry floor* (a unit where you monitor heart patients hooked up to monitors), after you identify a tachycardia or bradycardia, your next step is to make sure the patient doesn't have a *dysrhythmia* (dizz-*rith*-mia) — an abnormal heart rhythm. If you see an abnormal heart rhythm on the monitor, call the doctor immediately. You will likely be ordered to do a patient assessment, including taking the vital signs and obtaining an *electrocardiogram* (or EKG for short), to help the doctor know if a dysrhythmia is indeed present.

Many meds, including amiodarone, diltiazem (Cardizem), metoprolol (Lopressor), esmolol, and other *anti-arrhythmic* medications, like procainamide, either speed up or slow down the heart rate. You give some of these medications, like metoprolol, in single doses. You administer others, like esmolol and diltiazem, as continuous infusions. The following sections show you how to do dosage calculations for some of these heart-related meds.

Administering continuous infusions to treat dysrhythmia

You can be instructed to administer meds like esmolol and diltiazem as continuous infusions, particularly when the doctor judges a single dose to be insufficient for keeping a patient out of the abnormal heart rhythm.

You're taking care of a patient who has developed atrial fibrillation with a rapid ventricular response. (In other words, the heart muscles of the atria are contracting in a chaotic manner and the ventricle of the heart is trying to keep up with the chaotic atria by beating very fast.) He has a tachycardia, with a pulse of 120 beats per minute. You're instructed to administer diltiazem by first giving a 5 mg bolus followed by a diltiazem drip at 10 mg/hr.

You first reconstitute the med by injecting 50 mL of D5W into 250 mg of diltiazem for a final volume of 300 mL and a final concentration of 0.83 mg/mL (see Chapter 12 for more details on reconstituting meds). What volume, in mL, contains the initial 5 mg bolus? What's the infusion rate for the ordered dose of 10 mg/hr?

To answer these questions, use the ratio-proportion method and follow these steps:

1. **Set up the following proportion to calculate the volume in mL that you need to administer as the bolus:**

   $$\frac{0.83 \text{ mg}}{1 \text{ mL}} = \frac{5 \text{ mg}}{x \text{ mL}}$$

2. **Cross-multiply and solve.**

   $0.83x = 5$

   $x = 6.02$

   You administer a 6 mL IV bolus.

3. **Set up the following proportion to calculate the flow rate in mL/hr, given that the concentration is 0.83 mg/mL and the drip is ordered as 10 mg/hr:**

   $$\frac{0.83\text{ mg}}{1\text{ mL}} = \frac{10\text{ mg}}{x\text{ mL}}$$

4. **Cross-multiply and solve.**

   $0.83x = 10$

   $x = 12.05$

   The flow rate is 12 mL/hr.

A patient has developed *ventricular tachycardia.* (*V-tach,* or *VT,* is tachycardia that originates in one of the heart's ventricles. It can be a life-threatening dysrhythmia if not treated promptly.) After an initial bolus, you're asked to administer a continuous infusion of amiodarone 360 mg over 6 hours. The available concentration is 1.8 mg/mL. What's the flow rate for the 6-hour period?

To find out, use the ratio-proportion method and flow rate formula. Follow these steps:

1. **Set up the following proportion to calculate the total volume to be infused (in other words, how many mL contain 360 mg):**

   $$\frac{1.8\text{ mg}}{1\text{ mL}} = \frac{360\text{ mg}}{x\text{ mL}}$$

2. **Cross-multiply and solve.**

   $1.8x = 360$

   $x = 200$

   The 360 mg are contained in 200 mL.

3. **Calculate the flow rate using the flow rate formula we describe in the section "Raising a Shockingly Low Blood Pressure."**

   flow rate (mL/hr) = 200 mL ÷ 6 hr

   flow rate (mL/hr) = 33.33

   The infusion rate for the next 6 hours is 33 mL/hr.

Giving a little push

Sometimes to treat a tachycardia or a bradycardia, you may have to administer only one or two doses of a medication. This "push" (or bolus) is the opposite of giving a continuous infusion.

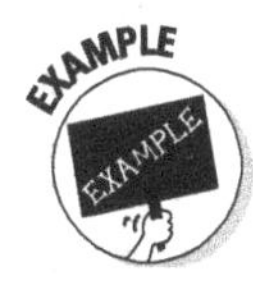

A patient develops significant bradycardia. You must administer atropine 1 mg IV. The vial you have available is at 0.4 mg/mL. How many mL do you give?

To find out, use the ratio-proportion method and follow these steps:

1. **Set up the following proportion to determine how many mL of a solution with a concentration of 0.4 mg/mL contain 1 mg:**

   $$\frac{0.4\text{ mg}}{1\text{ mL}} = \frac{1\text{ mg}}{x\text{ mL}}$$

2. **Cross-multiply and solve.**

   $0.4x = 1$

   $x = 2.5$

   You administer 2.5 mL of atropine.

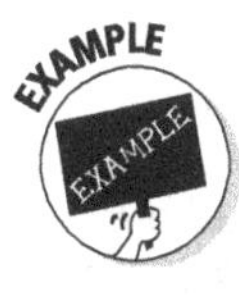

A patient has developed atrial fibrillation with a rapid ventricular response. You're asked to administer metoprolol 2.5 mg IV stat. Metoprolol is available in 5 mL ampules at a concentration of 1 mg/mL. How many mL do you give?

To find out, use the ratio-proportion method and follow these steps:

1. **Set up the following proportion to determine how many mL contain 2.5 mg:**

   $$\frac{1\text{ mg}}{1\text{ mL}} = \frac{2.5\text{ mg}}{x\text{ mL}}$$

2. **Cross-multiply and solve.**

   $1x = 2.5$

   $x = 2.5$

   You administer 2.5 mL of metoprolol. Because metoprolol comes in a 5 mL ampule, you give half the ampule.

Healing the heart attack: OH BATMAN!

One of the most critical conditions that you'll encounter in the ICU is treating a heart attack. In medical terminology, it's called a *myocardial infarction.* During his residency training, one of the authors (that's Rich, the doctor) learned this mnemonic to remember many of the meds required for treating a heart attack: OH BATMAN!

O = Oxygen

H = Heparin

B = Beta-blocker (for example, metoprolol, also known as Lopressor)

A = ACE Inhibitor

T = tPa (fallen by the wayside with the advent of percutaneous angioplasty)

M = Morphine

A = Aspirin

N = Nitroglycerin

Helping with Heparin

Heparin is one of the most common medications administered in a hospital setting. (We offer examples of infusing heparin intravenously in Chapter 11.)

Doctors order heparin to be given as continuous infusions to treat serious medical conditions, such as myocardial infarctions (MIs) and pulmonary embolisms (PEs). (In case you're wondering, an *MI* is a heart attack and a *PE* is a blockage of the main artery of the lung.) You also administer heparin subcutaneously to treat deep venous thrombosis (DVT). *DVT* is a condition in which a patient has a blood clot in a deep vein.

You're instructed to administer heparin subcutaneously 5,000 units q8h. If the vial contains 20,000 units/mL, how much, in mL, do you inject?

To answer this question, use the ratio-proportion method and follow these steps:

1. **Set up the following proportion:**

$$\frac{20{,}000 \text{ units}}{1 \text{ mL}} = \frac{5{,}000 \text{ units}}{x \text{ mL}}$$

2 **Cross-multiply and solve.**

$20{,}000x = 5{,}000$

$x = 0.25$

Inject 0.25 mL subcut every 8 hours.

This dose is common for DVT prophylaxis. You're likely to give this dose to many patients in the hospital.

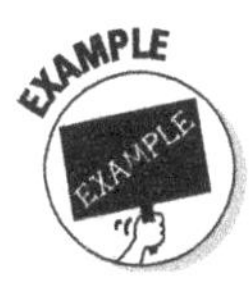

For a patient who has been admitted with a myocardial infarction, the doctor's orders state to administer heparin 25,000 units in 250 mL half-normal saline (½ NS) premixed solution at 80 units/kg bolus and then to administer a drip at 18 units/kg/hr. The patient weighs 250 pounds. What's the bolus dose, in mL? What's the infusion rate of the maintenance drip?

To answer these questions, first do some simple converting and then use the ratio-proportion method. Follow these steps:

1. **Use the conversion factor 1 kg = 2.2 lb to convert the patient's weight from lb to kg.**

   $x \text{ kg} = 250 \div 2.2$

   $x \text{ kg} = 113.6$

   The patient weights 114 kg.

2. **Multiply the bolus dose in units/kg by the patient's weight to calculate the initial bolus dose in units.**

   $x \text{ units} = \text{units/kg} \times \text{kg}$

   $x \text{ units} = 80 \times 114$

   $x \text{ units} = 9{,}120$

   The bolus must contain 9,120 units.

3. **Set up the following proportion to calculate the heparin bolus in mL, given that there are 25,000 units in 250 mL.**

   $$\frac{25{,}000 \text{ units}}{250 \text{ mL}} = \frac{9{,}120 \text{ units}}{x \text{ mL}}$$

4. **Cross-multiply and solve.**

   $25{,}000x = 250 \times 9{,}120$

   $25{,}000x = 2{,}280{,}000$

   $x = 91.2$

   Infuse a bolus of 91.2 mL.

5. **Multiply the maintenance drip dose in units/kg/hr by the patient's weight to get the units/hr of the drip.**

   x units/hr = units/kg/hr × kg

   x units/hr = 18 × 114

   x units/hr = 2,052

   You must infuse 2,052 units/hr for the maintenance drip.

6. **Set up the following proportion to calculate the infusion rate in mL/hr, given that there are 25,000 units in 250 mL.**

   $$\frac{25{,}000 \text{ units}}{250 \text{ mL}} = \frac{2{,}052 \text{ units}}{x \text{ mL}}$$

7. **Cross-multiply and solve.**

   $25{,}000x = 513{,}000$

   $x = 20.52$

   The infusion rate is 20.5 mL/hr.

Real-Life Practice: Calculating Flow Rates of Nitroglycerin and Furosemide

You're taking care of a patient admitted to the ICU for pulmonary edema and acute kidney failure. The patient has a nitroglycerin IV infusion 100 mg in 250 mL D5W running at 30 mcg/min. In order to promote a *diuresis* (increased formation of urine by the kidney), the doctor has also ordered a furosemide (Lasix) 80 mg IV bolus followed by a continuous infusion 500 mg in 50 mL at 40 mg/hr. What are the flow rates, in mL/hr, of the nitroglycerin and furosemide continuous drips?

To solve this problem, use the ratio-proportion method and follow these steps:

1. **Calculate the concentration of the nitroglycerin infusion in mcg/mL.**

   Remember that 1 mg = 1,000 mcg, so 100 mg = 100,000 mcg.

   $$\frac{100{,}000 \text{ mcg}}{250 \text{ mL}} = \frac{x \text{ mcg}}{1 \text{ mL}}$$

2. **Cross-multiply and solve.**

   $250x = 100{,}000$

   $x = 400$

   The concentration is 400 mcg/mL.

3. **Set up the following proportion to calculate the flow rate in mL/min.**

   $$\frac{400\text{ mcg}}{1\text{ mL}} = \frac{30\text{ mcg}}{x\text{ mL}}$$

4. **Cross-multiply and solve.**

   $400x = 30$

   $x = 0.075$

   The infusion rate of the nitroglycerin is 0.075 mL each minute.

5. **Convert the flow rate from mL/min to mL/hr.**

   flow rate (mL/hr) = flow rate (mL/min) × 60 min/1 hr

   flow rate (mL/hr) = 0.075 × 60

   flow rate (mL/hr) = 4.5

   The patient should get 4.5 mL/hr of nitroglycerin.

6. **Set up the following proportion to calculate the continuous furosemide infusion of 40 mg/hr in mL/hr:**

   $$\frac{50\text{ mL}}{500\text{ mg}} = \frac{x\text{ mL}}{40\text{ mg}}$$

7. **Cross-multiply and solve.**

   $500x = 2{,}000$

   $x = 4$

   The patient needs 4 mL/hr continuous infusion.

If you look at a drug reference, one of the major risks of furosemide (Lasix) is ototoxicity. (*Ototoxicity* is damage to the ear, especially the cochlea.) Too high a dose can cause vestibular symptoms that can manifest as impaired vestibulo-ocular reflex or balance problems (vertigo). Be sure that any furosemide dose doesn't exceed 4 mg/min.

Real-Life Practice: Finding the Initial Flow Rate for Nicardipine

Your patient was admitted to the critical care unit for a hypertensive crisis. The doctor's order says to start the patient on nicardipine 20 mg in 200 mL D5W at 5 mg/hr and to titrate the med to keep the systolic blood pressure at less than 180 mmHg. What's the initial flow rate in mL/hr?

To find out, use the ratio-proportion method and follow these steps:

1. **Set up the following proportion to calculate the flow rate of 5 mg/hr in mL/hr; ignore the hr unit.**

   $$\frac{20\text{ mg}}{200\text{ mL}} = \frac{5\text{ mg}}{x\text{ mL}}$$

2. **Cross-multiply and solve.**

   $$20x = 1{,}000$$

   $$x = 50$$

   The patient should receive nicardipine at 50 mL/hr.

Real-Life Practice: Determining the Flow Rate for Vasopressin

You must administer vasopressin 100 units in 100 mL NS at 0.01 unit/min to a patient in septic shock and titrate up to 0.04 units per minute (and no higher, according to the directions from a drug reference). What's the flow rate in mL/hr for 0.04 unit/min?

To find out, use the ratio-proportion method and the basic conversion formula (see Chapters 4 and 8). Follow these steps:

1. **Set up the following proportion to calculate the number of units in 1 mL of solution:**

   $$\frac{100\text{ mL}}{100\text{ unit}} = \frac{1\text{ mL}}{x\text{ unit}}$$

   $$100x = 100$$

   $$x = 1$$

The concentration is 1 unit/mL. Therefore, there are 0.04 units in 0.04 mL.

2. **Convert the flow rate from 0.04 mL/min to mL/hr.**

   flow rate (mL/hr) = flow rate (mL/min) × 60 min/1 hr

   flow rate (mL/hr) = 0.04 × 60

   flow rate (mL/hr) = 2.4

   The flow rate is 2.4 mL/hr.

Vasopressin has a very narrow therapeutic range when dosing for septic shock. Don't dose at a rate higher than 0.04 unit/min, because a higher dose can have serious adverse effects on the heart.

Chapter 18

Keeping a Patient Well-Nourished

In This Chapter

- Calculating your patient's caloric needs
- Figuring feeding rates through tubes versus veins
- Dosing and administering electrolytes
- Testing your calculation skills with some real-life dosing examples

Ingestion (taking in food) is an essential process of life. All life forms ingest food to survive, yet many people take eating for granted. Their relationship with food can be as simple as, "Am I hungry?" The medical professional, however, is much more serious and formal about food. For healthcare professionals, *food* is the collection of substances that promote growth, give energy, and sustain life.

Nutrition is essential for the treatment of any illness. It's more important than any medication because if a person doesn't receive the proper nutrition, he can't heal. Therefore, it's important that you monitor and record what your patients eat and drink with each meal. In addition, you need to record your patients' daily weight, as well as their inputs and outputs.

In this chapter, we show you how to stay aware of your patients' caloric needs, how to provide the nutrition, and how to replace the electrolytes that your patients may likely need. We explore the differences between tube feedings and intravenous nutrition, and we dig a little deeper into some of the most common electrolyte replacement therapies.

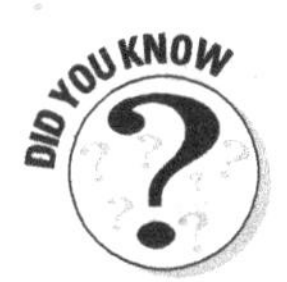

When Florence Nightingale went to the Crimea in 1854, she was mostly concerned with soldiers' nutrition. It wasn't until later, back in London, that she advocated for cleanliness.

Being Aware of a Patient's Caloric Needs

A doctor's order may ask you to do a calorie count for a pt (patient) or to record her food intake. So you need to be aware of the caloric requirements of the patients you're taking care of.

The *food calorie* (informally called the *calorie*) is a unit that indicates a food's energy value. One (1) food calorie is equal to 1,000 kcal (kilocalories). (When the United States goes completely metric, you'll no doubt have to change units, too — 1 kcal is equal to 4.2 kilojoules. In the meantime, nutrition is measured in kcal.)

Caloric requirements are based on kcal per kg of patient weight. For a person in the intensive care unit (ICU), the caloric goal is 35 kcal/kg. For a person on a general medical-surgical floor, the caloric goal is approximately 30 kcal/kg.

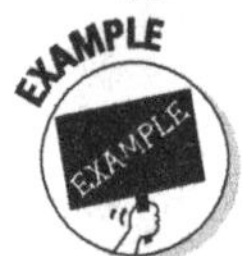

You're taking care of a pt in the ICU who weighs 140 pounds. The caloric goal is 35 kcal/kg. What's his estimated caloric need?

To solve this problem, use the basic conversion formula (desired unit = given unit × conversion factor) and follow these steps (see Chapter 4 for more on units and conversion):

1. **Convert lb to kg using the conversion factor 1 kg = 2.2 lb.**

   desired unit = given unit × conversion factor

   $$x \text{ kg} = 140 \text{ lb} \times \frac{1 \text{ kg}}{2.2 \text{ lb}}$$

   $$x \text{ kg} = \frac{140}{2.2}$$

   $$x \text{ kg} = 63.6$$

   The patient weighs 63.6 kg.

   To simplify things, you can also just divide the number of lb by 2.2 to get the kg equivalent.

2. **Calculate the patient's caloric need by multiplying the caloric goal by the patient's weight.**

   x = 35 kcal/kg × 63.6 kg

   x = 2,226 kcal

   The patient's total caloric need is 2,226 kcal.

The role of an RD in patient nutrition

A *registered dietitian* (sometimes called an *RD* or *nutritionist*) is a medical specialist who's an expert on food and nutrition. In terms of education, all RDs have a university degree, complete a lengthy internship, and pass a certification exam.

RDs can work in many places (for example, long-term care facilities, school districts, or prisons), but you're sure to find an RD on staff at every hospital and/or rehabilitation center. They often make recommendations about nutrition programs that doctors order. As a healthcare professional, you'll likely work regularly with your hospital's dietician.

RDs review hospital food for patients with low nutritional risk. A typical hospital menu includes meals that assist with weight loss and those that don't, as well as meal plans for diabetics, vegetarians, and those with special religious requirements. Hospitals also need to prepare liquid, pureed, and soft meals for patients as ordered by their doctors when necessary.

Many patients eat "regular" hospital meals, but others aren't able to do so. Fortunately, you can use other methods, like tube and IV feeding, to feed them. Check out the sections "Feeding through a Tube" and "Feeding through the Veins" for more details.

Remember: Although nutrition is primarily in the realm of the dietitian, the more you know, the better caretaker and patient advocate you'll be.

A patient is placed on a 2,400-calorie, low-sodium diet. You record that he ate only 50% of his breakfast, lunch, and dinner. What's his estimated caloric intake for the day?

This question is pretty straightforward. All you have to do is multiply the desired intake (2,400) by the percentage the patient consumed (50%, or 0.5), like so:

$$x = 2{,}400 \text{ kcal} \times 50\%$$

$$x = 2{,}400 \text{ kcal} \times 0.5$$

$$x = 1{,}200 \text{ kcal}$$

The patient consumed about 1,200 calories.

Feeding through a Tube

A *feeding tube* is a route of administration for getting nutrients into the patient. Doctors and dietitians often determine the goal rate for tube feedings by looking at the patient's total caloric needs. The goal rate is the desired rate of introducing nutrition into the patient, measured in mL/hr. The doctor orders tube feedings that start at a lower rate and slowly increase to the goal rate.

You can use different types of feeding tubes to get nutrients into a patient's stomach. Some tubes are used as temporary measures, often sufficing for a few days until a more permanent solution is sought. For example, *nasogastric intubation* is a procedure where a plastic tube (called a *nasogastric tube* or *NG tube*) goes into the patient's stomach through the nose and down the throat. Another temporary feeding arrangement uses the *Dobhoff feeding tube,* which is a thin plastic tube (thinner than the NG tube) that also goes into the patient's stomach through the nose and down the throat.

By contrast, other types of feeding tubes represent a more permanent solution and can last a long time, often for months, without needing replacement. One such tube is a *percutaneous endoscopic gastrostomy tube* (a *PEG tube*), which goes into the patient's stomach through the abdominal wall. It is often placed by a "stomach doctor" (called a *gastroenterologist*), but a general surgeon can place it as well.

Administering enteral nutrition

Enteral nutrition is the process of using the stomach and intestine for digestion; the term comes from the Greek word *enteron,* which means "intestine." When you administer enteral nutrition through a feeding tube, the doctor's orders often indicate changes in the rate of feeding. Calculating total volume over 24 hours, taking rate changes into account, is a common task, especially when you need to record total inputs and outputs for your patients.

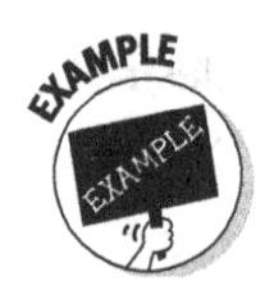

You're instructed to begin tube feedings with Jevity (a tube feeding formula from Abbott Nutrition) starting at 20 mL/hr. After 8 hours, the patient is tolerating the tube feeds, so the doctor's order says to increase the rate to 35 mL/hr. How many mL of tube feeds will the patient receive over 24 hours?

To solve this problem, follow these steps:

1. **Figure out the mL consumed at 20 mL/hr in the first 8 hours.**

   $x = 20 \text{ mL/hr} \times 8 \text{ hr}$

   $x = 160 \text{ mL}$

   The patient took in 160 mL in the first 8 hours.

2. **Figure out the mL consumed at 35 mL/hr in the remaining 16 hours.**

   $x = 35 \text{ mL/hr} \times 16 \text{ hr}$

   $x = 560 \text{ mL}$

   The patient will take in 560 mL in the remaining 16 hours.

3. **Add the two quantities together.**

   $x = 160 \text{ mL} + 560 \text{ mL}$

   $x = 720 \text{ mL}$

   The total volume of tube feeds for 24 hr is 720 mL.

Including free water flushes

Tube feeding is a great way to make sure patients who can't eat normally get the nutrition they need, but don't forget they have to drink, too! When a doctor orders a tube feeding at a certain rate, he also often orders water to be flushed through the tube at a certain frequency throughout the day — usually every 4 to 6 hours. In addition to the tube feeding itself, you record the volume of the *free water flushes,* as they're called, as part of the patient's total input.

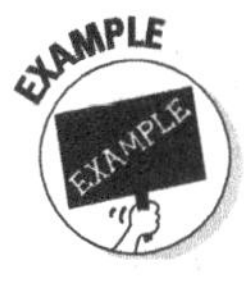

The patient from the preceding section received a total volume of 720 mL of Jevity in 24 hours. The doctor also orders free water flushes 150 mL q4h (every 4 hours) through the feeding tube. How much water do you administer over 24 hours? What's the total volume of feedings and water?

To find out, follow these steps:

1. **Figure out the total mL of free water flushes given in 24 hours.**

   $x = 150 \text{ mL/interval} \times 6 \text{ intervals}$

   $x = 900 \text{ mL}$

   You administer a total of 900 mL of free water in 24 hr.

2. **Calculate the total intake for 24 hr by adding the food and water inputs together.**

   $x = 720 \text{ mL} + 900 \text{ mL}$

   $x = 1{,}620 \text{ mL}$

   The total intake is 1,620 mL.

Feeding through the Veins

You can't give enteral nutrition to all your patients. For example, patients with a bowel obstruction can't digest nutrition regularly in their intestines. In these cases, the doctor may order parenteral nutrition (*parenteral* literally means "beside the intestine"). For these patients, you give the nutrients intravenously.

Doctors order the following two types of parenteral nutrition:

- **Total parenteral nutrition (TPN):** TPN solution is the most common type of parenteral nutrition. It's premade by the pharmacy and consists of dextrose, protein as amino acids, lipids, electrolytes, minerals, and trace elements. TPN comes in various standard solutions for normal, high-stress, and fluid-restricted patients.
- **Peripheral parenteral nutrition (PPN):** PPN has only one concentration of glucose and amino acids. Lipids can only be ordered in TPN.

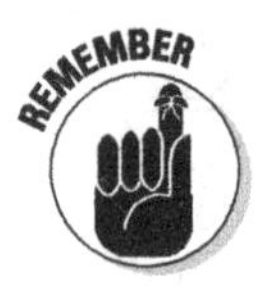

You can give PPN through a peripheral IV (hence the name), but you can't give TPN that way. TPN solutions are very concentrated and can be caustic and irritating to veins, so they require central access — either through a central venous catheter (CVC) or a peripherally inserted central catheter (PICC) line. (A PICC line is a central line, even though it has the word *peripheral* in its name.)

On the TPN/PPN order sheet, the doctor often determines the total volume to be infused and the duration of infusion, which means you need to calculate the infusion rate (flow rate). The calculations you use to find the flow rate of IV feeding are similar to those for other intravenous (IV) infusions (refer to Chapter 11 for more details).

The doctor orders 1.5 L (1,500 mL) of TPN to be infused over 24 hours. What's the infusion rate in mL/hr?

To find out, use the ratio-proportion method (see Chapter 8) and follow these steps:

1. **Set up the following proportion to calculate the infusion rate for 1 hour:**

$$\frac{\text{known equivalent}}{\text{known equivalent}} = \frac{\text{desired equivalent}}{\text{known equivalent}}$$

$$\frac{1{,}500 \text{ mL}}{24 \text{ hr}} = \frac{x \text{ mL}}{1 \text{ hr}}$$

2. **Cross-multiply and solve.**

$24x = 1{,}500$

$x = 62.5$

You infuse 62.5 mL/hr.

Replacing Low Electrolytes

One of the most common doctor's orders is replacing electrolytes that show up as low on lab tests. Examples of electrolytes include sodium, potassium, bicarbonate, magnesium, calcium, and phosphorus. Electrolytes may be low because of vomiting, diarrhea, or the use of diuretics.

Measuring in milliequivalents

Most electrolytes (except for phosphorus, which we discuss in the next section) are measured in milliequivalents (mEq). Electrolyte replacement solutions are usually premixed in a certain concentration. For example, a 1 L bag of 0.9% normal isotonic saline contains 154 mEq of Na^+ (sodium) and 154 mEq of Cl^- (chlorine) ions, while a 1 L bag of 0.45% NaCl (½ NS) contains 77 mEq of Na^+ and 77 mEq of Cl^- ions.

A *milliequivalent* (mEq) is one thousandth (0.001) of the gram equivalent of an ion. A *millimole* (mmol) is one thousandth (0.001) of the gram equivalent of a substance. You use the units mEq/L and mmol/L in dosing electrolytes. Both units are common in lab values, along with the unit mg/dL. For example, a normal lab value for sodium is 136–142 mEq/L and 136–142 mmol/L.

You're instructed to administer 1 L (1,000 mL) of normal isotonic saline over 6 hours. It contains 154 mEq/L sodium. What's the infusion rate? How many mEq of sodium have you given after 4 hours?

To solve this problem, use the ratio-proportion method (see Chapter 8) and follow these steps:

1. **Calculate the infusion rate over 1 hour by dividing the total mL infused by the total hours.**

   x = 1,000 mL ÷ 6 hr

   x = 166.67 mL/hr

   The infusion rate is 167 mL/hr.

2. **Calculate how many mL you give over 4 hours by multiplying by 4.**

   x = 167 mL/hr × 4 hr

   x = 668 mL

   After 4 hours, you've given 668 mL of fluid.

3. **Set up the following proportion to figure out how many mEq are in 668 mL:**

   $$\frac{154 \text{ mEq}}{1{,}000 \text{ mL}} = \frac{x \text{ mEq}}{668 \text{ mL}}$$

4. **Cross-multiply and solve.**

   $1{,}000x = 102{,}872$

   $x = 102.87$

   In 4 hours, you've given 103 mEq in 668 mL of solution.

The first part of this example, calculating the infusion rate, represents a common physician's order. The second part of this example, calculating how much sodium you have administered, is not something you will ever be asked to do. We included this problem to help you understand sodium replacement a little better.

Betting on bicarbonate

Sodium (Na) bicarbonate is measured in mEq. You can either add it to an existing IV containing saline or use it as an isolated bicarbonate infusion.

A doctor's order says "Begin D5 ½ NS with 75 mEq of Na bicarbonate at 100 mL/hr." What's the total mEq of Na^+ you will give?

In this example, you're adding 75 mEq of sodium bicarbonate to 1 L of D5 ½ NS, which has 75 mEq of sodium already. So to get the total mEq of sodium, all you have to do is add the two quantities together.

$x = 75 \text{ mEq} + 75 \text{ mEq}$

$x = 150 \text{ mEq}$

The total sodium is 150 mEq, which is about the same concentration as normal saline (154 mEq/L).

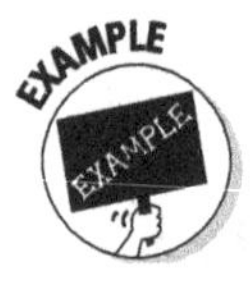

The doctor wants you to start 1 L (1,000 mL) of D5W with 100 mEq of Na bicarbonate at 150 mL/hr. What's the infusion time?

You know the quantity (1,000 mL) and the flow rate (150 mL/hr). To calculate the infusion time, just use the simple infusion time formula that we describe in Chapter 11.

infusion time (hr) = total volume (mL) ÷ flow rate (mL/hr)

$x = 1{,}000 \div 150$

$x = 6.67$

The infusion time is 6.67 hours, or 6 hr 40 min.

Except in rare circumstances, the dose of sodium (whether sodium chloride or sodium bicarbonate) should never exceed 154 mEq/L. A liter bag of "normal saline" has 154 mEq of sodium, and it's called an *isotonic* solution because its concentration of sodium is similar to that of blood (*iso* means "same" and *tonic* refers to "concentration").

Because IV fluids come in many varieties, you will see a lot of variation in the types of fluids that doctors order, and you should be on the lookout for problems. Call the doctor if you ever see an order like this: "D5NS with 75 mEq $NaHCO_3$ at 100 mL/hr." D5NS contains a very high concentration of sodium — 154 mEq of sodium chloride. When you add 75 mEq from the NaHCO3 (sodium bicarbonate), you get a total of 229 mEq, which is too high a sodium concentration and can be harmful to the patient.

No procrastinating on potassium

Potassium is one of the most common electrolytes you have to replace, in part because many patients in the hospital are on diuretics, like furosemide (Lasix), which can deplete the body of potassium. You can administer potassium orally or intravenously.

You're asked to administer 50 mEq of potassium gluconate elixir PO (orally). It comes in a concentration of 20 mEq/15 mL. How many mL do you give?

To find out, use the ratio-proportion method and follow these steps:

1. **Set up the following proportion to figure out how many mL contain 50 mEq:**

   $$\frac{20 \text{ mEq}}{15 \text{ mL}} = \frac{50 \text{ mEq}}{x \text{ mL}}$$

2. **Cross-multiply and solve.**

   $20x = 750$

   $x = 37.5$

   Give 37.5 mL orally.

You're asked to administer 20 mEq of potassium chloride (KCl) IV in 200 mL of normal saline (NS) over 3 hours. The potassium for intravenous administration has a concentration of 2 mEq/mL. How much KCl do you add to the NS? What's the infusion rate?

To solve this problem, use the ratio-proportion method (see Chapter 8) and the basic flow rate formula (see Chapter 11). Follow these steps:

1. **Set up the following proportion to determine how many mL of KCl contain 20 mEq:**

$$\frac{2 \text{ mEq}}{1 \text{ mL}} = \frac{20 \text{ mEq}}{x \text{ mL}}$$

2. **Cross-multiply and solve.**

   $2x = 20$

   $x = 10$

   Add 10 mL KCl to the 200 mL bag of NS.

3. **Use the following simple formula to determine the flow rate:**

   flow rate (mL/hr) = total volume (mL) ÷ designated time (hr)

   flow rate (mL/hr) = 210 mL ÷ 3 hr

   flow rate (mL/hr) = 70

   The flow rate is 70 mL/hr.

Note: KCl comes as a premixed solution in doses of 10 to 40 mEq. Physicians usually order 20 or 40 mEq KCl IV.

You're asked to administer 40 mEq KCl over 4 hours. It's available as a premixed infusion of 20 mEq in 100 mL normal saline. What's the infusion rate?

To find the infusion rate, use the ratio-proportion method and the basic flow rate formula. Follow these steps:

1. **Set up the following proportion to determine how many mL of KCl you need to give to make up 40 mEq:**

$$\frac{20 \text{ mEq}}{100 \text{ mL}} = \frac{40 \text{ mEq}}{x \text{ mL}}$$

2. **Cross-multiply and solve.**

   $20x = 4{,}000$

   $x = 200$

   You need to give 200 mL of the solution.

3. **Use the flow rate formula to determine the flow rate:**

   flow rate (mL/hr) = 200 mL ÷ 4 hr

   flow rate (mL/hr) = 50 mL/hr

   The flow rate is 50 mL/hr.

Because the total amount of potassium you need to infuse is 200 mL, which is more than the 100 mL container available, you have to infuse the 100 mL twice.

When administering potassium, be aware of the following:

- **Don't administer more than 10 mEq/hr.** The body needs time to adapt to the potassium load given. Giving more potassium at one time can be harmful.
- **Don't administer inadequately diluted potassium.** Potassium administered in too small a volume can be caustic and irritating to the vein. So you may notice that in the premixed potassium solutions, the higher the concentration of potassium being administered, the more fluid it's dissolved in. For example, it's relatively common to see 40 mEq KCl in a volume of 250 mL.

No milling about with magnesium

You can give magnesium as a continuous infusion for a patient with preeclampsia (see Chapter 14 for more details on this pregnancy-related condition).

As you work through the following examples, you probably think to yourself, "Wait a minute. I thought we were dealing mainly with mEq." Well, you're right. It turns out that 1 g of magnesium sulfate equals 8 mEq of magnesium sulfate. Doctors can be tricky, and you may see two different types of orders that really say the same thing. For instance, the order may say, "Administer magnesium sulfate 1 g IV over 3 hr," or it may say, "Administer magnesium sulfate 8 mEq IV over 3 hr." In other words, you say "tom-*ay*-to" and we say "tom-*ahh*-to."

The doctor's order says to administer 4 g magnesium sulfate IV over 3 hr. It's available as a premixed infusion of 4 g in 50 mL of normal saline. What's the infusion rate?

To solve this problem, all you have to do is use the simple flow rate formula we cover in Chapter 11.

flow rate (mL/hr) = 50 mL ÷ 3 hr

flow rate (mL/hr) = 16.7 mL/hr

You would program the infusion pump to a flow rate of 16.7 mL/hr.

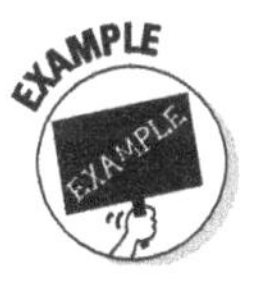

You must give 4 g magnesium sulfate over 4 hr. You know that 1 g of magnesium sulfate equals 8 mEq. How many mEq are you administering?

To find out, use the ratio-proportion method and follow these steps:

1. **Set up the following proportion:**

$$\frac{1\text{ g}}{8\text{ mEq}} = \frac{4\text{ g}}{x\text{ mEq}}$$

2. **Cross-multiply and solve.**

   $x = 32$

   A quantity of 4 g of magnesium sulfate is equivalent to 32 mEq.

Minding the millimoles when giving phosphorus

In contrast to the other electrolytes, phosphorus isn't dosed in mEq. Instead, it's dosed in millimoles (mmol). Unlike sodium, potassium, and other electrolytes, which exist in the body in only one *ionic form,* phosphorus can exist in the body in different "charged forms" (as phosphoric acid or phosphorous acid, for example). Phosphorus is commonly measured in mmol/L to accommodate those different forms. (It can also be measured in mg/dL, but doctors use mmoL.)

You're asked to administer 15 mmol sodium phosphate (NaH_2PO_4) in 100 mL normal saline intravenously over 6 hr. What's the infusion rate?

To find out, just use the simple flow rate formula we discuss in Chapter 11.

flow rate (mL/hr) = 100 mL ÷ 6 hr

flow rate (mL/hr) = 16.67 mL/hr

Rounding up, the flow rate is 17 mL/hr.

Keep the following in mind whenever you administer phosphorus intravenously:

- Phosphorus is usually administered as sodium phosphate or potassium phosphate when given IV.
- Phosphorus isn't usually given for less than 6 hours. If you give phosphorus too quickly, it can precipitate with or bind to the calcium in the blood, which can be life-threatening. Infusing over 6 hours gives the body enough time to adapt to the phosphorus load.

Real-Life Practice: Administering Furosemide and Replacing Lost Electrolytes

You're reviewing the doctor's admitting orders for a patient diagnosed with congestive heart failure (CHF). You're instructed to administer furosemide

(Lasix) 80 mg IV now and every 8 hours. Furosemide for injection is available in a concentration of 10 mg/mL. Because the patient's potassium and magnesium levels are low, you're also instructed to give KCl (potassium chloride) 30 mEq PO and magnesium sulfate 16 mEq over 4 hr. The KCl comes in a concentration of 20 mEq/15 mL, and the magnesium sulfate is a premixed solution of 2 g/100 mL NS. With magnesium sulfate, 1 g equals 8 mEq. How much liquid potassium should you give?

To solve this problem, use the ratio-proportion method and the flow rate formula. Follow these steps:

1. **Set up the following proportion to determine how many mL contain 80 mg of furosemide:**

   $$\frac{10 \text{ mg}}{1 \text{ mL}} = \frac{80 \text{ mg}}{x \text{ mL}}$$

2. **Cross-multiply and solve.**

   $10x = 80$

   $x = 8$

   Now you know that 8 mL of solution contain 80 mg of furosemide. Administer 8 mL now and 8 mL every 8 hours.

3. **Set up the following proportion to calculate how many mL are in 1 dose of 30 mEq KCl:**

   $$\frac{20 \text{ mEq}}{15 \text{ mL}} = \frac{30 \text{ mEq}}{x \text{ mL}}$$

4. **Cross-multiply and solve.**

   $20x = 450$

   $x = 22.5$

   Administer 22.5 mL of liquid potassium.

5. **Calculate the infusion rate for giving 16 mEq of magnesium sulfate over 4 hours, considering that the concentration of 2 g/100 mL = 16 mEq/100 mL.**

   flow rate (mL/hr) = 100 mL ÷ 4 hr

   flow rate (mL/hr) = 25 mL/hr

   The flow rate is 25 mL/hr.

Real-Life Practice: Calculating a Patient's Total Input

You're treating a patient who was started on Jevity tube feeding 24 hours ago. You've been increasing his feeding rate every 12 hours, as ordered by the doc. The patient had been at 10 mL/hr for the first 12 hours and is now at 15 mL/hr for the second 12 hours.

You're also administering free water flushes 50 mL every 6 hours. In addition to the tube feedings, the patient is on TPN, which will be continued until the patient reaches the goal rate on the tube feedings. The volume of TPN is 1,100 mL, to be administered over 24 hours. What's the total input for this patient for 24 hours?

To solve this problem, follow these steps:

1. **Calculate the total volume of Jevity tube feedings administered.**

   First, determine the volume for the first 12 hours and the second 12 hours, like so:

   10 mL/hr × 12 hours = 120 mL for the first 12 hours

   15 mL/hr × 12 hours = 180 mL for the second 12 hours

   Then add them together to find the total.

   120 mL + 180 mL = 300 mL

   The total volume for the tube feedings is 300 mL.

2. **Calculate the total volume of free water flushes administered.**

   The patient gets flushes every 6 hours, meaning that you administer 4 flushes over 24 hours.

   50 mL/flush × 4 flushes = 200 mL

   The total volume for free water flushes is 200 mL.

3. **Calculate the total input by adding the TPN volume, tube feeding volume, and flush volume together.**

   x = 1,100 mL (TPN) + 300 mL (tube feeds) + 200 mL (water flushes)

   x = 1,600 mL total input

   The total input is 1,600 mL.

Part V
The Part of Tens

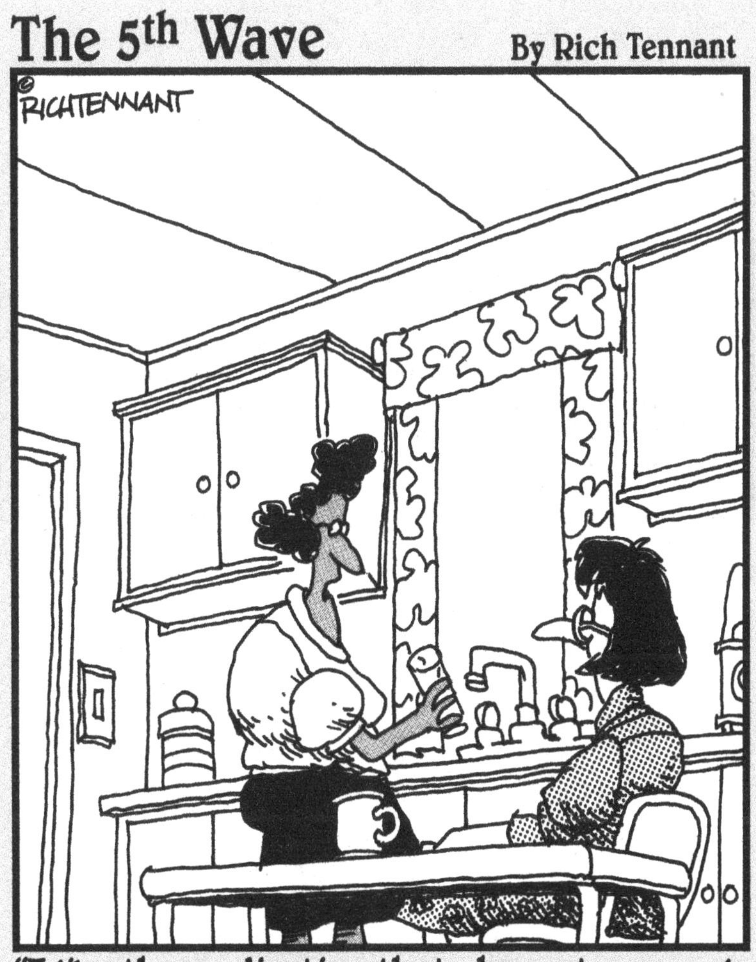

"I like the medication that shows two people in a rowboat, but Cliff likes the one with two people on a Roman holiday eating lasagna."

In this part . . .

The chapters in this part are brief and filled with useful information. Chapter 19 walks you through the ten dosage calculations you really need to know, and Chapter 20 lists ten bad dosing mistakes and shows you how to avoid them.

Chapter 19

Ten Essential Dosing Calculations

In This Chapter

- Converting from lb to kg and vice versa
- Mastering the metric system and calculating medical dosages in mg and mL
- Reviewing some important infusion-related calculations
- Doing basic parenteral and unit-based dosing calculations

As a healthcare professional, you need to get chummy with a few medical dosage calculations that you're sure to use every day. In this chapter, we walk you through ten specific calculations you really need to know.

Converting lb to kg and kg to lb

Patient weight conversion is an important first step in many dosing calculations. For example, you may need to calculate weight-based tube feeds to reach a calorie goal. For these types of calculations, you usually have to convert from lb to kg. On the other hand, when you discuss weight with a patient (or a child's parents), you need to covert from kg to lb.

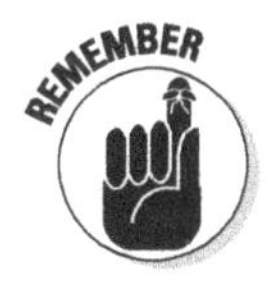

The shortcut conversion factors you need to know are

- lb = kg × 2.2
- kg = lb ÷ 2.2

You're taking care of a patient who weighs 140 lb. What's her weight in kg?

All you have to do is plug the given number into the following simple conversion equation and solve:

kg = lb ÷ 2.2

kg = 140 ÷ 2.2

kg = 63.6

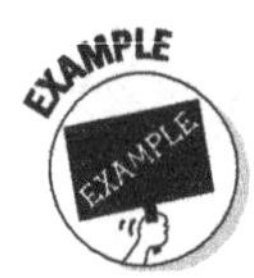

You're taking care of a patient who weighs 80 kg. What's his weight in lb?

The solution's the same as the preceding example, except you have to go from kg to lb. Just plug in the given numbers and solve:

$$lb = kg \times 2.2$$

$$lb = 80 \times 2.2$$

$$lb = 176$$

Converting mL to L and L to mL

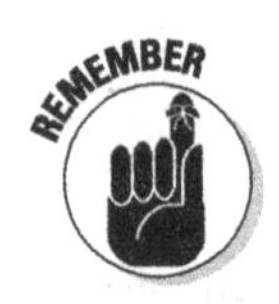

When you dose liquid volumes, you work mostly with the metric system, particularly mL and L.

The conversion factors you need to know are

- $mL = L \times 1{,}000$
- $L = mL \div 1{,}000$

You're asked to place a patient on a 1,350 mL fluid restriction. What's the equivalent in L?

To find out, just plug the given number into the following simple conversion equation and solve:

$$L = mL \div 1{,}000$$

$$L = 1{,}350 \div 1{,}000$$

$$L = 1.350$$

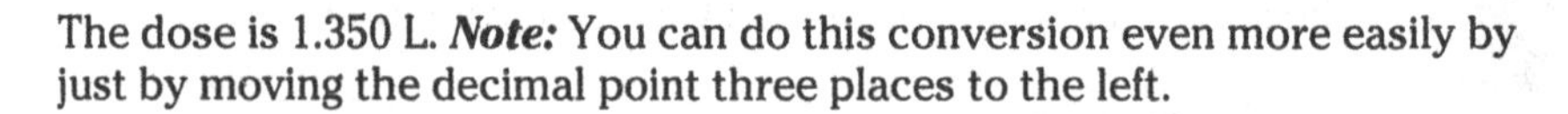

The dose is 1.350 L. ***Note:*** You can do this conversion even more easily by just by moving the decimal point three places to the left.

You calculate the patient's total input for your shift to be 1.863 L. What's the equivalent in mL?

Plug the given number into the following simple conversion equation and solve:

$$mL = L \times 1{,}000$$

$$mL = 1.863 \times 1{,}000$$

$$mL = 1{,}863$$

The patient's input is 1,863 mL. ***Note:*** Moving the decimal point three places to the right accomplishes the same conversion more easily.

Converting mg to g and g to mg

In medicine, most dosing of meds is by weight, and you most often convert between mg and g. Sometimes you need to convert between milligrams (mg) and micrograms (mcg).

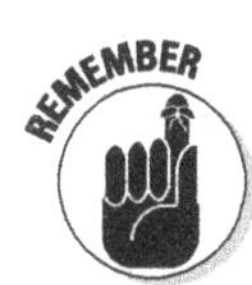

The conversion factors you need to know are

- mg = g × 1,000
- g = mg ÷ 1,000
- mcg = mg × 1,000
- mg = mcg ÷ 1,000

You can also convert these units by moving the decimal point three places to the right or three places to the left. To convert from large to small (g to mg, for example), move the decimal point three places to the right. To convert from small to large (mcg to mg, for example), move it three places to the left.

You're administering 750 mg vancomycin intravenously. What's the equivalent dose in g?

To find out, plug the given number into the following simple conversion equation and solve:

$$g = mg \div 1{,}000$$

$$g = 750 \div 1{,}000$$

$$g = 0.75$$

You administer 0.75 g of vancomycin.

Calculating the mg Dose of Oral Meds

To figure out how many tablets or capsules of a med to give, you must know the total dose needed and the mg content of 1 tablet or capsule of the med. Here's what it looks like in an equation:

$$\text{tablets} = \cancel{\text{mg}}\ (\text{ordered}) \times \frac{1\ \text{tablet}}{\cancel{\text{mg}}\ (\text{per tablet})}$$

The quantity you need is the ordered dose multiplied by a factor that shows the amount of the med in a single tablet. This equation is a variation of the formula method of dosage calculation (see Chapter 8 for more details).

The ratio-proportion method (which we discuss in Chapter 8) is equally good for dosing tablets and capsules, as the following example shows.

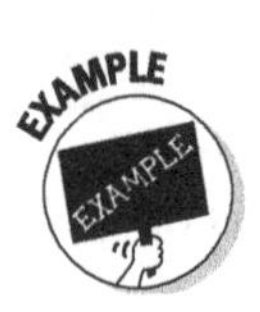

You're asked to give ciprofloxacin 750 mg PO bid for 5 days. The available tablets are 250 mg. How many tablets do you give with each dose?

To solve this problem, use the ratio-proportion method and follow these steps:

1. **Set up the following proportion:**

$$\frac{\text{known equivalent}}{\text{known equivalent}} = \frac{\text{known equivalent}}{\text{desired equivalent}}$$

$$\frac{250 \text{ mg}}{1 \text{ tablet}} = \frac{750 \text{ mg}}{x \text{ tablet}}$$

2. **Cross-multiply and solve.**

$250x = 750$

$x = 3$

Three tablets contain 750 mg.

Calculating the mL Dose of Liquid Meds

You administer many oral medications in oral suspension or liquid form. So you frequently convert the mg in a dose to the corresponding amount of liquid in mL. You can do so using the ratio-proportion method, like you do in the preceding section and example.

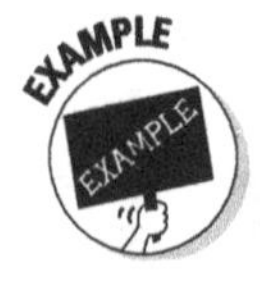

You're asked to administer ciprofloxacin 750 mg PO bid for 5 days. The ciprofloxacin is available in a liquid suspension at a concentration of 500 mg/5 mL. How many mL do you administer with each dose?

To find out, use the ratio-proportion method and follow these steps:

1. **Set up the following proportion:**

$$\frac{500 \text{ mg}}{5 \text{ mL}} = \frac{750 \text{ mg}}{x \text{ mL}}$$

2. **Cross-multiply and solve.**

   $500x = 3{,}750$

   $x = 7.5$

   Each dose is 7.5 mL.

Calculating Infusion Rates

Figuring out the infusion rate (also called the *flow rate*) is a regular activity any time you're administering meds intravenously. (See Chapter 11 for a lot more details about infusions.)

The infusion rate formula is

infusion rate (mL/hr) = total volume (mL) ÷ infusion time (hr)

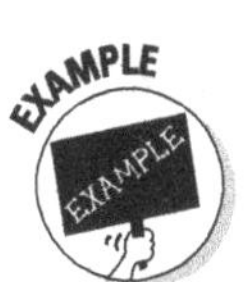

The doctor orders 1,000 mL of 0.9% saline to be infused over 24 hours. What's the infusion rate in mL/hr?

To solve this problem, all you have to do is plug the given numbers into the infusion rate formula and solve:

infusion rate (mL/hr) = 1,000 ÷ 24

infusion rate (mL/hr) = 41.67

The infusion rate is 41.7 mL/hr.

Calculating Infusion Times

The infusion time formula is a variation of the infusion rate formula; it looks like this:

infusion time (hr) = total volume (mL) ÷ flow rate (mL/hr)

The doctor orders 1,600 mL of 0.9% saline to be infused at 60 mL/hr. What's the total infusion time?

To find out, just plug the given numbers into the infusion time formula and solve:

infusion time (hr) = 1,600 ÷ 60

infusion time (hr) = 26.67

The infusion time is 26.67 hours (26 hours and 40 minutes).

Calculating Infusion Volumes

The infusion volume formula is a variation of the infusion rate formula; it looks like this:

total volume (mL) = infusion rate (mL/hr) × infusion time (hr)

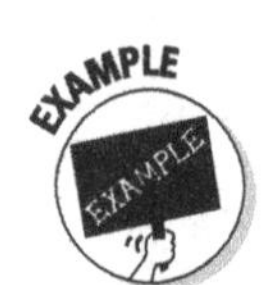

A patient is on Jevity tube feeding at 15 mL/hr. What volume of the substance does the patient intake in 24 hours?

To answer this question, plug the given numbers into the basic infusion volume formula and solve:

total volume (mL) = 15 × 24

total volume (mL) = 360

The volume of the Jevity is 360 mL.

Doing Parenteral Dosing Calculations

The key calculation for parenteral administration (both injection and intravenous) is determining the liquid volume (mL) that contains the desired amount of the med (in mg).

The ratio-proportion method offers the clearest, most accurate way to do these calculations (see Chapter 8 for more details).

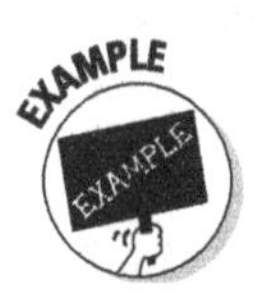

A patient develops significant bradycardia. You're asked to give atropine 1 mg IV. The available vial has a concentration of 0.4 mg/mL. How many mL do you give?

To find out, use the ratio-proportion method and follow these steps:

1. **Set up the following proportion:**

   $$\frac{0.4\text{ mg}}{1\text{ mL}} = \frac{1\text{ mg}}{x\text{ mL}}$$

2. **Cross-multiply and solve.**

   $0.4x = 1$

   $x = 2.5$

   The dose is 2.5 mL.

Doing Unit-Based Dosing Calculations

Two of the most common medications you give, insulin and heparin, are dosed in units. You need to calculate the relationship between units of medication and the volume (mL) containing the units.

The ratio-proportion method offers the clearest, most accurate way to do these calculations (see Chapter 8 for more details).

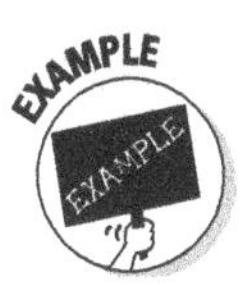

A patient has been admitted with a myocardial infarction. The doctor's order says to administer heparin 25,000 units in 250 mL half-normal saline (½ NS) premixed solution at 80 units/kg bolus and then administer at a drip of 18 units/kg/hr. The patient weighs 90 kg. What's the bolus dose?

To solve this problem, you need to do a little converting and then cross-multiplying with the ratio-proportion method. Follow these steps:

1. **Calculate the bolus in units.**

   total units = units/kg × kg

   total units = 80 units/kg × 90 kg

   total units = 7,200

2. **Set up the following proportion to determine how many mL contain 7,200 units:**

   $$\frac{25{,}000\text{ units}}{250\text{ mL}} = \frac{7{,}200\text{ units}}{x\text{ mL}}$$

3. **Cross-multiply and solve.**

$$25{,}000x = 250 \times 7{,}200$$

$$25{,}000x = 1{,}800{,}000$$

$$x = 72$$

The dose is 72 mL.

If you're extra careful, you can use a shortcut for this problem. Notice that the concentration of heparin is exactly 100 units/mL. Therefore, the 7,200 units have to be contained in 72 mL.

Chapter 20

Ten Ways to Avoid Common Dosing Mistakes

In This Chapter

- Double-checking medication names and dosage abbreviations
- Minimizing conversion errors
- Carefully calculating infusion rates and administration times
- Reviewing all patient allergies and the "rights" of medication administration
- Communicating with your fellow healthcare professionals

As a medical professional, your goal is to minimize dosing mistakes and medication errors whenever possible. In this chapter, you see ten techniques or behaviors that can help you do just that.

Watch Out for Meds That Sound Similar

Many medication names sound alike or are spelled similarly. So make sure you double-check the doctor's order for the correct drug name; otherwise, a dangerous drug error could happen. For example, Cerebyx and Celebrex have very similar pronunciations and spellings. The first medication is used to treat seizures; the second is an anti-inflammatory drug. (See Chapter 5 for a list of more drugs with similar names.)

If you have difficulty understanding a medication name from either a written order or a verbal order, clarify the order with the prescribing professional. The computer-based order-entry systems that many hospitals and medical facilities use today dramatically minimize the risk of errors related to medication names.

Avoid Ambiguous Abbreviations

Any healthcare professional who prescribes medications, transcribes them onto a Medication Administration Record (MAR), or administers them to patients must avoid writing or reading abbreviations that are incorrect or vague. Giving the wrong medication or the wrong dose (or giving it at the wrong time) because of an unacceptable abbreviation can be fatal!

To help you be as clear as possible when writing or reading abbreviations, use common and accepted abbreviations, such as *mL* rather than *cc,* or simply write out the word when the abbreviation may cause confusion, such as *units* rather than *U.* Don't use unacceptable or easily misinterpreted abbreviations. For example, don't write *QD* to mean "every day," because it may be misread as *OD.* Instead, write *daily.*

Check the Joint Commission's list of abbreviations (`www.jointcommission.org/Do_Not_Use_List_of_Abbreviations/`) and Chapter 5 for more on acceptable versus unacceptable dosage abbreviations.

You're taking care of a patient admitted to the hospital with an exacerbation of his emphysema. You read a medication order that states: "Administer M Sulfate 2 g IV now and every six hours." What's your next course of action?

You're unsure whether this order refers to magnesium sulfate ($MgSO_4$) or morphine sulfate (MSO_4), which is a narcotic. Because the med name is vague, you call the physician to clarify the medication order.

Assess a Med's Applicability

Make sure a medication is applicable to your patient before you administer it. Sometimes the prescribed medication is wrong, given the patient's current condition (for example, low BP or high BP). Similarly, elderly patients (or those with reduced liver or kidney function) may not benefit from the med or the dose prescribed by the doc (see Chapter 16 for more details). Before administering a medication, ask yourself, "Is this medication, at its current dose, okay for my patient?"

Building on the example in the preceding section, the doctor confirms that her order is for morphine sulfate because the patient was in discomfort at the time of her assessment. What do you do next?

You do a patient assessment before administering the medication and note that the patient has a reduced respiratory rate of 10 per minute and is lethargic but arousable. You also note that the patient is confused. Because of these changes in the patient's condition, you need to question the doctor about giving the medication.

You call the doctor with the patient's status, and she holds the medication order. You don't want to administer morphine to a patient in this state. The doctor reassesses the patient and evaluates the cause for the change in the patient's mental status.

Doctors often order medications like morphine sulfate and other pain medications with restrictions. For example, you may see the order "morphine sulfate 2 g IV PRN for pain, hold if respiratory rate <12 breaths per minute."

Minimize Metric Mistakes

In healthcare, you deal almost entirely with units of the metric system, especially mg, g, mL, and L. Converting from one quantity to another without double-checking your results can lead you to give the wrong dose! So you have to be careful whenever you're doing unit conversions (see Chapter 4 for more details).

Many computer-based order-entry systems and "smart" infusion pumps have built-in checks and balances, but you still need to double-check your math. Although all you have to do to convert from one quantity to another within the metric system is move the decimal point, make sure you move the decimal to the *correct* place. Remember the following:

- 1 kg = 1,000 g
- 1 g = 1,000 mg
- 1 mg = 1,000 mcg

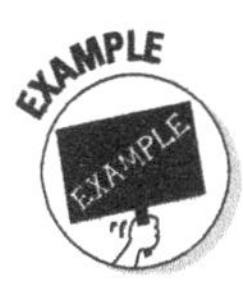

You're ordered to administer furosemide (Lasix) 40 mg IV daily. The furosemide is available in an infusion of 10 mg/mL. You administer 40 mL of furosemide. Was this the correct dose to be administered?

Although the answer is obvious, you can use the ratio-proportion method to verify how incorrect your dose was. Just follow these steps (see Chapter 8 for more on the ratio-proportion method):

1. **Set up the following proportion to determine how many mL contain 40 mg of furosemide:**

$$\frac{\text{known equivalent}}{\text{known equivalent}} = \frac{\text{known equivalent}}{\text{desired equivalent}}$$

$$\frac{10\text{ mg}}{1\text{ mL}} = \frac{40\text{ mg}}{x\text{ mL}}$$

2. **Cross-multiply and solve.**

   $10x = 40$

   $x = 4$

   You *should* have given 4 mL, not 40 mL. The patient received 10 times more furosemide than ordered. Make sure you don't read *mg* as *mL* — they're certainly not the same thing!

Check Infusion Rates

Watch out when you're dosing continuous infusions. If you're taking care of a patient with simultaneous infusions (for example, in a critical care unit), the potential for error increases. An example is a patient who requires pressor medications and continuous infusions to treat accelerated blood pressure. Other infusions, such as furosemide, insulin, and heparin, also require your increased attention. (See Chapter 11 for everything you need to know about infusions.)

A bad infusion rate calculation, especially one done with a wrong conversion, can often lead to the wrong dose being given.

You're ordered to administer a furosemide infusion at 20 mg/hr. The furosemide comes as 10 mg in 100 mL of normal saline (NS). You do the dosing calculation and program the pump to run the drip at 20 mL/hr. Is this correct?

To find out, use the ratio-proportion method and follow these steps:

1. **Set up the following proportion to determine how many mL contain 20 mg of furosemide:**

   $$\frac{10\text{ mg}}{100\text{ mL}} = \frac{20\text{ mg}}{x\text{ mL}}$$

2. **Cross-multiply and solve.**

   $10x = 100 \times 20$

   $10x = 2{,}000$

   $x = 200$

   You must give the dose of 20 mg/hr by infusing 200 mL/hr, not 20 mL/hr. Because of your calculation error, this patient got only one-tenth as much furosemide as he needed. This kind of error is easy to make with heparin and insulin infusions, too, so be extra careful when calculating infusion rates!

Avoid Measurement System Conversion Errors

When the doctor orders a med in a measurement system other than the metric system, you must be extra cautious that you don't make any conversion errors in your dosage calculations. For example, you must become skilled at converting from metric to household units (see Chapter 4 for more details). Ounce (oz), tablespoon (Tbsp), and teaspoon (tsp) doses are common in discharge instructions because these units are the most common units used in American households. Families need to know how to dose a recovering patient.

One very common dosing error occurs when doctors write orders in grains (a measurement in the apothecaries' system). (See Chapter 4 for more info on this archaic measurement system and for details on converting it to metric units.)

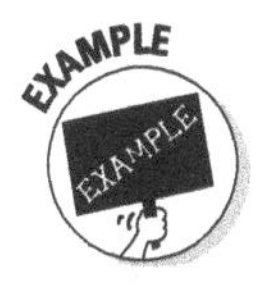

You're ordered to administer thyroid extract (Armour Thyroid) gr 1.5 PO daily. How many mg do you administer to the patient?

First, recognize that the order refers to grains (gr), not grams (g). You don't want to administer 1.5 g, because that dose would be far from therapeutic. Instead, follow these steps to convert gr to mg:

1. **Call the pharmacy or check a conversion calculator to find the conversion factor 1 gr = 65 mg.**
2. **Use that conversion factor to convert the dose of 1.5 gr to mg.**

   desired unit = given unit × conversion factor

   $$\text{mg} = \text{gr} \times 65\ \text{mg/gr}$$

   $$\text{mg} = 1.5\ \text{gr} \times 65\ \text{mg/gr}$$

   $$\text{mg} = 97.5$$

   You call the prescribing doctor for clarification; you are to instruct the patient to take 90 mg thyroid extract initially and to follow up with the doctor for further dosing adjustments. This example demonstrates why communication is so important, especially concerning a medication whose dosing you're not familiar with.

Rich, one of the authors, recommends calling the pharmacist after calculating gr-to-g doses, because grain doses aren't very common in medicine these days. (He himself would call the pharmacy when ordering this medication, just to double-check.)

Get the Timing Right When You Administer

In terms of timing, two potential medication administration errors stand out. First, you must make sure that the patient is getting the medication at the correct time and at the correct dosing frequency. For example, dosing a medication 3 times a day (tid) is different from every 8 hours. If you have any questions about dosing times, call the prescribing physician.

Second, make sure you don't administer the med too quickly. Certain medications, such as phenytoin (Dilantin), require a relatively slow infusion rate. Consult a drug reference or call the pharmacist if you have any questions regarding the infusion rate. (See Chapter 5 for more on verifying time-related dosage info.)

Review the Allergies and ADEs

Before you administer any med, review any allergies and adverse drug reactions the patient may have. Although the admitting physician and other members of the medical team have likely already done this review, you must do it, too.

Don't Forget the "Rights" of Medication Administration

To ensure patient safety and promote healing, never forget the six rights of medication administration. Give the *right patient* the *right medication* in the right way: *right dose/frequency, right time,* and *right route of administration.* And be sure to do the *right documentation* afterward. (See Chapter 6 for more details on these six rights of medication.)

Communicate!

One of the biggest errors that all medical professionals make is failing to communicate concerns or questions about medication administration and dosing to a physician or pharmacist. Not surprisingly, improving communication among medical professionals is one of the most important factors for improving patient safety, not only with medical dosing calculations but with all aspects of clinical care.

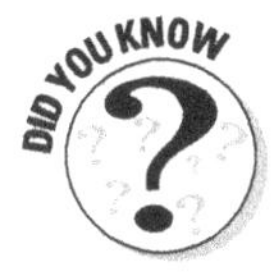

You know doctors "make the rounds" with medical residents and students. But did you know that many hospitals use interdisciplinary rounding? Often, particularly in critical care units, doctors, nurses, pharmacists, dieticians, and case managers make joint bedside rounds. Together, they review the patient's course, medication dosage, medication administration, medication necessity, and diet. Such rounding is great for patient care because it ensures that everyone's on the same page concerning the patient's plan of care and medication. In fact, interdisciplinary rounding may minimize errors, especially concerning medication.

Index

• Numerics •

• A •

• B •

• C •

• D •

• E •

• F •

• G •

• H •

• I •

• K •

• L •

• N •

• O •

• P •

• R •

• S •

• T •

• U •

e & Macs

For Dummies
0-470-58027-1

ne For Dummies,
Edition
0-470-87870-5

Book For Dummies, 3rd
on
0-470-76918-8

OS X Snow Leopard For
mies
0-470-43543-4

ness

keeping For Dummies
0-7645-9848-7

nterviews
ummies,
dition
-470-17748-8

mes For Dummies,
dition
-470-08037-5

ng an
e Business
ummies,
dition
-470-60210-2

Investing
ummies,
dition
-470-40114-9

ssful
Management
ummies
-470-29034-7

Computer Hardware

BlackBerry
For Dummies,
4th Edition
978-0-470-60700-8

Computers For Seniors
For Dummies,
2nd Edition
978-0-470-53483-0

PCs For Dummies,
Windows
7 Edition
978-0-470-46542-4

Laptops For Dummies,
4th Edition
978-0-470-57829-2

Cooking & Entertaining

Cooking Basics
For Dummies,
3rd Edition
978-0-7645-7206-7

Wine For Dummies,
4th Edition
978-0-470-04579-4

Diet & Nutrition

Dieting For Dummies,
2nd Edition
978-0-7645-4149-0

Nutrition For Dummies,
4th Edition
978-0-471-79868-2

Weight Training
For Dummies,
3rd Edition
978-0-471-76845-6

Digital Photography

Digital SLR Cameras &
Photography For Dummies,
3rd Edition
978-0-470-46606-3

Photoshop Elements 8
For Dummies
978-0-470-52967-6

Gardening

Gardening Basics
For Dummies
978-0-470-03749-2

Organic Gardening
For Dummies,
2nd Edition
978-0-470-43067-5

Green/Sustainable

Raising Chickens
For Dummies
978-0-470-46544-8

Green Cleaning
For Dummies
978-0-470-39106-8

Health

Diabetes For Dummies,
3rd Edition
978-0-470-27086-8

Food Allergies
For Dummies
978-0-470-09584-3

Living Gluten-Free
For Dummies,
2nd Edition
978-0-470-58589-4

Hobbies/General

Chess For Dummies,
2nd Edition
978-0-7645-8404-6

Drawing
Cartoons & Comics
For Dummies
978-0-470-42683-8

Knitting For Dummies,
2nd Edition
978-0-470-28747-7

Organizing
For Dummies
978-0-7645-5300-4

Su Doku For Dummies
978-0-470-01892-7

Home Improvement

Home Maintenance
For Dummies,
2nd Edition
978-0-470-43063-7

Home Theater
For Dummies,
3rd Edition
978-0-470-41189-6

Living the
Country Lifestyle
All-in-One
For Dummies
978-0-470-43061-3

Solar Power Your Home
For Dummies,
2nd Edition
978-0-470-59678-4

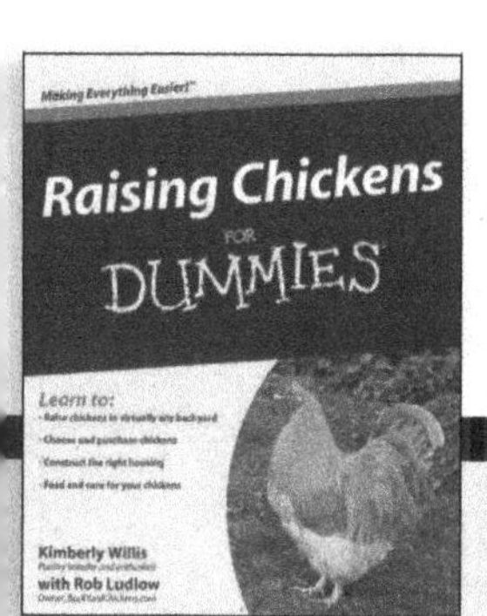

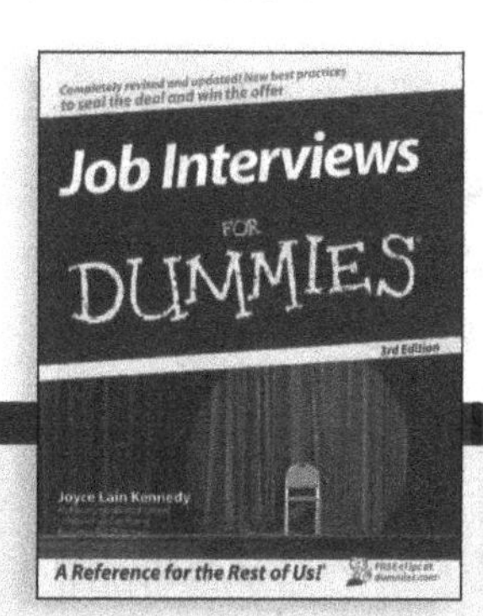

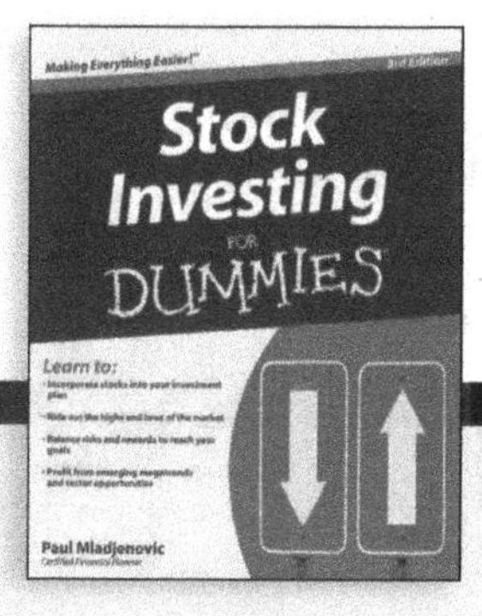

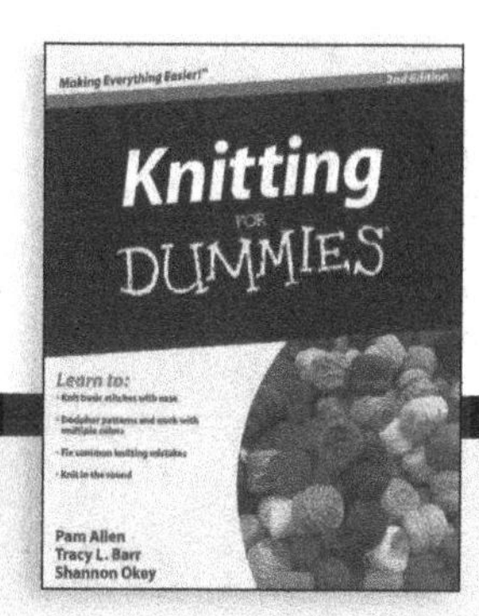

le wherever books are sold. For more information or to order direct: U.S. customers visit www.dummies.com or call 1-877-762-2974.
stomers visit www.wileyeurope.com or call (0) 1243 843291. Canadian customers visit www.wiley.ca or call 1-800-567-4797.

Internet

Blogging For Dummies, 3rd Edition
978-0-470-61996-4

eBay For Dummies, 6th Edition
978-0-470-49741-8

Facebook For Dummies, 3rd Edition
978-0-470-87804-0

Web Marketing For Dummies, 2nd Edition
978-0-470-37181-7

WordPress For Dummies, 3rd Edition
978-0-470-59274-8

Language & Foreign Language

French For Dummies
978-0-7645-5193-2

Italian Phrases For Dummies
978-0-7645-7203-6

Spanish For Dummies, 2nd Edition
978-0-470-87855-2

Spanish For Dummies, Audio Set
978-0-470-09585-0

Math & Science

Algebra I For Dummies, 2nd Edition
978-0-470-55964-2

Biology For Dummies, 2nd Edition
978-0-470-59875-7

Calculus For Dummies
978-0-7645-2498-1

Chemistry For Dummies
978-0-7645-5430-8

Microsoft Office

Excel 2010 For Dummies
978-0-470-48953-6

Office 2010 All-in-One For Dummies
978-0-470-49748-7

Office 2010 For Dummies, Book + DVD Bundle
978-0-470-62698-6

Word 2010 For Dummies
978-0-470-48772-3

Music

Guitar For Dummies, 2nd Edition
978-0-7645-9904-0

iPod & iTunes For Dummies, 8th Edition
978-0-470-87871-2

Piano Exercises For Dummies
978-0-470-38765-8

Parenting & Education

Parenting For Dummies, 2nd Edition
978-0-7645-5418-6

Type 1 Diabetes For Dummies
978-0-470-17811-9

Pets

Cats For Dummies, 2nd Edition
978-0-7645-5275-5

Dog Training For Dummies, 3rd Edition
978-0-470-60029-0

Puppies For Dummies, 2nd Edition
978-0-470-03717-1

Religion & Inspiration

The Bible For Dummies
978-0-7645-5296-0

Catholicism For Dummies
978-0-7645-5391-2

Women in the Bible For Dummies
978-0-7645-8475-6

Self-Help & Relationship

Anger Management For Dummies
978-0-470-03715-7

Overcoming Anxiety For Dummies, 2nd Edition
978-0-470-57441-6

Sports

Baseball For Dummies, 3rd Edition
978-0-7645-7537-2

Basketball For Dummies, 2nd Edition
978-0-7645-5248-9

Golf For Dummies, 3rd Edition
978-0-471-76871-5

Web Development

Web Design All-in-One For Dummies
978-0-470-41796-6

Web Sites Do-It-Yourself For Dummies, 2nd Edition
978-0-470-56520-9

Windows 7

Windows 7 For Dummies
978-0-470-49743-2

Windows 7 For Dummies, Book + DVD Bundle
978-0-470-52398-8

Windows 7 All-in-One For Dummies
978-0-470-48763-1

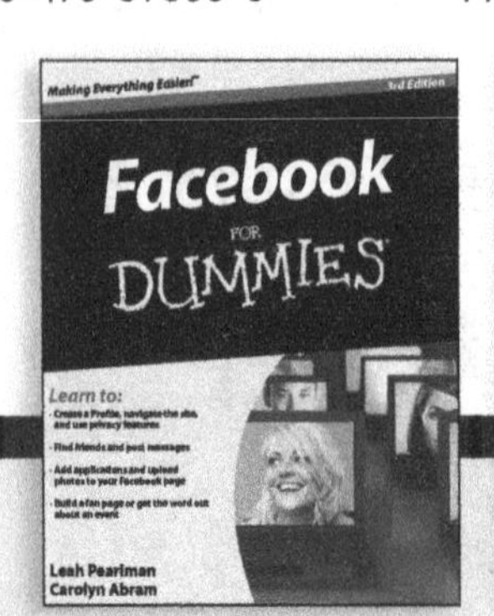

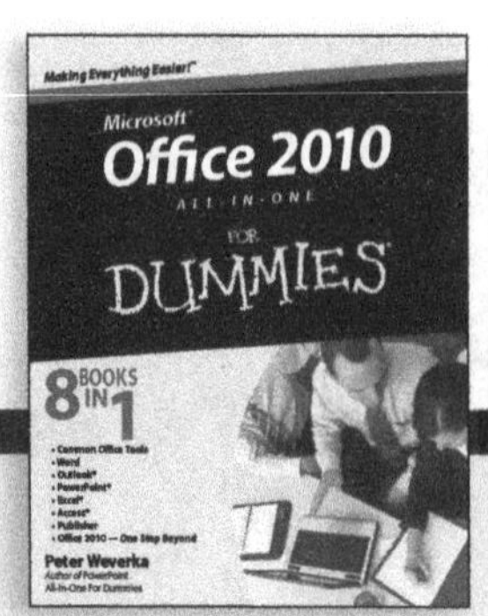

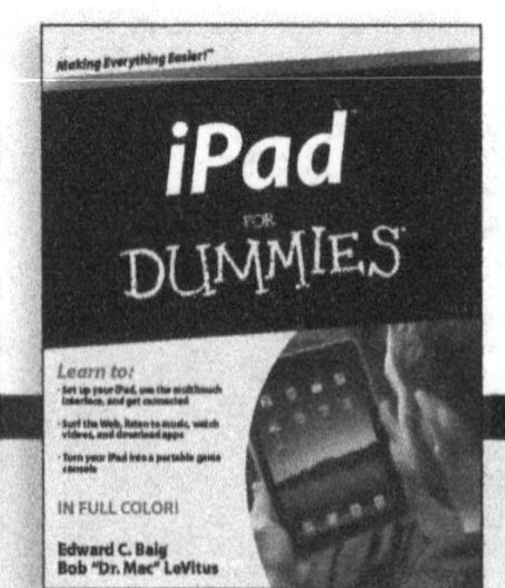

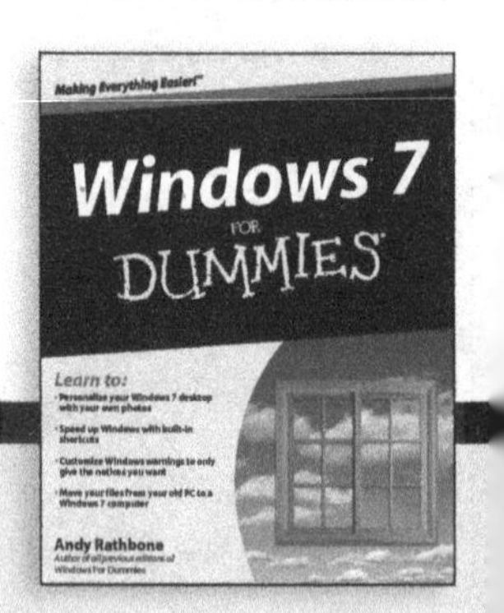

Available wherever books are sold. For more information or to order direct: U.S. customers visit www.dummies.com or call 1-877-76
U.K. customers visit www.wileyeurope.com or call (0) 1243 843291. Canadian customers visit www.wiley.ca or call 1-800-567-4797.

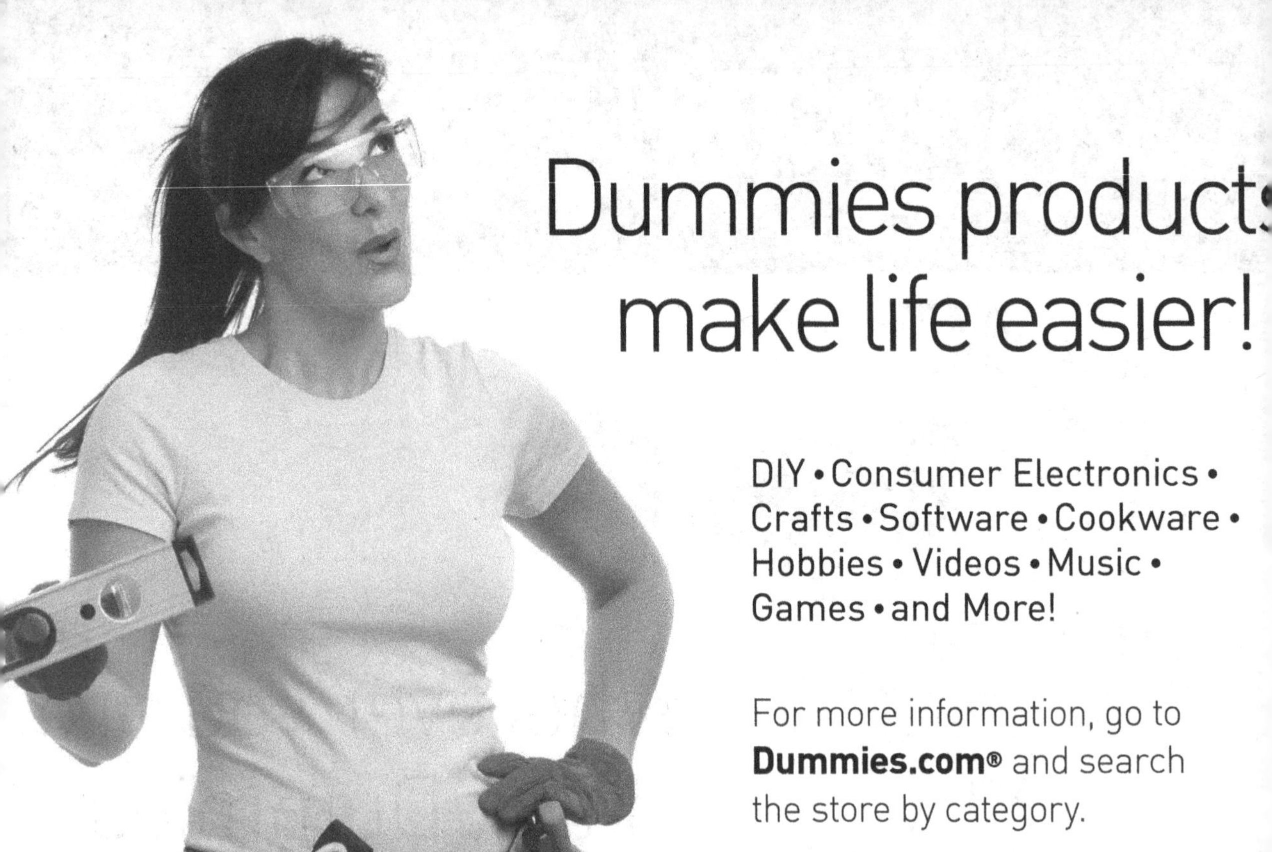
Dummies products
make life easier!
DIY • Consumer Electronics •
Crafts • Software • Cookware •
Hobbies • Videos • Music •
Games • and More!
For more information, go to
Dummies.com® and search
the store by category.

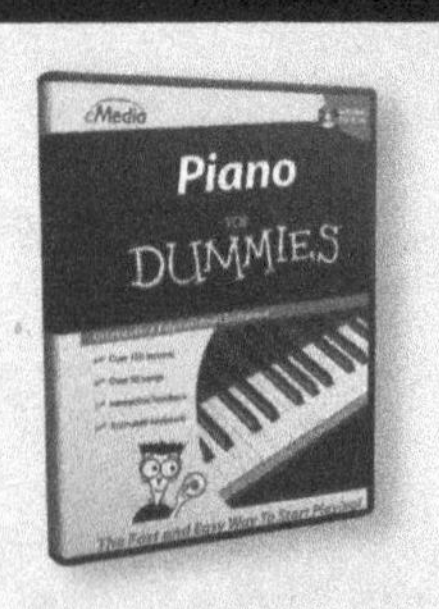
Piano
FOR
DUMMIES

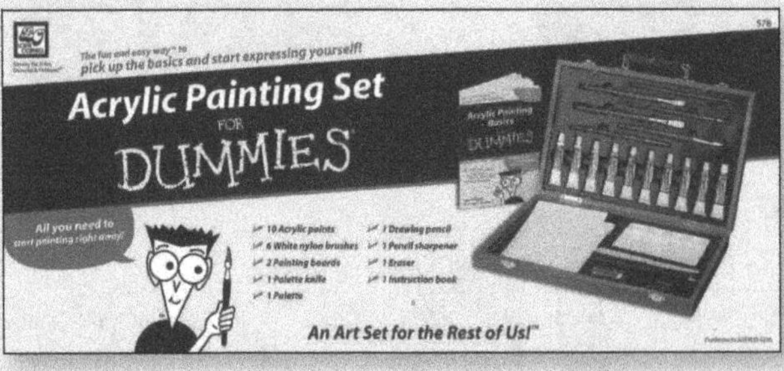
Acrylic Painting Set
FOR
DUMMIES
An Art Set for the Rest of Us!™

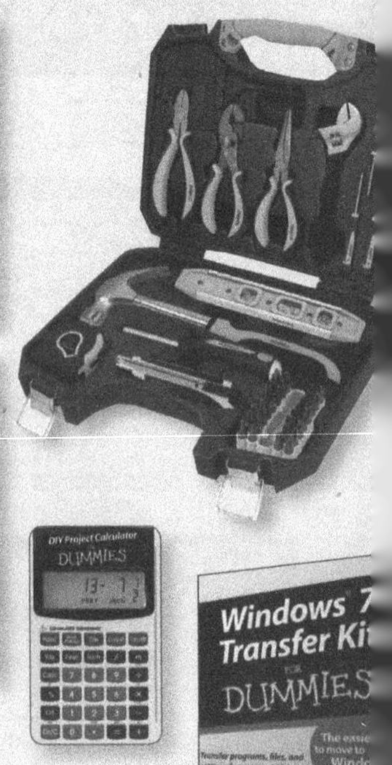
Windows 7
Transfer Ki
FOR
DUMMIES

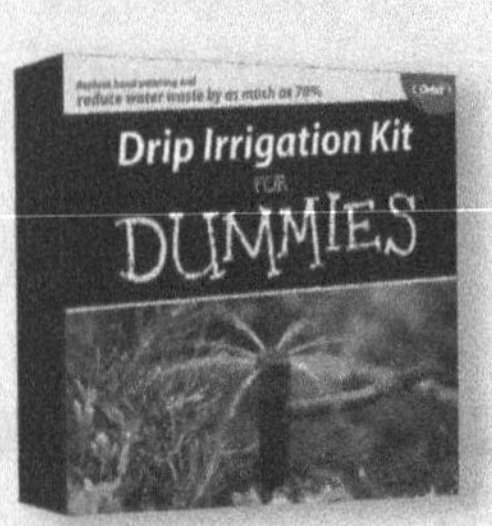
Drip Irrigation Kit
FOR
DUMMIES

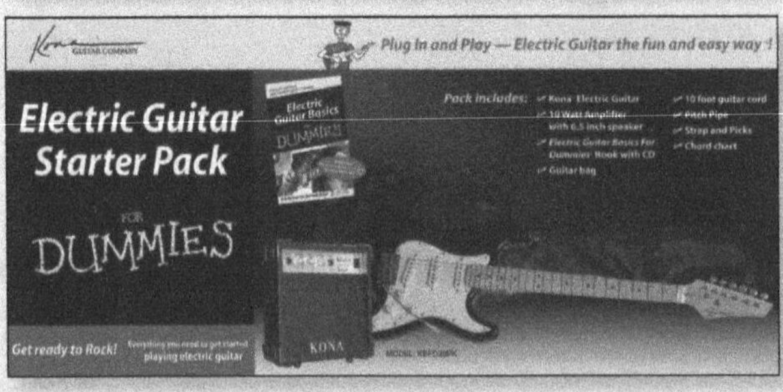
Plug In and Play — Electric Guitar the fun and easy way!
Electric Guitar
Starter Pack
FOR
DUMMIES
Get ready to Rock!

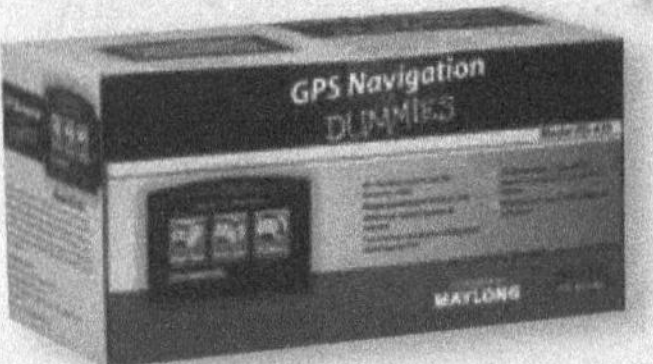
GPS Navigation

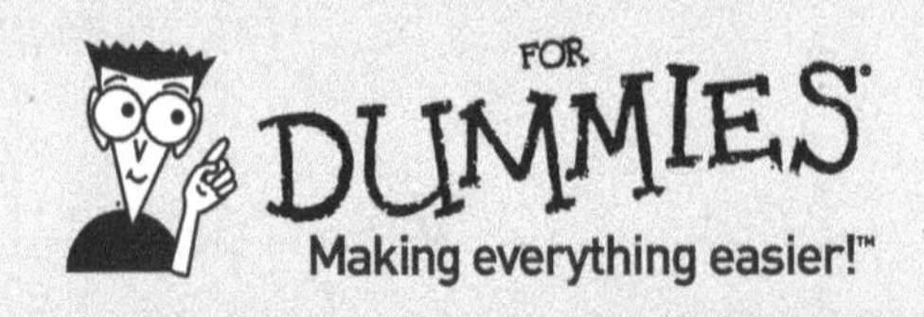
FOR
DUMMIES®
Making everything easier!™